The Right to Health

Theory and Practice

EDITOR:
GUNILLA BACKMAN

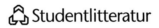
Studentlitteratur

Art. No 33824
ISBN 978-91-44-06780-3
Edition 1:1

© The authors and Studentlitteratur 2012
www.studentlitteratur.se
Studentlitteratur AB, Lund

Cover design by Francisco Ortega
Cover photo: Joseph Fitchett

Printed by Pozkal, Poland 2012

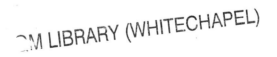

CONTENT

CONTRIBUTORS

Shahira Ahmed, MPH, is a doctoral student majoring in health systems at the Department of Global Health and Population, Harvard School of Public Health (HSPH). Her research interests include the social and cultural factors that influence health-seeking behaviour and health-care delivery, particularly in the context of HIV/AIDS. Previously, Shahira worked with the Program on International Health and Human Rights, HSPH, on a breadth of projects to operationalise human rights in public health policy, programming, and practice. She has also consulted with many international organisations, including UNAIDS, UNDP, UNFPA, and WHO, as well as civil society organisations, on the development of global and national health policy guidance documents. Originally from the Sudan, Shahira also researches and writes on the human rights, cultural, and health implications of female genital cutting.

Henry Ascher, MD, PhD, is associate professor in paediatrics and senior lecturer at the Nordic School of Public Health in Gothenburg, where he initiated the school's work on migration and health. Other areas of interest include child health, health and human rights, and inequities in health. He has also conducted clinical work at the Refugee Children Team. Henry is one of the founders of the Rosengrenska Clinic, a voluntary network of health workers with the aim to secure health care for undocumented migrants, and is chairman of the Working Group on Refugee Children in the Swedish Paediatric Association. Henry has been active in the public debate on refugees and health and the right to health for all, including undocumented migrants. He is a member of the advisory board of the Swedish Discrimination Ombudsman.

Gunilla Backman, MSc, MA, is health advisor (specific focus on health systems and the right to health) for conflict and post-conflict countries at the Swedish International Development Cooperation Agency. She is also a doctoral student at the London School of Hygiene and Tropical Medicine, where she is majoring in health systems, the right to health, and post-conflict countries. Prior to her present post, she worked as senior research officer to Paul Hunt, the UN Special Rapporteur on the Right to Health (2002–2008). Gunilla has also spent over ten years living and working in fragile states and post-conflict countries, including Bosnia and Herzegovina, Kosovo, El Salvador, the Republic of Nauru, East Timor, and Guatemala, where she held health management and coordination positions with WHO, UNDP, UNFPA, Médecins Sans Frontières, and the International Organization for Migration. Her teaching, research, and publications focus mainly on the right to health, health systems, and mental health, with a specific interest in fragile states and post-conflict countries. She holds post-graduate degrees in health service management (London School of Hygiene and Tropical Medicine) and human rights (University of Essex).

Sivan Bomze, MPH, is a doctoral student in sociology at Syracuse University. She has worked as a researcher for projects on social and health inequities; the right to health and social services; human rights as it relates to sexual orientation and gender identities; and social movements, social action, and social justice. She holds a degree in health policy from York University in Toronto, as well as an MPH in health promotion from the Dalla Lana School of Public Health at the University of Toronto.

Lisa Forman, LLB, MA, SJD, is the Lupina Assistant Professor in global health and human rights at the Dalla Lana School of Public Health and director of the Comparative Program on Health and Society at the Munk School of Global Affairs at Trinity College in the University of Toronto. Her research focuses on international human rights law relating to health, medicines, and trade. Lisa's current research focuses on the contribution of international human rights law to global health inequities, focusing in particular on the interactions between international human rights law and trade law related to medicines. Lisa is qualified as an attorney of the High Court of South Africa. She holds a BA and an LLB from the University of the Witwatersrand, a master's degree in human rights studies from Columbia University, and a doctorate in juridical science from the University of Toronto's Faculty of Law.

Lance Gable, JD, MPH, is an assistant professor of law at Wayne State University Law School, where he teaches public health law, bioethics and the law, torts, and other health law subjects. He is also a scholar with the Centers for Law and the Public's Health: A Collaborative at Georgetown and Johns Hopkins Universities, which is a Collaborating Center of WHO and the Centers for Disease Control and Prevention. Lance specialises in public health law, ethics, and policy; bioterrorism and emergency preparedness; mental health; international human rights; genetics and genomics; research ethics; and information privacy. He has helped develop course materials for the WHO Diploma in International Human Rights and Mental Health and has worked as a human rights consultant for the Pan American Health Organization. Lance received a JD from Georgetown University Law Center and a master's in public health from the Johns Hopkins Bloomberg School of Public Health.

Anand Grover, LLB, is the director of the HIV/AIDS Unit of Lawyer's Collective (India) and the current UN Special Rapporteur on the Right to Health, appointed by the Human Right Council in 2008. As a long-time, now senior, advocate in the Bombay High Court and Supreme Court of India, he has argued many significant human rights cases in India, including the first HIV case relating to employment law and the case that decriminalised voluntary sexual intercourse between consenting adults. In his first term as Special Rapporteur, he submitted reports to the Human Rights Council and General Assembly on the right to health and the following subjects: TRIPS, patents, and free trade agreements; criminalisation of HIV transmission, same-sex relations, and sex work; criminalisation of drug use; and the right to sexual and reproductive health, among others.

Sofia Gruskin, JD, MIA, is director of the Program on Global Health and Human Rights at the Institute for Global Health at the University of Southern California, and holds professorial appointments at the Keck School of Medicine and the Gould School of Law. She is also an adjunct professor of global health at the Harvard School of Pubic Health and serves as an associate editor for the *American Journal of Public Health*, *Global Public Health*, and *Reproductive Health Matters*. Sofia has extensive experience in research, training, policy, and programmatic work with nongovernmental, governmental, and intergovernmental organisations working in the fields of health and human rights around the world.

Rachel Hammonds, JD, is a researcher in the Public Health Department at the Institute of Tropical Medicine, Antwerp, and a member of the Law and Development Research Group at the University of Antwerp's Faculty of Law. She holds a BA in political science from McGill University and a JD from the University of Ottawa. Rachel is also a New York licensed attorney.

Hans V. Hogerzeil, MD, PhD, DSc, FRCP (Edin), is a medical doctor with a PhD in public health. He worked for five years as a mission doctor in India and Ghana and joined the WHO Action Programme on Essential Medicines in 1985. As director for WHO's Department of Essential Medicines and Pharmaceutical Policies (2004–2011), Hans was responsible for WHO's global policies, nomenclature, and standards on medicines, as well as for technical support to over one hundred countries in medicine access, quality, and rational use. He is the editor of numerous WHO books and has published over sixty scientific papers in peer-reviewed journals, including several on the right to health. In 1998, he received an honorary doctorate from the Robert Gordon University in Aberdeen.

Gorik Ooms, Lic.Jur, PhD, is a post-doctoral researcher in the Public Health Department of the Institute of Tropical Medicine, Antwerp. Since 2010, he has also been an adjunct professor of law at Georgetown University. For most of his professional career, he worked with Médecins Sans Frontières Belgium, of which he was the executive director between 2004 and 2008. Gorik received his law degree from the Catholic University of Leuven, Belgium, in 1989, and his PhD in medical sciences from the University of Ghent, Belgium, in 2008.

John Porter, MBBS, MD, MPH, is a professor of international health at the London School of Hygiene and Tropical Medicine. He trained in paediatrics before studying international public health in the UK and United States. His research work focuses on the control of infectious diseases, particularly TB, HIV, and leprosy, and he uses this perspective to gain access to themes around health systems, policy, and ethics. He has been teaching a course on ethics, public health, and human rights at the London School for the past ten years and is seeking to find novel ways of teaching ethics.

Helen Potts, MTH, PhD, is director of the Age Equality Unit at the Australian Human Rights Commission. She holds academic qualifications in human rights, public health, and law. She has extensive field experience in Australia,

8

Thailand, Papua New Guinea, the Democratic People's Republic of Korea, Cambodia, Uganda, Kenya, the UK, and the United States. Her areas of research include the relationship between the right to health and public health, accountability and the right to health, participation and the right to health, and the impact of culture and ethnicity on access to health services.

Jan Stjernswärd, MD, PhD, FRCP (Edin), LFS, earned his medical degree from the Karolinska Institute, where he also became an assistant professor in tumour biology and a specialist in radiotherapy/oncology. He was the first to use meta-analysis in the analysis of controlled clinical trials. Jan created one of the largest international clinical breast cancer groups (today known as the International Breast Cancer Study Group). As chief of WHO's Cancer and Palliative Care Unit (1980–1996), he reoriented WHO's global cancer programme so that existing knowledge could serve to benefit all, including those in developing countries, where the majority of cancer deaths were shown to be. Jan initiated the "WHO pain ladder," which became a global standard for pain control and the implementation of palliative care worldwide. He has served as advisor to several non-governmental organisations and has assisted numerous countries and their ministries of health in establishing national cancer control programmes and national palliative care programmes.

Daniel Tarantola, MD, is a visiting professorial fellow at the Faculty of Medicine of the University of New South Wales (UNSW). His earlier career, with WHO, was devoted to large-scale public health programmes (1974–1990). After leaving WHO in 1991, he joined the Harvard School of Public Health where, as a close collaborator of Jonathan Mann, he contributed to the conceptual development and launching of the health and human rights movement. From 1998 to 2004, Daniel re-joined WHO as a senior policy advisor to the director general and director of WHO's Department of Immunization, Vaccines and Biologicals. Between 2005 and 2010, he taught health and human rights at the UNSW School of Public Health and Community Medicine.

Sridhar Venkatapuram, MSc, MPhil, PhD, is a Wellcome Trust Research Fellow in ethics at the London School of Hygiene and Tropical Medicine, and an affiliated lecturer at Cambridge University. From 2008 to 2011, he worked with Sir Michael Marmot, chair of the WHO Commission on the Social Determinants of Health. Sridhar was an early health and human rights advocate as the first researcher at Human Rights Watch to examine HIV/AIDS and other health issues directly as human rights concerns. He also worked with the late Arjun Sengupta, the UN Special Rapporteur on the Right to Development, in conceptualising the philosophical and ethical framework for the right to development. He holds degrees in international relations, public health, sociology, and political philosophy.

Susan Wright, JD, MTS, studied law and theology at Harvard University and was a Fulbright Scholar at the University of Sarajevo, where she taught international humanitarian law. She worked for the UN Office of the High Commissioner for Human Rights and for Paddy Ashdown as the head of Rule of Law at the Office of the High Representative. In Sierra Leone, Susan was co-counsel for one of the accused being tried at the war crimes tribunal. Most recently, she led the Doctors of the World UK team, with a particular focus on human rights advocacy.

Alicia Ely Yamin, JD, MPH, is director of the Program on the Health Rights of Women and Children (the HRWC Program) at the François-Xavier Bagnoud Center for Health and Human Rights at Harvard University, which aims to promote rights-based approaches to women's and children's health in the context of strengthening effective and equitable health systems. She is also an adjunct lecturer on health policy and management at the Harvard School of Public Health, and an associated senior researcher at the Christian Michelsen Institute, Norway. She currently directs the HRWC Program from Tanzania, which facilitates greater field work in East Africa. Previously, Ali lived and worked in Latin America for over a decade. From 2007 to 2011, she was the Joseph H. Flom Fellow on Global Health and Human Rights at Harvard Law School. From 2008 to 2010, she also served as special advisor to Amnesty International's Demand Dignity Campaign in relation to maternal health. She holds degrees from Harvard College, Harvard Law School, and the Harvard School of Public Health.

Health and human rights have much in common. Both are concerned with the well-being of individuals, and both, in part, pertain to caring for those who suffer. The right to health synthesises these concerns and elevates the health of individuals and populations to the level of a universal human right. The right to health was first enunciated in 1948 in the Constitution of the World Health Organization. Today, the most authoritative pronouncement of the right is found in article 12 of the International Covenant on Economic, Social and Cultural Rights (ICESCR): the right of everyone to the highest attainable standard of physical and mental health.

The scope of the right to health is extensive. It encompasses medical care, the functioning of national health systems, and the underlying determinants of health, such as basic sanitation, adequate housing, and equality. For political and historical reasons, and because of its complex legal character, the right to health remained little more than a slogan in much of the world for more than fifty years. Since the 1990s, however, the international community has devoted more attention to economic, social, and cultural rights, including the right to health. In 2000, the United Nations (UN) Committee on Economic, Social and Cultural Rights, in close collaboration with the World Health Organization and others, adopted General Comment 14, which elaborates on article 12 of the ICESCR and clarifies what the right to health entails. In particular, General Comment 14 establishes a framework for the operationalisation of the right to health.

The promotion and protection of the right to health was further strengthened in 2002 with the establishment of the UN Special Rapporteur on the right of everyone to the highest attainable standard of physical and mental health. Although it is difficult to measure the direct impact of this "special procedure," few would disagree that it has helped raise awareness and clarify the content and contours of the right to health. The Special Rapporteurs have completed numerous reports, consultations, speeches, and analytical and methodological initiatives that operate to deepen our understanding of the right to health and to promote its adoption and protection globally. Paul Hunt, my predecessor and the first Special Rapporteur on the Right to Health, observed in one of his reports that there is a new maturity about the health and human rights movement.[1] I can only agree. Today, the movement seeks to engage in health-related policy making in a practical and constructive way, and to ensure the participation of affected communities at all levels of health-related decision making. This is all with a view towards achieving our primary goal: the effective implementation of the right to health for all without discrimination.

Although significant progress has been made, human rights workers must still strive to clarify and demonstrate the practical and operational dimensions of the right to health in order to help health workers achieve their professional objectives. Human rights workers must also recognise that the right to health cannot be realised without the interventions and insights of health workers.[2] The expertise of medical and public health professionals is integral to the fulfilment of the right to health.

It is absolutely imperative that health workers understand how human rights affect their work so that they can more effectively realise the right to health of their patients. At the same time, human rights workers must be willing to learn and understand the complex nature of health and the varied ways in which the right to health bears on the health sector. This is only possible, however, if the human rights and health communities work together. Each community must attempt to understand and appreciate the other's language, concepts, reasoning, and skills.

The critical importance of health systems is one of the primary themes of this important book. The right to health requires strong national health systems that are effective, responsive, of good quality, and accessible to all, just as strong health systems are fundamental if health outcomes are to improve and the Millennium Development Goals are to be reached.[3] Whether we are discussing maternal health, HIV, essential medicines, or palliative care, a functioning health system is necessary for both good health outcomes and the full realisation of the right to health.

The first of its kind, this student guide bridges health and human rights in theory and practice. It brings together leading experts in the fields of health and human rights in order to explore and demonstrate how the right to health can be and has been operationalised in practice. Health specialists and human rights specialists have jointly written most of the chapters, each of which has been reviewed by both experts and students alike. The final chapter takes stock of where we are and what is needed for the future.

The Right to Health: Theory and Practice fills a significant gap in the literature. It deepens our understanding of health and human rights and will likely stimulate new perspectives in the field; it promotes the practical application of the right to health; and it stresses that the right to health requires effective, integrated, and responsive national health systems that are accessible to all.

Anand Grover

UN Special Rapporteur on the Right to Health

NOTES

1   Paul Hunt, Report of the Special Rapporteur on the right of everyone to the enjoyment of the highest attainable standard of physical and mental health, Human Rights Council, U.N. Doc. A/HRC/4/28 (2007), para. 30.

2   By "health workers," I imply all those developing, managing, delivering, monitoring, and evaluating preventive, curative, and rehabilitative health in the private and public health sectors, including traditional healers.

3   World Health Organization. 2009. *Systems Thinking for Health Systems Strengthening.* Geneva: WHO.

ACKNOWLEDGMENTS

I would like to thank everyone who helped transform this project into a student guide. Firstly, I owe my gratitude to Professor Paul Hunt, former UN Special Rapporteur on the Right to Health (2002–2008), who believed in the usefulness of a law course demonstrating the practical application of the right to health, with health systems as a thread throughout, and in which each session would be taught by a health and human rights professional in order to make it more dynamic. Furthermore, he gave me the freedom to develop the course as I believed to be useful.

I am also grateful to Professor Sabine Michalowski for making it possible to run the course, which came to be named "Theory and Practice of Health and Human Rights," as part of the LLM in Health-Care Law and Human Rights at the University of Essex, UK.

I would also like to thank Peter Stoltz at Studentlitteratur, who believed in the idea of turning the LLM course into a book. Throughout the entire process, he has been there to guide, listen, and support, as well as to provide constructive criticism.

I would like to give a special thanks to all the authors. It has been a real honour to have had the opportunity to realise this student guide with some of the most renowned people in this field. Their expertise, dedication, and encouraging attitudes are reflected throughout this book. As I reviewed their chapters, questions and comments emerged, teaching me so much about their respective topics and about the meaning and rationale of the right to health. It has been an incredible learning experience. Most of the authors I have known or known of for years, and others I have had the honour of getting to know during the course of this project. Many of them were great inspirations during my years as a student, and assisted me in better understanding the contour and content of the human rights (the right to health) and health. I hope that their expertise will assist and inspire readers of this book as much as they have me.

Sincere thanks is also due to Pia Engstrand, who responded to queries that arose during the drafting process, and to the reviewers, not all mentioned here by name, who read the chapters with curiosity, enthusiasm, and thoroughness. It has been particularly interesting to see how health and human rights professionals, on the one hand, view a chapter, and then how post-graduate and PhD students, on the other, perceive it. Some of the many brilliant reviewers include Elisabeth Abiri, Onome Akopogheneta, Samuel D. Allen, Lena Andersson, Gustav Asp, Judith Bueno de Mesquita, Darlena David, Mariana Deniz-Hidalgo, Carl-Magnus Edenbrandt, Lars Ek, Elis Envall, Katherine Footer, Rajat Khosla, Anneka Knutsson Gunilla Krantz, Alexandra Lamb, Elisabeth Lönnemark, Guevara Catherine Mbema, Ian Mclellan, Joshua Mendelsohn Amelie Möller, Harriet Nwacheukwu, Lisa Oldring, Birgitta Rubenson, Egbert Sondorp, Lucy Stackpool-Moore, Milosz Swiergiel, Andrada Tomoaia-Cotisel, Karolina Tumoisto, Javier Velasquez, Richard Wild and Anders Ågård.

Morgan Stoffregen, the book's copyeditor, has been wonderful to work with. She is incredibly diligent, goes out of her way to lend support, and is always positive.

I am also very grateful to Joseph Fitchett, who gave his permission to use one of his many beautiful photos for this book's cover.

Gunilla Backman

AAAQ The AAAQ framework is a right-to-health tool for evaluating governments' compliance with the right to health. AAAQ stands for availability, accessibility (which has four overlapping dimensions: non-discrimination, physical accessibility, economic accessibility, and information accessibility); acceptability (respectful of medical ethics and culturally appropriate); and good quality.

AIDS Acquired immune deficiency syndrome or acquired immunodeficiency syndrome (AIDS) is a disease of the human immune system caused by the human immunodeficiency virus (HIV). *See HIV.*

Alma-Ata Declaration (1978) The Alma-Ata Declaration expressed the need for urgent action by all governments, all health and development workers, and the world community to protect and promote the health of everyone in the world. It was the first international declaration to highlight the importance of primary health care. Since then, the primary health care approach has been accepted by WHO member countries as a key to achieving "Health for All." The Alma-Ata Declaration also viewed both health and community participation as fundamentally rooted in social justice and human rights.

Catastrophic health expenditure Catastrophic health expenditure occurs when a household must reduce its basic expenditures over a certain period of time or sacrifice other basic needs in order to cope with the medical expenses, including out-of-pocket fees for services, of one or more of its members. There is currently no consensus on the catastrophic threshold; WHO states that it is equal to or above 40% of a household's capacity to pay.

Committee on Economic, Social and Cultural Rights (ESCR Committee) The UN Committee on Economic, Social and Cultural Rights is the body responsible for monitoring state parties' compliance with the International Covenant on Economic, Social and Cultural Rights. *See General Comment 14; human rights treaty bodies; International Covenant on Economic, Social and Cultural Rights; state party.*

Community-based approach A "community" can be described as a group of
people that recognises itself or is recognised by outsiders as sharing common
cultural, religious, or other social features, backgrounds, or interests, and that
forms a collective identity with shared goals.

A community-based approach is a way of working in partnership with the
community. It recognises the resilience, capacities, skills, and resources of
persons of concern, builds on these to deliver protection and solutions, and
supports the community's own goals.

General comments The human rights treaty bodies publish their interpretations
of the content of human rights provisions, in the form of "general comments"
on thematic issues. All treaty bodies have issued general comments, with the
exception of the UN Committee on Migrant Workers, which has not yet issued
any. The UN Committee on the Elimination of Racial Discrimination and the
UN Committee on the Elimination of Discrimination against Women refer to
their comments as "general recommendations." *See General Comment 14.*

General Comment 14 In 2000, the ESCR Committee presented General
Comment 14, which interprets the content of "the right of everyone to the
enjoyment of the highest attainable standard of physical and mental health"
(right to health), as laid out in article 12 of the International Covenant on
Economic, Social and Cultural Rights. *See Committee on Economic, Social
and Cultural Rights; general comments; human rights treaty bodies; right to the
enjoyment of the highest attainable standard of physical and mental health.*

Health system WHO's definition of a health system is "all organizations, people
and actions whose *primary intent* is to promote, restore or maintain health." It
encompasses health care and efforts to influence the determinants of health,
and includes both public and private providers. *See WHO health system
building blocks.*

HIV The human immunodeficiency virus (HIV) causes acquired immunodeficiency syndrome (AIDS), a condition in humans in which progressive failure
of the immune system allows life-threatening opportunistic infections and
cancer to thrive. *See AIDS.*

Human development While there is no firm agreement on the key dimensions
of human development, some areas considered central to human development
include social progress, growth with equity, participation and freedom,
sustainability, and human security. This book defines human development
as the transformation of the social, economic, and political conditions that
determine people's living standards, life opportunities, and quality of life.
Development is not necessarily "more" (growth) or "bigger" (larger scale). It is
a change to "better," defined as an improvement in individual and social living

standards and security (welfare) in general, and improved access to resources (incomes and employment), life claims, and opportunities in particular.

Human rights impact assessment   A human rights impact assessment is the process of predicting the potential consequences of a proposed policy, programme, or project on the enjoyment of human rights. The objective of the assessment is to inform decision makers and the people likely to be affected so that they can improve the proposal to reduce potential negative effects and increase positive ones. Human rights impact assessments are a relatively recent concept.

Human rights treaty bodies   UN human rights treaty bodies are committees of independent experts that monitor implementation of the core international human rights treaties. They are created in accordance with the provisions of the treaty that they monitor. They also issue "general comments" interpreting rights within their respective treaties. There are currently nine human rights treaty bodies. (Also referred to as "committees," "treaty bodies," and "treaty monitoring bodies.") *See Committee on Economic, Social and Cultural Rights; general comments.*

International Bill of Human Rights   The International Bill of Human Rights encompasses the Universal Declaration of Human Rights (1948); the International Covenant on Economic, Social and Cultural Rights (1966); and the International Covenant on Civil and Political Rights (1966) and its two protocols. (Also referred to as the "International Bill of Rights," which is the term used in this book.) *See Universal Declaration of Human Rights; International Covenant on Civil and Political Rights; International Covenant on Economic, Social and Cultural Rights.*

International Covenant on Civil and Political Rights (ICCPR)   Adopted in 1966, this international treaty protects individuals' civil and political rights. *See International Bill of Human Rights; state party.*

International Covenant on Economic, Social and Cultural Rights (ICESCR)   Adopted in 1966, this international treaty protects individuals' economic, social, and cultural rights. *See International Bill of Rights; state party.*

Millennium Development Goals (MDGs)   In 2000, 189 nations made a promise to free people from extreme poverty and multiple deprivations. This pledge, which took the form of eight Millennium Development Goals, was to be achieved by 2015. The eight goals are (1) eradicate extreme poverty and hunger; (2) achieve universal primary education; (3) promote gender equality and empower women; (4) reduce child mortality; (5) improve maternal health; (6) combat HIV/AIDS, malaria, and other diseases; (7)

ensure environmental sustainability; and (8) develop a global partnership for development. *See human development.*

Right of everyone to the enjoyment of the highest attainable standard of physical and mental health More often referred to by its abbreviations, "the right to the highest attainable standard of physical and mental health" or "the right to health," this fundamental human right is enshrined in a number of international and regional human rights treaties, as well as many national constitutions. The right to health encompasses not just health care but also the underlying determinants of health, both of which should be affordable to all without discrimination. In addition, this right is concerned with disadvantaged groups, participation, and accountability. For the right to health to be realised, there needs to be a functioning health system, accessible to all without discrimination. *See underlying determinants of health.*

Rights-based approach The official term by the Office of High Commissioner for Human Rights is "human rights-based approach." It is a conceptual framework that is normatively based on international human rights standards and operationally directed to promoting and protecting human rights. It seeks to analyse obligations, inequalities, and vulnerabilities and to redress discriminatory practices and unjust distributions of power that impede progress and undercut human rights. (This book uses the term "rights-based approach.")

State party A state party to a treaty is a country that has ratified or acceded to that particular treaty and is therefore legally bound by the instrument under international law.

UN Special Rapporteurs Appointed by the UN Secretary-General, Special Rapporteurs are individuals who act independently of governments and who bear a specific mandate from the UN Human Rights Council to examine, monitor, advise, and publicly report on human rights situations in specific countries or on a thematic issue. Special Rapporteurs undertake a variety of activities, including presenting annual reports to the Human Rights Council and the General Assembly, monitoring, identifying general trends, undertaking country visits and communicating with states and other concerned parties with regard to alleged cases of human rights violations, and receiving complaints. One of these Special Rapporteurs is the Special Rapporteur on the Right to Health, whose work focuses on the right to physical and mental health; this book, when referring to a UN Special Rapporteur, is usually referring to this particular mandate holder.

Underlying determinants of health Underlying determinants influence health outcomes and the realisation of the right to health. They include, for example, housing, gender equality, nutrition, employment, and education. Fulfilment of the underlying determinants is required to improve overall physical and mental health. *See right of everyone to the enjoyment of the highest attainable standard of physical and mental health.*

Universal Declaration of Human Rights Adopted in 1948 by the UN General Assembly, this human rights instrument is at the foundation of modern international human rights law. *See International Bill of Human Rights.*

WHO health system building blocks WHO describes six clearly defined health system "building blocks" that together constitute a system: service delivery; health workforce; information; medical products, vaccines, and technologies; financing; and leadership and governance. *See health system.*

INTRODUCTION

GUNILLA BACKMAN

Health (medicine and public health) and human rights law (the right to health) are two very powerful and influential professional areas. Their objectives are similar: to improve the well-being of the whole population and to ensure that everyone, without discrimination, has access to good-quality health services. To realise these objectives, a strong health system is necessary. At the heart of "the right to health"[1] is a functioning health system accessible to all without discrimination. An equitable and efficient health system is also central to improving the health and well-being of the population, including realising the Millennium Development Goals. In addition, the realisation of this right is dependent on other human rights (e.g., the right to information, the right to food, and freedom from torture), for all human rights are interrelated and interdependent. Finally, respect for and realisation of underlying determinants (e.g., education, gender, water and sanitation) also influence to what extent, or if at all, the right to health is realised.

Although the right to health has matured in the last decade and there has been an increased understanding of its meaning—including the development and testing of practical tools (such as indicators and impact assessments) by health and human rights workers, as well as courts' use of the human rights framework to determine whether violations have taken place in the health sector—human rights are still frequently associated with "naming and shaming." While "naming and shaming" has an important role to play, human rights—and in this case, the right to health—are more than that. The argument that the right to health is also practical is poorly understood and has been difficult to convey. Health workers and policy makers often ask questions such as, if human rights (e.g., the right to health) are practical, what are the tools and how do I use them? Will a rights-based approach improve the health and well-being of the people? What is the evidence?

The reasons for this continued disconnect (or, rather, difficulty in conveying the practical aspect of the right to health) are many—for example, history, politics, and, in particular, misunderstandings between health and human rights professionals due to different professional languages and frames of reference.

Health workers tend to overlook the laws (domestic but especially international) that govern their work and by which they are bound. The tools and instruments that come with these laws could be beneficial to advancing their purpose and could assist in improving the delivery and quality of their services. For example, the health sector might overlook the principles of participation and accountability when developing health services and programmes; this could lead to the services not being culturally acceptable to the people and, as a result, the people not accessing the services. This analysis, admittedly simplistic, is meant to show that improving people's health and well-being depends on numerous factors; not only do health services need to be staffed with qualified health professionals and equipped with the relevant vaccines, medications, and technologies, but there are also underlying determinants that affect health outcomes.

Human rights workers, on the other hand, often lack a strong understanding of how human rights law—and the law in general—affects (positively or negatively) health services and the overall health system. For example, human rights organisations might lobby for free access to medication but overlook the link with laboratory testing that goes in tandem with some medications; or they might win a legal case granting the right to expensive drugs outside the essential medicines list but fail to consider the implications that such a decision could have for other health services or interventions. At the same time, human rights litigation does have a critical accountability role to play; for example, a court case might be needed to ensure that health services are structured in such a manner that everyone, without discrimination, can receive a certain treatment or medication. Both professions have a tendency to overlook the impact that their work has on the overall health system. Irrespective of their differences, both fields are very strong, with valuable skills and knowledge; if working together, they can be strengthened even further.

One of the main motivations behind this student guide is to show how different disciplines (health, human rights, law, and ethics) and perspectives are interrelated and how they affect one another. Nothing in health and human rights takes place in a silo, and every intervention made in the health sector affects the overall health system. This book also seeks to demonstrate the practical applications of the right to health as well as the benefits of having different disciplines analyse, interpret, and bring attention to various aspects of the same health issue. Listening to and considering these divergent perspectives can strengthen analysis and improve the planning and quality of a programme or project. Yet, in order to take advantage of the different perspectives, as well as prevent frustration, it is important to better comprehend each discipline, including its history, foundation, and politics. For example, we should understand why the right to health stresses principles such as health plans, non-discrimination, and participation; why the health sector is concerned with issues such as cost-efficiency; and what the concept and role of ethics is. But this book also seeks to demonstrate that many aspects claimed or acknowledged by these professions to be necessary to improve people's health and well-being (such as participation) are actually quite similar or even the same.

Ultimately, the aim of this book is to provide health and human rights students and professionals, with a basic understanding of human rights (specifically the right to health), health (medicine/public health), and ethics and law. It seeks to demonstrate how the characteristics of each field, broadly defined, interact or can interact with one another to improve health outcomes and strengthen health systems. It is not possible to go into each field in great detail; and the focus has been on public health, broadly defined, rather than medical interventions. The aim is not to justify whether or not human rights tools should be applied, for this question has been answered: the meaning and tools of the right to health are now so well developed and tested that they cannot be ignored by practitioners or policy makers. The key is to show what these tools are, how to apply them, and, if not applied, what the consequences could be.

This book's structure is based on the post-graduate law course "Theory and Practice of Health and Human Rights," which was developed and taught at the University of Essex, UK, in 2007–2008. When Professor Paul Hunt gave me permission to develop this course, I used the book by Rebecca Cook, Bernard M. Dickens, and Mahmoud F. Fathalla, *Reproductive Health and Human Rights: Integrating Medicine, Ethics, and Law* (Oxford University Press, 2003), as my inspiration.

The "right-to-health course," as it came to be known, was well received by human rights students at the University of Essex. The structure was later tested, in a greatly condensed form, on medical and public health students at the Karolinska Institute, the University of Gothenburg, King's College, the University of Essex, Lund University, and the Nordic School of Public Health. The feedback by the students studying health was also positive to the structure of the course.

This book does not offer a comprehensive analysis but rather highlights some of the many issues of concern regarding the right to health. The topics, pragmatically selected, are to a great extent the same as those used in the course.[2] These topics were some of the areas that the former UN Special Rapporteur on the Right to Health[3] paid particular attention to during his mandate and whose contours and content were deepened as a result, with the assistance of many experts around the world. The exceptions are chapters 2, 5, and 11, which were not part of the course but have been added to this book, as they are considered pertinent in understanding the fields of both health and human rights. For example, chapter 2 highlights international assistance and the controversies surrounding it—a key issue in human rights; and with today's increasing focus on accountability, looking at this international dimension is particularly important. Chapter 5 brings attention to ethics—critical to understanding health; and chapter 11 on palliative care was introduced to reflect the changes in demographics and disease patterns, and to show that the same attention we pay to birth should be paid to the end of life.

The chapters have been written by experts in their respective fields. As in the law course, where health and human rights professionals sometimes jointly taught a class, certain chapters have been co-authored by a health professional and a human rights professional. The reason for this, both with the course and this book, was an attempt to properly reflect the health and human rights perspectives and to use a language with which both fields feel comfortable.

All of the chapters were reviewed by health and human rights workers and by post-graduate students in health and human rights (or students with a strong interest in health and human rights). The aim of these reviews was twofold: first, to ensure the quality of each chapter and, second, to guarantee that each chapter was written in a way that both the health profession and the human rights profession could understand. The students played an especially critical role because they not only helped improve the quality of each topic but also helped ensure that the chapters were organised in a "student friendly" way.

The book is structured to take the reader from theory to practice. Section I provides the theoretical foundation and section II operationalises the theory. Each chapter in section II begins with a case—not a court case but a case from the health sector—after which it introduces that chapter's specific topic and then analyses the topic/case from various perspectives: public health and medicine, ethical and legal, and the right to health. An attempt has been made to include case studies from both developed and developed countries, as violations and neglect of human rights are an issue for all countries, not just developing ones. The thread throughout the book is health systems.

The first section begins with chapter 1 (Forman and Bomze), which takes the reader through the international human rights legal system and the origins, development, and content of the right to health, bringing attention to tools such as reporting, litigation, indicators, and impact assessments. Chapter 2 (Hammonds and Ooms) introduces readers to two influential philosophical theories—nationalism and cosmopolitanism—that are central to addressing issues of international political arrangements and explores these theories' potential to advance our understanding of the importance of health-related international obligations. Chapter 3 (Potts) looks at PHC and its relationship to the right to health. It briefly explores the history of public health, highlights the similarities between the right to health and PHC, and shows that the adoption of the right to health as a means of implementing PHC offers one way to ensure greater success in primary health care. Chapter 4 (Backman) provides a brief introduction to a large number of highly complex and wide-ranging issues regarding health systems and the right to health. It introduces health systems and their relationship with the right to health and explores the features that health systems should have in order to be respectful of the right to health. Chapter 5 (Porter and Venkatapuram) expands on the relationship between ethics and the right to health. It provides a brief understanding of ethics and its role in relation to the right to health and health systems.

Section II takes the theory presented in section I and applies it practice. Chapter 6 (Yamin) uses a case from Peru to examine aspects of maternal mortality from a rights-based perspective. It highlights the many issues that underpin the failure to care for women in pregnancy and childbirth—issues related but not exclusive to gender inequalities and the functioning or lack of health systems. Chapter 7 (Gruskin and Ahmed) looks at the HIV epidemic, using a case from Vietnam. The authors stress that HIV is best analysed and addressed through the application of a rights-based approach. Chapter 8 (Gable) brings attention to the millions of people around the world who are affected by mental health problems and are largely neglected by public health. This chapter illustrates how the achievement of good mental health presents one of the most important and compelling challenges for both global public health and the enjoyment of the right to health and other human rights. Chapter 9 (Hogerzeil) focuses on essential medicines as part of the right to health. Despite being part of one of the World Health Organization's health system building blocks and a core obligation of the right to health, essential medicines are still widely unavailable. Chapter 10 (Wright and Ascher) uses the cases of the UK and Sweden to explore the situation of undocumented migrants, illustrating that developed countries, too, fall short of their human rights obligations. It highlights some of the barriers that migrants face in accessing health services, as well as some of the progress that has been made in using the right to health as a tool to increase this access. Chapter 11 (Backman and Stjernswärd) looks at palliative care and the issues that many patients face during their last stages of their life, whether due to age or a terminal illness. Using Sweden as a case study, it examines the discrimination and neglect faced by these patients, as well as strategies to improve access to and the quality of palliative care in both developed and developing countries.

Section II could have been structured in many different ways. It could have analysed the case studies starting with their legal aspects, then the right to health, followed by ethics, and finally medicine and public health. This would have stressed that international human rights law is overarching and that what has been ratified by a state at the international level should be incorporated into the national constitution. In turn, the contents of a country's constitution should be reflected in its national health plan, which should then be translated into health programmes and projects. On the other hand—and this is the structure that the book finally adopted—section II could have also started with the national perspective, first by examining what is taking place at the health service level (medicine/public health), looking at the relevant gaps, then moving on to what ethics and national laws say, and finally exploring what the state has committed to at the international level. Irrespective of the order of the analysis, it is hoped that the reader will uncover the interrelationship between medicine and public health, ethics and law, and the right to health—and understand that the issues are firmly grounded in the law.[4]

The book's conclusion is written by Daniel Tarantola, who, with his deep experience and expertise in this field, provides a personal reflection on the topic and highlights what the future holds. As Tarantola states, readers of this book, who represent the next generation of health and human rights workers, "have an enormous opportunity to bring a human face to the panoply of ideological and technological forces that are now reshaping our world."

It is hoped that this book, by illustrating the important role that the right to health plays in improving people's well-being, will help them achieve this task.

NOTES

1   The full term is "the right of everyone to the enjoyment of the highest attainable standard of physical and mental health." Throughout this book, the short version— "the right to health"—will be used.

2   Neglected tropical diseases is unfortunately not included in this book, although it was part of the course.

3   The official name for this position is Special Rapporteur on the right of everyone to the enjoyment of the highest attainable standard of health. Throughout this volume, the shorthand "Special Rapporteur on the Right to Health" will be used.

4   An attempt has been made to cross-reference the chapters throughout the book. However, it is worth nothing that the chapter on ethics is cross-referenced only one or two times; this is so because each chapter in section II contains a brief sub-section on ethics, and in order to avoid being repetitive it was decided to cross-reference chapter 5 only when a very specific aspect is highlighted.

THE FOUNDATION

International Human Rights Law and the Right to Health: An Overview of Legal Standards and Accountability Mechanisms

LISA FORMAN AND SIVAN BOMZE

INTRODUCTION

This chapter introduces readers to the international human rights law system and the origins, development, and content of the right to health. It explores primary human rights instruments addressing the right to health, as well as key developments of the normative content of the right to health, including declarations and programmes of action; General Comment 14 of the UN Committee on Economic, Social and Cultural Rights (ESCR Committee), which extensively interprets the right to health in international law; and international procedures, such as the Optional Protocol to the International Covenant on Economic, Social and Cultural Rights and the creation of the UN Special Rapporteur on the Right to Health. It then highlights practical mechanisms that can be used to hold governments accountable for realising this right, particularly the Special Rapporteur, regional and domestic litigation, civil society participation, and new human rights tools such as indicators and impact assessments.

AN INTRODUCTION TO INTERNATIONAL LAW AND HUMAN RIGHTS

INTERNATIONAL LAW

International law can be defined as "a body of rules and principles which are binding upon states in their relations with one another" (Brierly 1978, p. 1). While international law originally was concerned with governing the relations between states, since World War II states have signed multiple human rights treaties extending the protection of international law to individuals (Dugard 2001, p. 1). These human rights treaties have seen millions of people become the "beneficiaries of international law" (Dugard 2001, p. 1).

International law is created primarily in two ways—namely, treaties (binding legal agreements between states) and customary law (rules that evolve over time, becoming commonly accepted through continuous practice).[1] Both of these sources share the common feature of being created through state consent; in other words, they are not imposed on states by any central lawmaking body (Dugard 2001, p. 3). Not all aspects of international law are legally binding. For example, a large portion of international law—including declarations, codes of practice, recommendations, guidelines, standards, charters, and resolutions—is understood as "soft law." Although soft law, by definition, is not legally binding, there remains a strong expectation that the international community will respect and follow its provisions (Aust 2010). Moreover, some soft law instruments can "harden" into binding law over time.

Historically, states were the only subjects of international law. However, a growing body of international soft law is devoted to defining the rights and responsibilities of non-state actors, such as individuals, non-governmental organisations (NGOs), and private transnational corporations. Nonetheless, international law remains largely state-centric, viewing states as the dominant actors within the international system who, accordingly, carry the bulk of duties generated by international law.

INTERNATIONAL HUMAN RIGHTS LAW

While earlier human rights instruments exist (e.g., the 1776 U.S. Declaration of Independence and the 1789 French Declaration of the Rights of Man), modern conceptions of human rights gained real force in the twentieth century, in the wake of gross violations during World War I and World War II (Henkin 1990). The UN was formed in the immediate aftermath of World War II, premised in part on the determination to reaffirm faith in "fundamental human rights, in the dignity and worth of the human person, in the equal rights of men and women and of nations large and small."[2] The international human rights law system can be understood to have formally come into existence in 1948 with the Universal Declaration of Human Rights, which established the normative foundations of the modern international human rights system, articulated by a broad range of civil, political, economic, social, and cultural rights.[3] Since 1948, these rights have been further developed by more than one hundred human rights instruments, including not simply treaties but also UN resolutions, declarations, conferences, and programmes of action. In addition to the development of a comprehensive international human rights system at the UN level, regional human rights systems have developed in Africa, the Americas, and Europe. Since then, human rights law has become the fastest growing field in international law (Mutua 2001). Indeed, the field has grown so dramatically since 1945 that we are currently said to be living in the "age of rights" (Henkin 1990), with international human rights viewed as having become "constitutive elements of modern and 'civilized' statehood" (Risse et al. 1999, p. 234).

Within this system, human rights are understood as the basic rights and freedoms to which all human beings are entitled by virtue of being human. As Sofia Gruskin and Daniel Tarantola explain in more practical terms, human rights define globally, nationally, and locally "what governments can do to us, cannot do to us, and should do for us" (2005, p. 8). Within international human rights law, human rights are rooted in "recognition of the inherent dignity and of the equal and inalienable rights of all members of the human family" and are seen as "the foundation of freedom, justice and peace in the world."[4]

A wide range of human rights are viewed as necessary to assure these aspirations. Accordingly, international human rights law recognises several categories of rights, including civil and political rights (including the rights to be free from torture, to equality before the law, and to free expression, movement, and association) and economic, social, and cultural rights (including the rights to social security, to work, to education, and to participation in cultural life). The right to health is considered a social right falling within the latter category. A third category deals with collective rights (such as the rights to development, to the environment, and to self-determi-nation). Despite being categorised in this way, within international human rights law all human rights are understood to be indivisible, interrelated, and interdependent.[5] While the right to health is a free-standing right, it is closely linked to many other human rights, including the rights to life, to non-discrimination, to privacy, to water, and to education, as well as the freedoms of association, assembly, and movement.

CONTROVERSIES OVER HUMAN RIGHTS

Social acceptance of human rights has progressed considerably since Jeremy Bentham's famous critique of the French Declaration of the Rights of Man as "nonsense upon stilts" (quoted in Waldron 1987). Nonetheless, contemporary human rights remain subject to extensive critique, including with regard to their efficacy and universality. The latter claim is a primary critique, holding that rather than reflecting truly universal values, international human rights law reflects Western liberal values, such that this body of law constitutes the globalisation of culturally embedded and geographically specific values of the West (Panikkar 1996, p. 75; de Sousa Santos 2002, p. 178). Indeed, critics argue that the inherent liberalism of international human rights law may pose significant challenges to achieving transformative change, given liberalism's prioritisation of individual freedom, particularly the right to property, over other social interests (Otto 1997, p. 7; de Sousa Santos 2002, p. 178). Certainly, as this chapter will illustrate, this critique is somewhat undercut by international human rights law's increasingly extensive protection of economic, social, and cultural rights. Moreover, while it is true that human rights are individual entitlements, many rights impose duties on governments that benefit the collective. This is particularly true of the right to health, which, while certainly entrenching individual entitlements, is relatively meaningless without a corresponding health system to enable its fulfilment. These and other controversies provide important context for this chapter's discussion of the right to health and for understanding possible institutional and structural factors contributing to its non-realisation.

THE RIGHT TO HEALTH IN INTERNATIONAL LAW

EVOLUTION OF THE RIGHT TO HEALTH

The origins of the right to health can be found in nineteenth-century Europe, with the emergence of a public health movement and recognition of economic, social, and cultural rights (Toebes 1999, p. 7). Increasingly poor working and living conditions associated with the Industrial Revolution in England fomented a broader recognition of state responsibility for population health, including for improving health care for the poor (Toebes 1999, pp. 10–11). At the same time, a series of international sanitary conferences were held to coordinate the prevention of transmissible disease at the international level (Toebes 1999, p. 12). These earlier developments paved the way for a broader recognition of social rights, coalescing after Franklin D. Roosevelt's "Four Freedoms Speech" in 1941, which identified freedom from want as one of the four freedoms necessary to create a secure world (Roosevelt 1941). These developments set the context for an explicit recognition of the right to health within the new UN.

THE RIGHT TO HEALTH WITHIN THE UN

The first formal articulation of state duties concerning health can be found in the 1945 Charter of the UN, which states that one of the UN's objectives is to promote "solutions of international economic, social, health, and related problems."[6] In pursuance of this objective, in 1946 the World Health Organization (WHO) was created as a specialised agency of the UN. The Constitution of the World Health Organization was the first international document to recognise an individual right to health; according to the Constitution's preamble, "the enjoyment of the highest attainable standard of health is a fundamental right of every human being without distinction," and governments are responsible "for the health of their peoples which can be fulfilled only by the provision of adequate health and social measures."[7] The Constitution does not, however, provide clarity or guidance on what constitutes "adequate" measures—a definition further complicated by the document's broad definition of health as "a state of complete physical, mental and social well-being and not merely the absence of disease or infirmity" (preamble).

The Universal Declaration of Human Rights (1948)

Two years after WHO adopted its Constitution, the right to health was further developed in the non-binding yet iconic Universal Declaration of Human Rights, which articulates a broad range of civil, political, economic, social, and cultural rights.[8] Its primary provision on health is found in article 25(1), which states in part that "everyone has the right to a standard of living adequate for the health and well-being of himself and of his family, including food, clothing, housing and medical care and necessary social services." The inclusion of medical care within the minimum socio-economic conditions necessary for health advances the definition of health by providing potential parameters for achieving the highest attainable standard of health. Nonetheless, the combination of health with other social rights in article 25 is very broad and vague, without providing any textual explanation of health (Toebes 1999, p. 40).

As a declaration, the Universal Declaration was meant to act as "a common standard of achievement" and not as a binding human rights treaty (preamble; Glendon 2002). However, the Universal Declaration is widely understood to have become customary international law, imposing universal obligations (i.e., obligations that apply to all states globally) for its realisation (International Law Association 1994, pp. 525–569; McDougal et al. 1980, pp. 273–274; Sohn 1982, p. 16).[9]

In 1966, the UN attempted to codify the Universal Declaration's provisions in two distinct international human rights treaties: the International Covenant on Economic, Social and Cultural Rights (ICESCR) and the International Covenant on Civil and Political Rights (ICCPR).[10] Together with the Universal Declaration, these instruments form what is known as the International Bill of Rights.

The UN's original intention was to create one new treaty that would codify the Universal Declaration; however, this idea was scuppered by the ideological and geopolitical conflicts of the Cold War, which ensured that the two primary categories of rights—civil and political rights on the one hand and economic, social, and cultural rights on the other—were kept separate. The ideological roots of this division assured that civil and political rights came to be associated with liberal democracy while economic, social, and cultural rights came to be associated with communism. Indeed, even today, lingering ideological opposition to the right to health is often rooted in the misconception that this right is inherently communist or socialist by nature, and therefore incompatible with liberal and capitalist democracy.

The International Covenant on Economic, Social and Cultural Rights (1966)

Amongst numerous human rights instruments protecting health, the ICESCR contains the most authoritative formulation of this right. Article 12 recognises the right of everyone to the enjoyment of the highest attainable standard of physical and mental health. While repeating the broad definition of the right to health contained in the WHO Constitution, article 12 also prescribes specific steps that states must take in order to fully realise this standard of health. For example, state parties should take steps to reduce the stillbirth rate and infant mortality; to improve all aspects of environmental and industrial hygiene; to prevent, treat, and control epidemic, endemic, occupational, and other diseases; and to create conditions that assure medical services and attention to all in the event of sickness. Notably, under article 2 of the ICESCR, states also agree with regard to all economic, social, and cultural rights

> to take steps, individually and through international assistance and cooperation, especially economic and technical, to the maximum of [their] available resources, to achieve progressively the full realization of Covenant rights by all appropriate means, including particularly legislation.

By telling states to take steps according to the "maximum of [their] available resources," this provision appears to delimit state obligations to realise the expansive promise of article 12's right to health. Read together, articles 2 and 12 give little indication of the scope of the highest attainable standard of health or of states' obligations to progressively realise this right. The task of elaborating this scope and duties fell to the various institutions created within the UN, as discussed below.

International Covenant on Civil and Political Rights (1966)

While the ICCPR does not specifically address health, it protects numerous rights that are directly or indirectly relevant to health. These include the rights to life (art. 6), privacy (art. 17), liberty and security (art. 9), and equality (art. 26), as well as the protection of minorities (art. 27). Moreover, the UN Human Rights Committee—an independent body of experts charged with monitoring implementation of the ICCPR and thus further interpreting the treaty's provisions—has interpreted the right to life as requiring states to take positive measures to reduce infant mortality and increase life expectancy, especially with respect to eliminating malnutrition and epidemics.[11] The

Committee's interpretation gives practical force to the theoretical indivis-ibility of all human rights and, indeed, to the centrality of health to the realisation of many other human rights, including those within the civil and political realm. It is important to note that in contrast to the economic, social, and cultural rights laid out in the ICESCR, the civil and political rights in the ICCPR are not subject to progressive realisation, meaning that state duties to realise these rights are immediate and not limited by a country's financial capacity.

The Right to Health in Subsequent International Treaties

Since the development of the International Bill of Rights, there has been a tremendous growth in international human rights treaties providing explicit protection to vulnerable groups, such as racial minorities, women, children, and people with disabilities. Several of these treaties develop the right to health and apply it to their focus populations. In so doing, each new treaty has incrementally developed the scope and content of the right to health. The 1969 International Convention on the Elimination of All Forms of Racial Discrimination, in its discussion of general measures to prohibit racial discrimination, obligates state parties to guarantee everyone's right to public health and medical care.[12] This Convention is notable in that it not only identifies medical care as an individual entitlement but also suggests a collective right to public health. The 1979 Convention on the Elimination of All Forms of Discrimination against Women similarly expands on the right to health, demanding that state parties undertake measures to ensure women's equal access to health-care services, particularly appropriate services for "pregnancy, confinement and the post-natal period, granting free services where necessary, as well as adequate nutrition during pregnancy and lactation."[13] Although this Convention has a narrower focus than either the ICESCR or the International Convention on the Elimination of All Forms of Racial Discrimination, since it refers only to health-care services and not to underlying health determinants (Toebes 1999, p. 55), it does fill a significant lacuna in the right to health, which previously did not specifically address women's reproductive rights.

The 1989 Convention on the Rights of the Child contains the most extensive identification of specific state obligations regarding health.[14]

This treaty is also distinctive since 193 countries have ratified it, giving it an effectively universal reach. In article 24(1), state parties recognise children's right to health, including facilities for the treatment of illness and rehabilitation of health, and strive to ensure that no child is deprived of his or her right to access such health-care services. States also undertake to reduce infant and child mortality, to combat disease and malnutrition, and to emphasise primary health care in the provision of necessary medical assistance and health care to all children (art. 24(2)). Like the ICESCR and the International Convention on the Elimination of All Forms of Racial Discrimination, this Convention reflects an inclusive understanding of the right to health as encompassing both medical care and the underlying determinants of health (Toebes 1999, p. 59). The effect is to restate the principles of the right to health with respect to children (Toebes 1999, p. 59).

The newest international human rights treaty is the 2006 Convention on the Rights of Persons with Disabilities, which aims to protect people with disabilities from a variety of social and political obstacles that may impair their full and equal participation in society.[15] The Convention includes a number of articles that directly or indirectly concern health, including people with disabilities' right to access health facilities (art. 9) and their "right to the enjoyment of the highest attainable standard of health without discrimination on the basis of disability" (art. 25). Notably, the treaty introduces a new human right related to health—namely, the right of people with disabilities to habilitation and rehabilitation, which obligates states to take steps to ensure that people with disabilities achieve maximum independence and full physical, mental, social, and vocational ability (art. 26) (see chapter 8).

The Right to Health in Regional Human Rights Treaties

The right to health is also recognised in each of the three regional human rights systems. These systems developed at different times following the creation of the UN and the drafting of the International Bill of Rights. In 1950, the Council of Europe moved to adopt the European Convention on Human Rights, only two years after the Universal Declaration was drafted.[16] In contrast, the American Convention on Human Rights was adopted in 1969 and the African Charter on Human and Peoples' Rights in 1981.[17] The reasons for the staggered introduction of these regional systems are varied, including because "for a long time, regionalism in the matter of human rights was not popular at the United Nations: there was often a tendency to regard it as the expression of a breakaway movement" (Vasak and Alston 1982, p. 451). Indeed, it was only in 1966 that the UN General Assembly began to consider actively encouraging the development of regional mechanisms, and only in 1977 that it formally appealed to states to establish regional machinery where it did not yet exist for the promotion and protection of human rights (Steiner and Alston 2000, p. 564).

In Africa, the African Charter protects every individual's right to enjoy the "best attainable state of physical and mental health" and calls on states to take necessary measures to protect the health of their people and to ensure that they receive medical attention when they are sick (art. 16). The African Charter on the Rights and Welfare of the Child, another regional treaty, specifies every child's right to enjoy the best attainable state of physical, mental, and spiritual health, with states agreeing to undertake a range of measures, including ensuring the provision of necessary medical assistance and health care to all.[18] In Europe, health rights are contained in the European Social Charter (the system's social rights treaty, which supplements the civil rights protected in the European Convention on Human Rights).[19] In the Inter-American system, the Protocol of San Salvador provides that "everyone shall have the right to health, understood to mean the enjoyment of the highest level of physical, mental and social well-being."[20] Like the European system, the Protocol's social rights supplement the civil rights protected in the American Convention on Human Rights. While there is no regional human rights system in Asia, in 1998 over two hundred NGOs from the region drafted a "people's charter" of Asian human rights, which includes several health-related provisions.[21] In addition, in the Middle East, the Cairo Declaration on Human Rights in Islam provides that "everyone shall have the right to medical and social care, and to all public amenities provided by society and the State within the limits of their available resources."[22] Figure 1.1 illustrates the key regional and international instruments that protect the right to health.

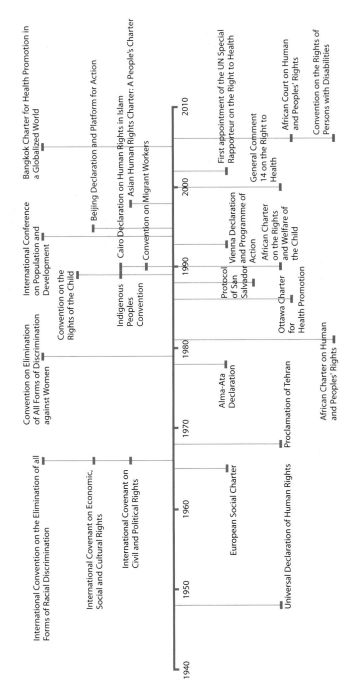

FIGURE 1.1 Timeline of major human rights instruments protecting the right to health.

PIVOTAL STEPS IN THE DEVELOPMENT OF THE RIGHT TO HEALTH

DECLARATIONS AND CONFERENCES ON HEALTH

In addition to being developed through legally binding treaties, the right to health has been significantly advanced during the last three decades through a series of international health conferences focused on clarifying and further developing governmental duties around the right. The imperative to develop this right was advanced by an emerging understanding of the relationship between health and human rights, animated by the HIV and AIDS pandemics, women's health issues, and gross violations of human rights globally, including in the Balkans and Great Lakes of Africa (Gruskin and Tarantola 2005, p. 1). The 1978 International Conference on Primary Health Care, one of the most important and earliest of these conferences, issued the ground-breaking Alma-Ata Declaration,[23] which declared primary health care the principal vehicle for achieving health for all by the year 2000 (see chapter 3). The Declaration reflected a paradigmatic shift in which health was viewed not simply as the outcome of biomedical interventions but also as the result of underlying determinants (Lawn et al. 2008, p. 919) and as fundamentally rooted in social justice and human rights. Thus, the first paragraph of the Declaration reaffirms that "health is a fundamental human right and that the attainment of the highest possible level of health requires the action of many other social and economic sectors in addition to the health sector." The notion of human rights is reflected similarly in the Declaration's recognition that "governments have a responsibility for the health of their people which can be fulfilled only by the provision of adequate health and social measures," particularly primary health care (para. v). The Declaration defines primary health care as "essential health care" to be made universally accessible in a participatory and affordable way (para. vi). The Alma-Ata Declaration's emphasis on primary health care as "essential health care" played an influential role in the ESCR Committee's later elaboration of states' core duties regarding essential elements of health care (discussed below; see chapter 4).

Elaborating on Alma-Ata's definition of health, the Ottawa Charter for Health Promotion set a framework for understanding and addressing the social conditions that influence and ultimately determine health, including "peace, shelter, education, food, income, a stable eco-system, sustainable resources, social justice, and equity."[24] These conditions move health beyond the health sector to a phenomenon infused with moral and social values inextricably linked to all public sectors and players. Towards this end, the Charter proposes that actions on health include intersectoral policy development, individual and community empowerment, and restructuring health services towards preventative rather than curative services.

Subsequent international health conferences have reinforced and expanded this emphasis on primary health care and the social determinants of health. At the 1994 International Conference on Population and Development (ICPD) held in Cairo, 179 states agreed to achieve a number of health-related goals, marked for the first time by global indicators, by 2004.[25] At the 1995 Fourth World Conference on Women held in Beijing, 189 states endorsed the Beijing Declaration and Platform for Action, which while focused primarily on women's health, reinforced and advanced key definitions later applied to the international human right to health.[26] For example, building on ICPD, states committed to increasing women's access to appropriate, affordable, and quality health care and services. The 1993 World Conference on Human Rights produced the Vienna Declaration and Programme of Action, which is viewed as an important consensus statement on human rights.[27] In the Declaration, 171 states proclaimed the protection and promotion of human rights and fundamental freedoms as the first responsibility of governments (para. 1). The Declaration also recognises the right to health, including in relation to environmental degradation, women, and vulnerable groups, such as migrant workers (paras. 11, 18, 24, 41).

The Bangkok Charter for Health Promotion in a Globalized World was released at the 6th Global Conference on Health Promotion in 2005 to update the 1986 Ottawa Charter by "addressing the determinants of health in a globalized world through health promotion."[28] Accordingly, the Charter proposes advocating for health based on human rights and solidarity; investing in policies, actions, and infrastructure to address the determinants of health; and assuring policy coherence across governmental departments, the UN, and other organisations, including the private sector (p. 3). While the Bangkok Charter explicitly recognises the right to health and the importance of health advocacy based on human rights, it has been criticised for diminishing health promotion goals from striving for social justice to simply improving social opportunities (People's Health Movement 2005; Porter 2007).

These declarations and conferences have served a number of important functions, including influencing international and national policy making and generating consensus-based global indicators of achievement.[29] They not only provide consistency in health policies across countries and guide national and international bodies in enforcing health rights, but have also elevated global health issues (such as HIV pandemics) to the top of the global agenda (see chapter 7).[30]

GENERAL COMMENT 14 ON THE RIGHT TO HEALTH

The most significant advancement in the interpretation of article 12 of the ICESCR is reflected in a general comment written by the ESCR Committee in 2000, referred to as General Comment 14.[31] The ESCR Committee is a group of independent experts tasked with monitoring states' implementation of the ICESCR; like other human rights treaty bodies, from time to time the Committee publishes "general comments" in which it interprets specific provisions of the ICESCR. General Comment 14 provides the most authoritative international interpretation of the right to health by extensively interpreting its normative scope and identifying state obligations and correlative violations. The Comment makes several important conceptual advances, including identifying entitlements, essential elements of the right to health, and states' core obligations, as well as general duties to respect, protect, and fulfil the right to health. It is notable that the Committee explicitly draws from international conferences—including Alma-Ata, ICPD, and Beijing—in specifying these essential elements and minimum core obligations

Entitlements

One of the most important advances of General Comment 14 is in the ESCR Committee's pragmatic interpretation of the right to health, which the Committee argues to be an inclusive right that includes the rights to both health care and the underlying determinants of health (including food, housing, access to water and adequate sanitation, safe working conditions, and a healthy environment) (para. 4). General Comment 14 notes that the right to health is not a right to be healthy but rather an entitlement to a system of health protection that provides equality of opportunity for people to enjoy the highest attainable standard of health, and which includes a variety of facilities, goods, services, and conditions necessary to realise this standard (paras. 8, 9) (see chapter 4). It also emphasises that non-discrimination is a key entitlement and duty under this right; it prohibits discrimination in access to health care and underlying determinants of health on multiple grounds, including race, sex, language, religion, national or social origin, physical or mental disability, health status (including HIV and AIDS), sexual orientation, and civil, political, social, or other status (para. 18). Practically assuring non-discrimination in health and health services requires that data be disaggregated according to these prohibited grounds of discrimination (paras. 16, 20, 57).

Essential Elements of the Right to Health: Availability, Accessibility, Acceptability, and Quality

The normative specificity of the right to health is aided considerably by the ESCR Committee's recognition that while the highest attainable standard of health and the health system will vary from country to country depending on national resources, the right must contain certain essential elements irrespective of a country's developmental levels (paras. 1, 12).

General Comment 14 identifies as essential elements of the right to health that health-care facilities, goods and services, and the social determinants of health should be available, accessible, acceptable, and of good quality (AAAQ) (see box 1.1). These elements provide an important analytical framework to state and non-state actors alike in assessing what adequate compliance with this right requires practically, including in the context of health systems.

> ## BOX 1.1
>
> ### THE AAAQ FRAMEWORK
>
> **Availability** requires sufficient quantities of functioning public health and health-care facilities, goods, and services within a state, irrespective of a country's developmental level.
>
> **Accessibility** encompasses a range of factors determining access, including discrimination, physical access, economic affordability, and information accessibility.
>
> **Acceptability** requires that health care be provided with attention to the criteria of medical ethics; cultural, gender, and age-related sensitivity; and confidentiality.
>
> Lastly, health facilities, goods, and services are expected to be scientifically and medically appropriate and of good **quality**.
>
> *Source*: Committee on Economic, Social and Cultural Rights, General Comment 14, U.N. Doc. E/C.12/2000/4 (2000), para. 12.

Core Obligations

Allied to the concept of essential elements is the identification of core obligations under the right to health. General Comment 14 holds that "a State party cannot, under any circumstances whatsoever, justify its non-compliance with the core obligations ... which are non-derogable" (para. 47). It specifies that "states parties have a core obligation to ensure the satisfaction of, at the very least, minimum essential levels of each of the rights," which include

- providing non-discriminatory access to health facilities, goods, and services, especially for vulnerable or marginalised groups
- ensuring access to the minimum essential food, which should be nutritionally adequate and safe, to ensure freedom from hunger
- ensuring access to basic shelter, housing, and sanitation, as well as an adequate supply of safe and potable water

- providing essential drugs as defined under the WHO Action Programme on Essential Drugs (see chapter 9)
- ensuring the equitable distribution of all health facilities, goods, and services
- adopting and implementing a national public health strategy and plan of action addressing the health concerns of the whole population, with particular attention to vulnerable and marginalised groups (see chapter 4)

General Comment 14 also indicates that as obligations of comparable priority, states must take measures to prevent, treat, and control epidemic and endemic diseases, and to ensure reproductive, maternal (prenatal as well as postnatal), and child health care (paras. 44(a)–(b)).

In addition to being related to the essential elements of the right to health, the concept of core obligations also allies strongly with the notion of primary health care as essential care, as originally promoted in the Alma-Ata Declaration. The core obligations concept thus provides a rights-based approach to systemic deprivation, suggesting that where large numbers of people are deprived of realisation of their basic needs, this should be viewed as a human rights problem and a potential violation of the right to health (Forman 2009).

Progressive Realisation

In General Comment 14, the ESCR Committee interprets progressive realisation as requiring states to take immediate action and effective movement towards realising the right to health, including by guaranteeing the non-discriminatory exercise of rights and by taking deliberate, concrete, and targeted steps towards full realisation (para. 31). This means that while states can justify some health-care deficiencies, they cannot justify the failure to work towards rectifying them. The intent of these clarifications is to provide states with greater guidance in fulfilling their duties of progressive realisation regarding the right to health, and to counter any perceptions that progressive realisation enables a state to indefinitely delay taking action.

Respect, Protect, and Fulfil

General Comment 14 provides further guidance on state obligations through its analytical framework of duties to respect, protect, and fulfil rights (para. 33).

Respecting human rights requires governments not to interfere with the right to health, including through policies that are discriminatory (para. 34) or that contravene article 12 standards and are likely to cause unnecessary morbidity and preventable mortality (para. 50).

Protecting rights requires states to take measures to ensure equal access to health services provided by third parties, including controlling the marketing of health goods and services by third parties (para. 35).

Fulfilling human rights requires states to give "sufficient recognition to the right to health in the national political and legal systems, preferably by way of legislative implementation, and to adopt a national health policy with a detailed plan for realizing the right to health" (para. 36). State obligations to fulfil a specific right arise "when individuals or a group are unable, for reasons beyond their control, to realize that right themselves by means at their disposal" (para. 37). States violate their obligation to fulfil the right to health when they fail to take all necessary steps to ensure its realisation, such as by failing to adopt a national policy to ensure the right to health for everyone or by spending insufficient funds or misallocating public resources, resulting in the non-enjoyment of the right to health, especially by vulnerable or marginalised individuals or groups (para. 52).

General Comment 14 holds that in determining whether particular actions violate the right to health, it is important to distinguish non-compliance arising from unwillingness from that arising from inability (para. 47). Thus, a state that is unwilling to use the maximum of its available resources to realise this right would be in violation (para. 47). While General Comment 14 does not specifically indicate the kind of resources that must be allocated to health, it is important to note that the ICESCR's drafters intended the "maximum of available resources" to refer "to both the resources existing within a State and those available from the international community though international cooperation and assistance."[32]

Limitations of Rights in Service of Public Health

In General Comment 14, the ESCR Committee indicates that when governments cite public health issues as reasons for restricting human rights, they bear the burden of justifying these measures as compatible with the nature of such rights and solely for the purpose of promoting general welfare in a democratic society. While states are permitted to limit rights under strictly defined circumstances, the purpose of these limitations is to "primarily to protect the rights of individuals rather than to permit the imposition of limitations by states" (para. 28). Accordingly, such limitations must be "in accordance with the law, including international human rights standards, compatible with the nature of the rights protected by the Covenant, in the interest of legitimate aims pursued, and strictly necessary for the promotion of the general welfare in a democratic society" (para. 28). In line with the UN Siracusa Principles on the Limitation and Derogation of Rights,[33] the Committee indicates that such limitations must be proportional—in other words, "the least restrictive alternative must be adopted where several types of limitations are available" (para. 29). Moreover, the Committee indicates that even where such limitations are permitted, they should be of limited duration and subject to review.

International Obligations: International Assistance and Cooperation

While state obligations under the right to health encompass largely domestic duties, they also extend to state action internationally, as chapter 2 explores in more detail. In the present chapter's general overview of the right to health, we will point simply to General Comment 14's reiteration that states must respect the right to health in other countries and must protect the right by preventing third parties from violating it elsewhere if states can influence them by legal or political means (para. 39). In particular, "depending on the availability of resources, States should facilitate access to essential health facilities, goods and services in other countries, where possible and provide the necessary aid when required" (para. 39). The international community has a collective responsibility to address disease, since some diseases are easily transmissible beyond state borders (para. 40). In this regard, developed countries have a special responsibility and interest in assisting poorer developing ones (para. 40).

SPECIAL RAPPORTEUR ON THE RIGHT TO HEALTH

In 2002, the UN Human Rights Council (which replaced the now defunct UN Commission on Human Rights) appointed Paul Hunt as the first Special Rapporteur on the Right to Health, with the mandate of promoting the development and realisation of this right globally. The creation of this position (see box 1.2) reflects an important recognition within the UN of the importance of the right to health and has enabled considerable international attention on the development of this right. The Special Rapporteur on the Right to Health has three main objectives:

- to promote and encourage the promotion of the right to health as a fundamental human right
- to clarify specific elements and the general content of the right to health
- to identify good practices at the community, national, and international levels for the operationalisation of the right to health, and to receive individual complaints, which the Rapporteur is to follow up on and make publicly available once a year (University of Essex Human Rights Centre 2008)

The Special Rapporteur fulfils this mandate by undertaking country missions and other visits, transmitting communications with governments regarding alleged violations of the right to health, and submitting annual reports to both the Human Rights Council and the General Assembly. These reports detail activities performed under the mandate and include information on particular issues relevant to the right to health, such as poverty, international trade, health systems, mental health, access to medicines, neglected diseases, HIV and AIDS, maternal mortality, indicators, and sexual and reproductive health (OHCHR 2010). In addition, the Special Rapporteur undertakes country missions, which to date include Peru (2004), Uganda (2005 and 2007), Israel (2006), Lebanon (2006), Colombia (2007), India (2007), Sweden (2007), Australia (2009), and Guatemala (2010). In addition, the Special Rapporteur has completed missions to international organisations and non-state actors that play a role in the realisation of the right to health, such as the World Trade Organization (2003), the World Bank (2007), the International Monetary Fund (2007), and GlaxoSmithKline (2008).[34] The aim of such visits is to obtain first-hand information on the right to health, report findings, and propose recommendations for improvement of priority issues (OHCHR 2010; University of Essex 2008). These missions are particularly significant since they expand international human rights law beyond its state-centric orientation, which traditionally has a limited application to non-state actors such as international organisations and corporations; in addition, these missions increase understanding of the right to health and improve its practical application.

The establishment of the Special Rapporteur procedure has provided an important platform for advancing the priority of the right to health within international law and the global political arena. It has also contributed to the development of new right-to-health tools, such as human rights indicators (see Backman et al. 2008).

BOX 1.2

SPECIAL RAPPORTEURS ON THE RIGHT TO HEALTH

Mr. Paul Hunt (New Zealand)
August 2002–July 2008
Paul Hunt is a professor of law and a member of the Human Rights Centre at the University of Essex, UK, as well as an adjunct professor of law at the University of Waikato, New Zealand.

Mr. Anand Grover (India)
August 2008–current
Anand Grover is a practising lawyer in the High Court of Bombay and the Supreme Court of India, and director of the Lawyers Collective in India.

PRACTICAL TOOLS FOR REALISING ACCOUNTABILITY UNDER THE RIGHT TO HEALTH

Increased legal understanding of the right to health has led to the development of practical tools and frameworks for realising this right, including by assuring that duty-bearers are held accountable. While these include traditional human rights tools—such as country reporting, litigation, and "naming and shaming"—they have also expanded to more programmatic or systemic approaches, such as participation and rights-based approaches. This section describes various accountability mechanisms for realising the right to health, including international, regional, and domestic procedures, as well as practical tools such as rights-based indicators and social participation. It does not suggest that accountability mechanisms are not practical, nor that practical tools do not contribute towards monitoring and realising accountability. Instead, this section adopts an understanding of accountability mechanisms and practical tools as interrelated and synergistic.

ACCOUNTABILITY MECHANISMS: INTERNATIONAL, REGIONAL, AND DOMESTIC

Accountability is not simply an aspirational by-product of human rights—it is "a distinctive, complex and central feature of human rights" (Potts 2008, p. 7). In relation to human rights, accountability is often associated with certain strategies, often litigation and "naming and shaming." However, account-ability is considerably broader than these strategies (critical as they are within the human rights arena). As Helen Potts argues,

> Accountability in the context of the right to health is the process which provides individuals and communities with an opportunity to understand how government has discharged its right to health obligations. Equally it provides government with the opportunity to explain what it has done and why. Where mistakes have been made, accountability requires redress. It is a process that helps to identify what works, so it can be repeated, and what does not, so it can be revised. (2008, p. 7)

Potts identifies five categories of accountability mechanisms at the national, regional, and international levels: namely, judicial, quasi-judicial, adminis-trative, political, and social mechanisms (2008; see box 1.3). Some of the more important of these mechanisms are discussed below. It is worth noting that almost all of these mechanisms are triggered by the claims of individuals and advocacy movements against states as the primary duty-bearers in interna-tional law—pointing to the key role played by civil society in the realisation of rights.

ACCOUNTABILITY MECHANISMS

- Judicial accountability mechanisms include judicial review of executive acts and omissions, constitutional redress, statutory interpretation, and public interest litigation.
- Quasi-judicial mechanisms include national, regional, and international human rights bodies.
- Administrative mechanisms include human rights impact assessments.
- Political mechanisms include parliamentary reviews of budgetary allocations, as well as the use of public funds, democratically elected health councils, and health-care commissions.
- Social mechanisms include the involvement of civil society in budget monitoring, health centre monitoring, public hearings, and social audits.

Source: Potts (2008)

International Accountability Mechanisms

Each of the international human rights treaties has a quasi-judicial treaty committee, comprised of independent experts, appointed as a monitoring and interpretive body. These human rights treaty bodies (also referred to as committees) release concluding observations assessing country compliance and produce "general comments" interpreting rights within their respective treaties. Treaty reporting and concluding observations (explained below) offer an important mechanism for state accountability and public participation, and are the primary way that human rights treaty bodies monitor governments' compliance with their treaty obligations. When a country ratifies a treaty, it agrees to submit regular reports on a basis determined by that treaty. These "country reports" provide an update to the treaty's monitoring body on how the state is complying with its obligations. Human rights treaty bodies can also receive information on a particular country's human rights situation from other sources, including NGOs, intergovernmental organisations, and the media—these reports, called "shadow reports," make the reporting process an open and transparent forum for assessing governmental action. The treaty body then examines both the country report and any shadow reports submitted, after which it publishes "concluding observations" that identify concerns about non-compliance and recommend action to enable improved implementation. Reporting is neither adversarial nor adjudicative but rather intended to operate as a "constructive dialogue" to assist governments (Alston 1997, p. 20). Indeed, there is a relatively low incidence in concluding observations of findings of violations, and a high incidence of recommendations concerning progressive steps to be taken (Lyon 2003, p. 37). However, where committees note their "concern" about particular acts or omissions by the state, as they often do, this is generally indicative of a treaty violation (Alston 1997)—providing important support to both domestic and regional judicial interpretation of comparable rights protections, as well as to individual complaints before the treaty bodies.

Within the UN system, most human rights treaties allow individual complaints to be lodged against state parties alleging the violation of treaty rights. For example, individuals in countries that have ratified the ICCPR can lodge complaints with the Human Rights Committee, the body tasked with overseeing governments' compliance with that treaty. There is presently no mechanism under the ICESCR for adjudicating individual complaints of violations of ICESCR rights, although an optional protocol to initiate this procedure at the CESCR has been under discussion at the UN since 1996. The ICESCR Optional Protocol will allow state parties to the ICESCR to recognise the competence of the CESCR to consider individual complaints.[35] Once it comes into operation, the mechanism will provide an important mechanism at the international level for assuring accountability with the right to health and for further developing the right to health.

With respect to individual complaints, a committee's decision is seen as an authoritative legal interpretation of the treaty in question.[36] Furthermore, states are expected to implement these decisions and provide appropriate remedies (Bayefsky 2002). It must be noted, however, that the decisions of human rights treaty bodies are not legally binding, reflecting a partial weakness in their utility. Nonetheless, the individual complaint mechanism can and does have normative influence and produces concrete outcomes. For example, in *Sandra Lovelace v. Canada*, Sandra Lovelace Nicolas lodged a complaint with the Human Rights Committee alleging that the Canadian government had violated her rights protected under the ICCPR.[37] Under Canadian law, Ms. Lovelace lost her aboriginal status when she married a non-aboriginal man; under the same legislation, however, a man would not have lost his status by marrying a non-aboriginal woman. In its decision, the Human Rights Committee found Canada to be in violation of the ICCPR. The Committee's decision subsequently had a significant impact domestically. For example, in 1985 the Canadian government amended the Indian Act to eliminate gender discrimination in determining Indian status and to restore the status of aboriginal women who had previously lost status.

Finally, in addition to the human rights treaty bodies, the Special Rapporteur on the Right to Health is an example of an international quasi-judicial accountability mechanism. Individuals, groups, communities, or representatives of affected people can send information to the Special Rapporteur alleging violations of the right to health (International Federation of Health and Human Rights Organisations 2009, p. 23). If the information is considered reliable, the Special Rapporteur may request information from the government in question or comment on the alleged violation. While these communications are confidential, the Special Rapporteur publishes summaries of their content in his or her annual reports.

Regional Accountability Mechanisms

Regional human rights bodies offer important venues for enforcing the right to health. These bodies include the European Court of Human Rights, the Inter-American Commission on Human Rights, the Inter-American Court of Human Rights, the African Commission on Human and Peoples' Rights, and the African Court on Human and Peoples' Rights. In both the European and Inter-American systems, decisions other than advisory opinions are legally binding. Furthermore, in contrast to the international human rights treaty bodies, the European and Inter-American systems offer oral hearings, appointed legal counsel, and far more detailed remedies (Bayefsky 2002, pp. 173–174). The African system introduced an African Court on Human and Peoples' Rights in 2006 with the capacity to issue advisory opinions and binding judgments (see box 1.4).

Rather than directly applying the rights in the European Social Charter, the European Court of Human Rights has interpreted certain civil rights, including the rights to life and to be free from inhuman and degrading treatment, to include health protections. For example, in *D v. United Kingdom*, the Court held that deporting someone with advanced AIDS back to St.

Kitts, where antiretrovirals were not available, would violate the European Convention on Human Rights' prohibition against inhuman or degrading treatment.[38] However, the Court has denied similar claims since then.

The Inter-American human rights system has been used extensively by people living with HIV to claim access to treatment on the basis of the rights to health and life. In the 2001 case of *Jorge Odir Miranda Cortez et al. v. El Salvador,* people living with HIV sought an interim order from the Inter-American Commission on Human Rights for El Salvador's government to provide antiretroviral therapies on an interim basis while the merits of their claim were being assessed.[39] Their claim alleged that the government of El Salvador had violated their rights to life and health by failing to provide them with antiretroviral therapies. The Commission granted an interim order requesting government to provide antiretroviral therapies to the petitioners pending the determination on the merits of the case, and also declared the complaint to be admissible, as a preliminary step to considering the merits of the case itself. Shortly thereafter, the El Salvadoran Supreme Court ordered the Salvadoran Social Security Institute to provide Cortez with antiretroviral therapies, so that it was no longer necessary to proceed with the complaint before the Inter-American Commission. This decision appears to have been largely motivated by the pressure exerted through the Commission's decision (UNAIDS and Canadian HIV/AIDS Legal Network 2006, p. 71). Notably, the government introduced legislation the same year affirming the right of every person living with HIV to "health care, medical, surgical and psychological treatment," and took preventive measures to impede the spread of the virus, which have been attributed to the influence of the interim order of the Commission and the order of the Supreme Court (UNAIDS and Canadian HIV/AIDS Legal Network 2006, p. 71).

SERAC V. NIGERIA[40]

In *SERAC v. Nigeria*, the African Commission on Human and Peoples' Rights held that the Ogoni people of Nigeria had suffered violations of their right to health and right to a general satisfactory environment because of the government's failure to prevent pollution and ecological degradation resulting from oil extraction by a multinational corporation, and for its violent attacks on Ogoni protesters against Shell. The Commission ordered the Nigerian government to cease attacks on the Ogoni people, to investigate and prosecute those responsible for attacks, to provide compensation to victims, to prepare environmental and social impact assessments in the future, and to provide information on health and environmental risks to communities affected by oil operations.

Domestic Accountability Mechanisms

Several mechanisms that operate primarily at the domestic level can be used to hold states accountable for realising the right to health. Three of these are explored below: litigation, right-to-health-based indicators and impact assessments, and rights-based participation in health. These mechanisms make an important contribution to ensuring the progressive realisation of the right to health in a non-discriminatory manner. However, it is important to note that in order for these tools to work, a range of state and non-state institutions often must play a role—including courts, ombudspersons, human rights commissions, non-governmental organisations, and the media.

Litigation. The past two decades have seen a significant increase in national-level cases involving the right to health, including in low- and middle-income countries (Gloppen 2008, p. 21). These cases have focused on a wide range of issues, such as access to health services and medication; discriminatory labour practices; various aspects of public health; and the basic determinants of health (e.g., food, water, shelter, and a healthy environment) (Gloppen 2008, p. 21). One of the best examples is from South Africa, where constitutional protections of the rights to health and life, along with international law, provided the basis for civil society groups to file a case before the Constitutional Court claiming access to medicine for the prevention of mother-to-child transmission (PMTCT) of HIV; in its decision, the Court ordered the establishment of a national perinatal programme.[41] In South Africa today, a national PMTCT programme provides medicines in over 96% of governmental clinics (Statistics South Africa 2010, p. 5).

Similarly successful litigation in Latin America illustrates how respect for and promotion of human rights can lead to both improved access to health care and increased budgetary allocations for health (Singh et al. 2007). For example, in *Mariela Viceconte v. Ministry of Health*, civil society groups argued that 3.5 million people living in an area affected by Argentine haemorrhagic fever lacked adequate access to preventive medical services to guard against infection.[42] While the government argued that it lacked an adequate vaccine supply and therefore could not launch a massive immunisation campaign, the court ruled that the government was legally obliged to intervene. The court made the ministers of health and economy personally liable for producing vaccines within a given time schedule. As a result of the case, Argentina's government developed a plan to deliver basic medicines to those in need within five years of the ruling (Singh et al. 2007, p. 525).

Certainly, "successful" cases that favour individual or group claimants at the expense of collective interests may not be conducive to good public health. Yet as the South African case on perinatal HIV transmission attests, individual and group claims can benefit collective health interests and potentially assist in reducing systematic disparities in health-care access (Forman 2011). Moreover, as the Colombian case discussed in box 1.5 illustrates, successful claims can also have systemic impacts on health system restructuring.

BOX 1.5

COLOMBIAN CONSTITUTIONAL COURT

The **Colombian Constitutional Court** handed down a landmark judgment in July 2008 ordering extensive restructuring of Colombia's health system.[43] The Court saw it necessary to step in because "the organs of government responsible for … the regulation of the health system have not adopted decisions that guarantee the right to health without having to seek recourse through the *tutela*" (Yamin and Parra-Vera 2009, p. 0148).

In 1991, the Constitutional Court was created, together with the complaint mechanism known as the *tutela*, which was created to protect individual rights by enhancing the public's access to the courts. In 1993, the country's health-care system underwent major reform, with the establishment of a two-tier system of provision and benefits. With the new *tutela* mechanism, patients could now turn to the courts to secure treatments and services that the health system had previously denied them. The Court's 2008 judgment, which was based on a compilation of these *tutelas*, reaffirmed that courts can play a significant role in enforcing access to health and social services, even when there are substantial resource implications for the state.

In its decision, the Court elaborated on Colombia's obligations with regard to health, including the following:

- accountability for ensuring the right to health
- progressive realisation of the right to health
- transparency, access to information, and evidence-based decision making that incorporates or allows for participatory action

The Colombian case reinforces the role that courts can play in setting health policy and shows that increasing citizens' access to the courts may, under certain circumstances, enhance the protection of the right to health, as well as potentially promote equity, transparency, and accountability within the health system itself.

Source: Yamin and Parra-Vera (2009)

Right-to-health indicators and impact assessments. Rights-based approaches, which seek to operationalise the concepts and standards of human rights, illustrate how rights may guide policies and programmes seeking health equity. Rights-based approaches to policy and programming mandate the incorporation of core human rights principles (e.g., non-discrimination, participation, and accountability), demand a focus on poor and marginalised groups, and require explicit reference to international human rights instruments. Indeed, Gunilla Backman et al. suggest that in the same way that the right to a fair trial has advanced a well-functioning court system, the right to health "can help to establish health systems that are reasonably equitable" (2008, p. 15). Accordingly, Backman and colleagues explored data from 194 countries, as well as related law, scholarship, and health indicators, to identify the right-to-health features of health systems. They proposed seventy-two indicators to guide researchers and policy makers in achieving health equity, strengthening health systems, and realising the right to health (see box 1.6 for examples of these indicators).

BOX 1.6

SELECT RIGHT-TO-HEALTH INDICATORS FOR HEALTH SYSTEMS

Recognition of the right to health
1. Number of international and regional human rights treaties recognising the right to health ratified by the state
2. Do the state's constitution, bill of rights, or other statutes recognise the right to health?

National health plan
17. Does the state have a comprehensive national health plan encompassing public and private sectors?

Participation
23. Is there a legal requirement for including the participation of marginalised groups in the development of the national health plan?

Medicines
28. Is access to essential medicines or technologies, as part of the fulfilment of the right to health, recognised in the constitution or national legislation?

Monitoring, assessment, accountability, and redress
65. Infant mortality rate
66. Mortality rate of children under five
67. Maternal mortality ratio

National financing
45. Is the per capita government expenditure on health greater than the minimum required for a basic effective public health system?

---

46. What is the proportion of households with catastrophic health expenditures?

47. Total government spending on health as percentage of GDP

48. Total government spending on military expenditure as percentage of GDP

Source: Backman et al. (2008)

Right-to-health impact assessments are another important mechanism that can guide realisation of the right to health. Health impact assessments have been carried out for several decades in a variety of sectors, particularly in relation to the economic, social, and environmental impacts of governmental policies (Harrison 2009, p. 1). Their primary objective is to predict the health consequences of governmental decisions and inform decision making accordingly (Kemm 2003). While a traditional health impact assessment looks at the health effects of a given policy, a right-to-health impact assessment focuses on the implications for realisation of the right to health—and does so by explicitly adopting standards on the right to health drawn from international human rights law. In a 2006 paper, Gillian MacNaughton and Paul Hunt developed a methodology for a general right-to-health impact assessment grounded in international human rights standards that seek the progressive realisation of rights, promote equality and non-discrimination, ensure meaningful participation by all, and ensure accountability. This tool has been adapted to address the impact of trade-related intellectual property rights on access to medicines, and is currently the focus of research by an interdisciplinary team that hopes to implement it in test countries globally (see box 1.7). Such tools offer the potential to ensure better realisation of the right to health and to ensure that governmental action in other domains, such as trade and commerce, does not unreasonably restrict individuals' right to health.

BOX 1.7

RIGHT-TO-HEALTH IMPACT ASSESSMENT OF TRADE-RELATED INTELLECTUAL PROPERTY RIGHTS

This right-to-health impact assessment tool provides a method for public officials and civil society to measure, evaluate, and moderate any negative impacts that trade-related intellectual property rights might have on access to affordable medicines. Based on the growing trend of health impact assessments as a critical human rights and health equity tool, a right-to-health impact assessment would consist of five key steps:

- a preliminary check on the potential impact of trade-related intellectual property rights
- the development of an assessment plan
- the collection of information
- an analysis of rights
- finalisation with a report that includes methods of implementation, evaluation and monitoring

Source: Human Rights Impact Resource Centre (2011)

Participation. Participation is a core component of the right to health. The right to health is interested not only in outcome but also process. Therefore, the right to health requires the active and informed participation of diverse actors in developing and implementing health policy (Potts 2008). As Potts suggests, the participation of individuals and groups in monitoring and developing health policy is an important component of the accountability process. There are a wide variety of participatory methods, including regional and national conferences, permanent or time-bound forums, local health committees and teams, focus groups, citizen's juries, public meetings, budgetary oversight, and local committee elections (Potts 2008, p. 20). As box 1.8 illustrates, rights-based citizen participation in health services can improve the delivery of these services.

BOX 1.8

RIGHTS-BASED CITIZEN MONITORING OF HEALTH SERVICES
IN PERU

In 2004, CARE–Peru implemented a rights-based programme to
improve the health of the poor, with a particular emphasis on improving
the relationship between citizens and the state and on ensuring
greater accountability on the part of health workers. The programme
implemented a variety of strategies to achieve these outcomes, including
strengthening citizens' monitoring of health services in the Piura and
Puno regions. A national NGO (Forosalud), the Regional Ombudsman's
Office, and networks of community Quechua and Aymara women
created a strategic alliance whereby forty-seven women were selected to
monitor local health authorities and ensure that the health rights of local
populations, including women and Quechua people, were realised. The
monitoring is reported to have resulted in a "distinct improvement in the
quality of health service provision" (Potts 2008, p. 36).

Source: Potts (2008, pp. 35–36)

CONCLUSION

This chapter has sought to introduce readers to the international human
rights law system; the origins, development, and content of the right to health;
and methods for ensuring the realisation of this right by state and non-state
actors. It has also sought to illustrate the increasingly specific content of
this right, as developed by mechanisms such as General Comment 14 and
the Special Rapporteur on the Right to Health. As cases from the domestic
level indicate, courts are increasingly being used to hold governments
accountable for protecting the right to health. Moreover, innovative new
mechanisms like right-to-health indicators and impact assessment offer
states guidance for realising this right and provide civil society with practical
tools for monitoring governments' progress. This legal background and these
practical strategies lay an important groundwork for understanding the
contribution that the right to health can make to improving health outcomes
and health systems.

REFERENCES

Alston, P. 1997. "The Purposes of Reporting." In *Manual on Human Rights Reporting*, United Nations, U.N. Doc. HR/PUB/91/1 (Rev. 1), 19–24.

Aust, A. 2010. *Handbook of International Law.* 2nd ed. Cambridge: Cambridge Univ. Press.

Backman, G., P. Hunt, R. Khosla, et al. 2008. "Health Systems and the Right to Health an Assessment of 194 Countries." *The Lancet* 372 (9655): 2047–2085.

Bayefsky, A. F. 2002. *How to Complain to the UN Human Rights Treaty System.* Ardsley Park: Transnational Publishers, Inc.

Brierly, J. L. 1978. *The Law of Nations: An Introduction to the International Law of Peace.* 6th ed. New York: Oxford Univ. Press.

Dugard, J. 2001. *International Law: A South African Perspective.* 2nd ed. Lansdowne: Juta Law.

Forman, L. 2009. "What Future for the Minimum Core? Contextualizing the Implications of South African Socioeconomic Rights Jurisprudence for the International Human Right to Health." In *Global Health and Human Rights: Legal and Philosophical Perspectives*, ed. J. Harrington and M. Stuttaford, 62–80. New York: Routledge.

—. 2011. "Making the Case for Human Rights in Global Health Education, Research and Policy." *Canadian Journal of Public Health* 102 (3): 207–209.

Glendon, M. A. 2002. *A World Made New: Eleanor Roosevelt and the Universal Declaration of Human Rights.* New York: Random House.

Gloppen, S. 2008. "Litigation as a Strategy to Hold Governments Accountable for Implementing the Right to Health." *Health and Human Rights* 10 (2): 21–36.

Gruskin, S., and D. Tarantola. 2005. "Health and Human Rights." In *Perspectives on Health and Human Rights*, ed. S. Gruskin, M. A. Grodin, G. J. Annas, and S. P. Marks, 1–61. New York: Taylor & Francis Group.

Harrison, J. 2009. "Conducting a Human Rights Impact Assessment of the Canada-Colombia Free Trade Agreement: Key Issues." Background paper prepared for Canada's Coalition to End Global Poverty Policy Group.

Henkin, L. 1990. *The Age of Rights.* New York: Columbia Univ. Press.

Human Rights Impact Resource Centre. 2011. "Right to Health Impact Assessment of Trade-Related Intellectual Property Rights." Accessed 9 November 2011. http://www.humanrightsimpact.org/rthia/home.

Hunt, P. 2006. "The Human Right to the Highest Attainable Standard of Health: New Opportunities and Challenges." *Transactions of the Royal Society of Tropical Medicine and Hygiene* 100: 603–607.

Hunt, P., and G. MacNaughton. 2006. "Impact Assessments, Poverty and Human Rights: A Case Study Using the Right to the Highest Attainable Standard of Health." Health and Human Rights Working Paper Series No. 6, World Health Organization and UNESCO.

International Federation of Health and Human Rights Organisations. 2009. *The UN Special Rapporteur on the Right to Health: A Guide for Civil Society.* Utrecht: International Federation of Health and Human Rights Organisations.

International Law Association. 1994. "Final Report on the Status of the Universal Declaration of Human Rights in National and International Law." In *Report of the 66th Conference, Buenos Aires, Argentina, 14–20 August 1994.* London: International Law Association.

Kemm, J. 2003. "Perspectives on Health Impact Assessment." *Bulletin of the World Health Organization* 81 (6): 387.

Lawn, J., J. Rohde, S. Rifkin, et al. 2008. "Alma-Ata 30 Years On: Revolutionary, Relevant and Time to Revitalize." *The Lancet* 372 (9642): 917–927.

Lyon, B. 2003. "Discourse in Development: A Post-Colonial Theory 'Agenda' for the UN Committee on Economic, Social and Cultural Rights." Villanova Public Law and Legal Theory Working Paper Series, Working Paper No. 2003–9.

McDougal, M. S., H. D. Lasswell, and L-C. Chen. 1980. *Human Rights and World Public Order.* New Haven: Yale Univ. Press.

Mutua, M. W. 2001. "Book Review and Note: Theory and Reality in the International Protection of Human Rights, by J. Shand Watson." *American Journal of International Law* 95 (1): 255–256.

OHCHR (Office of the UN High Commissioner for Human Rights). 2010. "Special Rapporteur on the right of everyone to the enjoyment of the highest attainable standard of physical and mental health." Accessed 10 September 2011. http://www2.ohchr.org/english/issues/health/right/index.htm.

Otto, D. 1997. "Rethinking Universals: Opening Transformative Possibilities in International Human Rights Law." *Australian Yearbook of International Law* 18: 1–36.

Panikkar, R. 1996. "Is the Notion of Human Rights a Western Concept?" In *Human Rights Law,* ed. P. Alston, 75–102. New York: New York Univ. Press.

People's Health Movement. 2005. "Submission from PHM on the Fifth Draft, 24 June 2005 of the Bangkok Charter for Health Promotion." Accessed 10 September 2011. http://www.phmovement.org/pha2/issues/bangkok_charter.php.

Porter, C. 2007. "Ottawa to Bangkok: Changing Health Promotion Discourse." *Health Promotion International* 22 (1): 72–79.

Potts, H. 2008. *Accountability and the Right to the Highest Attainable Standard of Health*. Colchester: Univ. of Essex. http://www.essex.ac.uk/human_rights_centre/research/rth/docs/HRC_Accountability_Mar08.pdf.

Roosevelt, F. D. 1941. "Four Freedoms Speech." Accessed 10 September 2011. http://history.acusd.edu/gen/WW2Text/wwt0047.

Risse, T., S. C. Ropp, and K. Sikkink, eds. 1999. *The Power of Human Rights: International Norms and Domestic Change*. Cambridge: Cambridge Univ. Press.

Singh, J. A., M. Govender, and E. J. Mills. 2007. "Do Human Rights Matter to Health?" *The Lancet* 370 (4): 521–527.

Sohn, L. 1982. "The New International Law: Protection of the Rights of Individuals Rather than States." *American University Law Review* 32 (1): 1–16.

de Sousa Santos, B. 2002. *Toward a New Legal Common Sense: Law, Globalization and Emancipation*. 2nd ed. London: Butterworths Lexis Nexis.

Statistics South Africa. 2010. *Mid-Year Population Estimates 2010*. Pretoria: Statistics South Africa. http://www.statssa.gov.za/publications/P0302/P03022010.pdf

Steiner, H. J., and P. Alston, eds. 2000. *International Human Rights in Context: Law, Politics, Morals*. Oxford: Clarendon Press.

Toebes, B. C. A. 1999. *The Right to Health as a Human Right in International Law*. Antwerp: Intersentia.

UNAIDS (Joint UN Programme on HIV/AIDS) and Canadian HIV/AIDS Legal Network. 2006. *Courting Rights: Case Studies in Litigating the Human Rights of People Living with HIV*. Geneva: UNAIDS.

University of Essex Human Rights Centre. 2008. "An Introduction to the Work of the Special Rapporteur." Accessed 10 September 2011. http://www.essex.ac.uk/human_rights_centre/research/rth/rapporteur.aspx

Vasak, K., and P. Alston, eds. 1982. *The International Dimensions of Human Rights*. Paris: UNESCO.

Waldron, J., ed. 1987. *Nonsense Upon Stilts: Bentham. Burke and Marx on the Rights of Man*. London: Methuen.

Yamin, A.E., and O. Parra-Vera. 2009. "How Do Courts Set Health Policy? The Case of the Colombian Constitutional Court." *PLoS Medicine* 6 (2): 0148–0150.

NOTES

1 Customary international law refers to the creation of international law through state practice over time that occurs out of a sense of legal obligation (*opinio juris*). Both elements (state practice and *opinio juris*) are necessary for a customary rule of international law to be considered to have formed.

2 Charter of the United Nations, 26 June 1945, 59 Stat. 1031, entered into force 24 October 1945, preamble.

3 Universal Declaration of Human Rights, G.A. Res. 217A (III), U.N. Doc A/810 at 71 (1948).

4 Ibid., preamble.

5 Vienna Declaration and Programme of Action, World Conference on Human Rights, 25 June 1993, U.N. Doc A/Conf.157/23 (1993).

6 Charter of the United Nations, *supra* note 2, art. 55.

7 Constitution of the World Health Organization, signed 22 June 1946.

8 Universal Declaration, *supra* note 3.

9 Proclamation of Teheran, Final Act of the International Conference on Human Rights, Teheran, 22 April–13 May 1968, U.N. Doc. A/CONF. 32/41 at 3 (1968), art. 2.

10 International Covenant on Economic, Social and Cultural Rights, G.A. Res. 2200A (XXI), 21 U.N. GAOR Supp. (No. 16) at 49, U.N. Doc. A/6316 (1966), 993 U.N.T.S. 3, entered into force 3 January 1976; International Covenant on Civil and Political Rights, G.A. Res. 2200A (XXI), 21 U.N. GAOR Supp. (No. 16) at 52, U.N. Doc. A/6316 (1966), 999 U.N.T.S. 171, entered into force 23 March 1976.

11 Human Rights Committee, General Comment 6, U.N. Doc. HRI/GEN/1 (1982), para. 5.

12 International Convention on the Elimination of All Forms of Racial Discrimination, G.A. Res. 2106 (XX), Annex, 20 U.N. GAOR Supp. (No. 14) at 47, U.N. Doc. A/6014 (1966), 660 U.N.T.S. 195, entered into force 4 January 1969, art. 5(e)(iv).

13 Convention on the Elimination of All Forms of Discrimination against Women, G.A. Res. 34/180, 34 U.N. GAOR Supp. (No. 46) at 193, U.N. Doc. A/34/46 (1979), entered into force 3 September 1981, arts. 12(1)–(2).

14 Convention on the Rights of the Child, G.A. Res. 44/25, Annex, 44 U.N. GAOR Supp. (No. 49) at 167, U.N. Doc. A/44/49 (1989), entered into force 2 September 1990.

15 Convention on the Rights of Persons with Disabilities, G.A. Res. 61/106, Annex I, U.N. GAOR, 61st Sess., Supp. No. 49, at 65, U.N. Doc. A/61/49 (2006), entered into force 3 May 2008.

16 Convention for the Protection of Human Rights and Fundamental Freedoms, 213 U.N.T.S. 222, entered into force 3 September 1953.

17 American Convention on Human Rights, O.A.S. Treaty Series No. 36, 1144 U.N.T.S. 123, entered into force 18 July 1978, reprinted in Basic Documents Pertaining to Human Rights in the Inter-American System, OEA/Ser.L.V/II.82 doc.6 rev.1 at 25 (1992); African [Banjul] Charter on Human and Peoples' Rights, OAU Doc. CAB/LEG/67/3 rev. 5, 21 I.L.M. 58 (1982), entered into force 21 October 1986.

18 African Charter on the Rights and Welfare of the Child, OAU Doc. CAB/LEG/24.9/49 (1990), entered into force 29 November 1999, art. 14.

19 European Social Charter, 529 U.N.T.S. 89, entered into force 26 February 1965, arts. 11, 13.

20 Additional Protocol to the American Convention on Human Rights in the Area of Economic, Social and Cultural Rights, "Protocol of San Salvador," O.A.S. Treaty Series No. 69 (1988), entered into force 16 November 1999, reprinted in Basic Documents Pertaining to Human Rights in the Inter-American System, OEA/Ser.L.V/II.82 doc.6 rev.1 at 67 (1992), art. 10.

21 Asian Human Rights Charter: A People's Charter, declared in Kwangju, South Korea, on 17 May 1998, arts. 3(2), 7(1), 9(3).

22 Cairo Declaration on Human Rights in Islam, 5August 1990, U.N. GAOR, World Conference on Human Rights, 4th Sess., Agenda Item 5, U.N. Doc. A/CONF.157/PC/62/Add.18 (1993), art. 17.

23 Declaration of Alma-Ata, International Conference on Primary Health Care, Alma-Ata, USSR, 6–12 September 1978.

24 Ottawa Charter for Health Promotion, First International Conference on Health Promotion, 21 November 1986, Ottawa, Canada, WHO/HPR/HEP/95.1, p. 1.

25 Programme of Action, International Conference on Population and Development, 5–13 September 1994, U.N. Doc. A/CONF.171/13 (1995), ch. VII, objective 8(3).

26 Beijing Declaration and Platform for Action, Fourth World Conference on Women, 4–15 September 1995, U.N. Doc. A/CONF.177/20 & Add.1 (1995).

27 Vienna Declaration and Programme of Action, *supra* note 5.

28 Bangkok Charter for Health Promotion in a Globalized World, Sixth Global Conference on Health Promotion, 7–11 August 2005, Bangkok, Thailand.

29 Paul Hunt, Report of the Special Rapporteur on the right of everyone to the enjoyment of the highest attainable standard of physical and mental health, Commission on Human Rights, U.N. Doc. E/CN.4/2003/58 (2003), para. 14.

30 Ibid., paras. 12, 14.

31 Committee on Economic, Social and Cultural Rights, General Comment 14, U.N. Doc. E/C.12/2000/4 (2000).

32 Committee on Economic, Social and Cultural Rights, General Comment 3, U.N. Doc. E/C.12/1991/23 (1990), para. 13.

33 Economic and Social Council, Siracusa Principles on the Limitation and Derogation Provisions in the International Covenant on Civil and Political Rights, U.N. Doc. E/CN.4/1985/4, Annex (1985).

34 For details on the presentations, projects, and reports by the Special Rapporteur, see http://www.essex.ac.uk/human_rights_centre/research/rth/index.aspx (for Paul Hunt, 2002–2008) and http://www2.ohchr.org/english/bodies/chr/special/themes.htm (for Anand Grover, 2008–current).

35 The Optional Protocol was adopted by the UN General Assembly on 10 December 2008, was opened for signature on 24 September 2009, and will enter into force when

it has been ratified by ten parties. As of November 2010, the Optional Protocol was signed by thirty-five state parties and ratified by three.

36 Commission on Human Rights, Report of the open-ended working group to consider options regarding the elaboration of an optional protocol to the International Covenant on Economic, Social and Cultural Rights on its first session, U.N. Doc. E/CN.4/2004/44 (2004), para. 42.

37 *Sandra Lovelace v. Canada*, Communication No. 24/1977, U.N. Doc. CCPR/C/OP/1 at 10 (1984).

38 *D. v. United Kingdom* (1997), European Court of Human Rights, 24 EHRR 423.

39 *Jorge Odir Miranda Cortez et al. v. El Salvador*, Case 12.249, Report No. 29/01, Inter-American Commission on Human Rights, Annual Report 2000, OEA/Ser./L/V/II.111, Doc. 20 Rev. 200.

40 *Social and Economic Rights Action Centre (SERAC) and Another v. Nigeria*, African Commission on Human and Peoples' Rights, (2001) AHRLR 60.

41 *Minister of Health and Others v. Treatment Action Campaign and Others*, Constitutional Court of South Africa, 2002 (5) SA 721 (CC).

42 *Mariela Viceconte v. Ministry of Health and Social Welfare*, Case No. 31.777/96 (1998), Argentina.

43 Sentencia T-760/2008, Colombian Constitutional Court, 31 July 2008.

CHAPTER 2

Realising the Right to Health: Moving from a Nationalist to a Cosmopolitan Approach

RACHEL HAMMONDS AND GORIK OOMS

INTRODUCTION

A mere sixty-eight countries account for 97% of the annual deaths of children under five (UNICEF 2008b), making the lottery of where a child is born one of the world's greatest injustices. Despite the "Health for All" ideals of the 1978 Alma-Ata Declaration,[1] health has remained largely an area in which all countries, save for those requiring temporary assistance from the international community,[2] are encouraged to be self-sufficient.

The first decade of the new millennium saw increased attention to global health and the launch of different initiatives engaging the international community in advancing the right to health for all. These developments include the Millennium Development Goals (MDGs), three of which directly address health goals,[3] and the launch of global health initiatives, such as the Global Fund to fight AIDS, Tuberculosis and Malaria and the Global Alliance for Vaccines and Immunisation (GAVI Alliance). Such developments could be seen as an expression of a cosmopolitan view of the right to health: one embracing the joint roles of national governments and the international community in achieving the right to health for all. So far, however, donors' willingness to provide open-ended international assistance seems to be limited to communicable diseases.

Is this willingness to provide open-ended assistance—but only for the fight against communicable diseases—in line with the right to health? The answer depends on whether we adopt a nationalist (i.e., limited to national solidarity) or a cosmopolitan (i.e., embracing international solidarity) view of human rights and justice. As this chapter argues, international human rights instruments do provide some guidance, leaning towards a cosmopolitan view. Yet this interpretation contradicts current international assistance practice, which leans towards a nationalist approach. Can the philosophical underpinnings of the right to health help to resolve these issues?

Global health scholar Jennifer Prah Ruger claims, "One would be hard pressed to find a more controversial or nebulous human right than the right to health—a right that stems primarily, although not exclusively, from Article 12 of the International Covenant on Economic, Social and Cultural Rights" (2006, p. 273). She further argues that although health activists have used the right to health to push for greater global health equity, they and international human rights scholars have largely ignored its philosophical and conceptual underpinnings, instead focusing their attention on governmental obligations to protect, respect, and fulfil human rights and public health. Ruger's assessment is that this was mistaken, and her contribution to a philosophical justification of the right to health essentially challenges international human rights scholars to address often-neglected questions, including how to approach the delineation of multiple-stakeholder responsibility for human rights obligations, as well as how to best achieve accountability and enforcement (Ruger 2006, 2009). Answering these questions in depth is beyond the scope of this chapter; however, this chapter takes Ruger's critique as a challenge and looks beyond the field of law for guidance in responding to the question of obligations related to global health justice. This chapter introduces readers to two influential philosophical theories— nationalism and cosmopolitanism—that are central to addressing issues of international political arrangements, and explores these theories' potential to advance our understanding of the importance of health-related international obligations.

The first part of this chapter introduces the theories of nationalism and cosmopolitanism and outlines how these two perspectives can affect approaches to realising the right to health globally. The second part surveys the legal grounds underpinning international legal obligations tied to the right to health. The third part reviews recent developments in global health, focusing in particular on the global struggle for access to HIV treatment and the upsurge in attention to health systems strengthening. The fourth part briefly addresses the reluctance of many human rights lawyers to discuss the philosophical underpinnings of human rights, and examines one approach that emerges from the Universal Declaration of Human Rights.[4]

The conclusion suggests areas for further research and activism to ensure that the right to health is truly a right for all.

NATIONALISM AND COSMOPOLITANISM

The disproportionately devastating impact of global health inequalities between developed and developing regions is reflected in global health indicators, including, for example, the fact that 99% of maternal deaths worldwide occur in the developing world (UNICEF 2008a; see chapter 6). Defining the respective roles and responsibilities of the national and international communities in responding to global health inequalities such as maternal mortality provokes wide disagreement among academics, politicians, and other key stakeholders. This section will introduce two influential philosophical theories of justice—nationalism and cosmopolitanism—to see what insights they bring to our understanding of the nature of obligations relating to the right to health and to understand why different groups support different approaches.

For the purposes of this discussion, nationalism is a philosophical school of thought positing that nations are the frameworks for organising social contracts; nationalism thus values "consent of the governed" within a state more highly than the extraterritorial consequences of consensual positions (e.g., the consequences of not providing assistance to other states). It also espouses the view that members of a nation owe greater duties to fellow members than to non-members—in other words, national partiality. This nationalist view is reflected in the highly influential social contract theory of John Rawls (1971, 1999) and has held sway in the international system since the 1648 Peace of Westphalia that many scholars argue established the principles of state sovereignty and non-interference in the affairs of other nations.

One of Rawls's key contributions to discussions of justice is his articulation of the difference principle. The difference principle holds that inequalities in the distribution of goods in a society are acceptable only if they benefit the least well-off members of society (e.g., allowing entrepreneurs to keep a substantial share of their gains if that incentivises a blossoming economy from which all members society benefit). He argued that individuals operating behind a "veil of ignorance" (i.e., individuals unaware of their position in society) would choose to maximise the prospects of the least well-off members of society; and therefore, a society organised according to the difference principle would be acceptable for all, stable, and functional. For Rawls, principles of justice are relational and thus rooted in the national level; most of them do not apply to the global level. The nationalist approach discourages states from entering into most international treaties—for example, while arms-control treaties to limit war are acceptable, those entailing the global redistribution of resources certainly are not. There is no platform where "consent of the governed" can be reached among all citizens of the world about collective efforts to distribute or redistribute goods (e.g., to realise essential social rights worldwide).

Cosmopolitans argue that universal values exist and that considerations of justice do not stop at national boundaries (Beitz 1999). According to Kok-Chor Tan, "Cosmopolitanism, as a normative idea, takes the individual to be the ultimate unit of moral concern and to be entitled to equal consideration regardless of nationality and citizenship" (2004, p. 198). For cosmopolitans, certain features of nationalism—namely, self-determination, national partiality, and national solidarity—are antithetical to cosmopolitan justice. If, at present, no platform exists where "consent of the governed" can be reached among all citizens of the world about collective efforts to distribute or redistribute goods, then such a platform should be created.

THE LEGAL FRAMEWORK

In thinking about the right to a health, a social right, and the implications of accepting that such a right may give rise to national *and* international legal obligations, it is necessary to outline the legal basis of the claims and obligations associated with this right (see chapter 1). The discussion in this section will focus on international human rights law emerging from UN bodies. While these instruments do not provide clear answers to many important questions, including how to delineate responsibility for obligations, they lean towards a more comprehensive view of the nature of obligations— that is, a cosmopolitan rather than nationalist view.

The 1945 Charter of the UN, a formal and authoritative basis for international human rights law, establishes the foundation for future declarations and treaties with respect to international cooperation.[5] Article 55(c) of the Charter notes that the UN shall promote "universal respect for, and observance of, human rights and fundamental freedoms for all without distinction as to race, sex, language or religion." Article 56 refers explicitly to the duties of international member states to achieve the purposes set out in article 55.

The 1948 Universal Declaration of Human Rights covers a broad range of rights, including economic, social, cultural, civil, and political rights. These rights were legally enshrined in the two principal UN human rights treaties, the International Covenant on Civil and Political Rights and the International Covenant on Economic, Social and Cultural Rights (ICESCR).[6] The ICESCR, adopted in 1966, and later UN conventions, including the 1989 Convention on the Rights of the Child, further clarify the nature of different rights and serve as the legal bases for the right to health, in addition to establishing international norms. Article 12 of the ICESCR broadly frames the concept of the right to health. This right has been refined in later conventions and through the jurisprudence of the UN Committee on Economic, Social and Cultural Rights (ESCR Committee), including the Committee's General Comment 14 on the right to health, discussed below (see chapter 1).[7]

With respect to obligations, article 2(1) of the ICESCR holds that "each State Party to the present Covenant undertakes to take steps, *individually and through international assistance and co-operation*, especially economic and technical, to the maximum of its available resources" (emphasis added), linking the binary nature of the obligation to the issue of resource constraints. In addition, article 23, a general provision with a declaratory character, establishes that state parties agree on the importance of "international action" for achieving the rights laid out in the ICESCR.[8]

Later conventions have been more explicit in affirming the need for international cooperation concerning the right to health (see chapter 1). For example, with regard to children's right to health, article 23(4) of the Convention on the Rights of the Child affirms that "States Parties undertake to promote and encourage international cooperation with a view to achieving progressively the full realization of the right recognized in the present article. In this regard, particular account shall be taken of the needs of developing countries."[9]

General Comment 14 acts as an authoritative interpretative guide to the right to health by further clarifying norms and addressing the scope of the right and the importance of international cooperation in achieving the right (see chapter 1). Whereas the language of article 2(1) of the ICESCR does not distinguish between national and international obligations—countries are bound "to take steps, individually and through international assistance and co-operation"—General Comment 14 further delineates the scope of national and international obligations in its discussion of core obligations, as explored below.

Unlike civil and political rights, many aspects of social rights (such as the right to health) are to be realised in a progressive manner, over time, and in accordance with available resources.[10] In its General Comment 3, the ESCR Committee notes that "the concept of progressive realization constitutes a recognition of the fact that full realization of all economic, social and cultural rights will generally not be able to be achieved in a short period of time."[11] However, the concept of progressive realisation should never be misinterpreted to justify endless delays in realising social rights, as such an interpretation would deprive social rights of any meaningful value. Thus, the Committee clarifies in paragraph 9 that state parties have "an obligation to move as expeditiously and effectively as possible." Further, to counter the interpretation that "progressive realisation" might imply no immediate obligations, the Committee emphasises a series of concepts and principles that define the nature of states' obligations, including the principle of non-retrogression (a state should not take steps backwards), the principle of non-discrimination, and the concept of core content.

This section focuses on the concept of core content, as it is a key element of international human rights law that gives rise to obligations concerning global health justice, and, as such, might be used to clarify legal obligations arising from the right to health. The ESCR Committee has defined the core content of the right to health through its definition of the core obligations that arise from that right.[12] According to the Committee, these core obligations are not subject to the principle of progressive realisation; rather, they are of immediate effect. In its General Comment 14, the Committee affirms that "a State party cannot, under any circumstances whatsoever, justify its non-compliance with the core obligations … which are non-derogable" (para. 47). In essence, these core obligations establish a minimum package of health services that all people in the world are entitled to enjoy immediately and that all states must provide, irrespective of available resources. They include obligations to ensure access to essential health facilities, goods, and services on a non-discriminatory basis and to develop and implement national public health plans that address the health needs of the entire population, including the promotion of the preconditions of health, through transparent and participatory processes.[13] Essential health services include the provision of essential drugs, as defined by the World Health Organization (WHO) (see chapter 9).

For most health practitioners in low-income countries, this definition sounds like a wild dream. Low-income countries are simply too poor to provide a basic package of health services for all, which WHO estimates to cost US$40 per person per year (Carrin, Evans, and Xu 2007, p. 652).[14] Given the legal principle of *ultra posse nemo obligatur*—the idea that individuals (and, by extension, countries) cannot be obligated beyond what they are able to do—does it make sense to define core obligations that are unaffordable for low-income countries? It does if we read the definition in conjunction with article 2(1) of the ICESCR, which states that "each State Party to the present Covenant undertakes to take steps, *individually and through international assistance and co-operation*, especially economic and technical, to the maximum of its available resources" (emphasis added). In other words, when assessing low-income countries' abilities to fulfil their core obligations, one should consider not only these countries' national resources but also resources received through international assistance. As Paul Hunt, who served as UN Special Rapporteur on the Right to Health from 2002 to 2008, remarked at the May 2000 Committee session in which General Comment 14 was drafted,

> If the Committee decided to approve the list of core obligations, it would be unfair not to insist also that richer countries fulfil their obligations relating to international cooperation under article 2, paragraph 1, of the Covenant. The two sets of obligations should be seen as two halves of a package.[15]

If the right to health is meaningless without the realisation of at least its core content, and if some countries lack the resources needed to realise the core content of the right to health, then the right to health itself cannot exist without international obligations to provide assistance. Without international obligations to provide assistance—without global responsibility, that is—the right to health is not a right but a privilege reserved for those born outside of the world's poorest communities.

Such a global obligation does not mean, however, that low-income countries have an unconditional and unlimited claim to international assistance in order to realise the core content of the right to health. As international human rights scholar Philip Alston has noted, "The correlative obligation would, of course, be confined to situations in which a developing country had demonstrated its best efforts to meet the [Millennium Development] Goals and its inability to do so because of a lack of financial resources" (2005, p. 778).

Arguing that the right to health is a universal right does not imply that all people have the right to the same health-care system or social determinants of health. Any claim to international assistance would be a conditional one, reserved for countries that demonstrate their best efforts.[16] Thus, while the primary legal obligation rests with the nation state, it is clear that the international community has a legal obligation to assist in realising at least the core content of the right to health for the world's poorest people.

PRINCIPLES IN ACTION

This section reviews recent developments in global health, arguing that there has been an upswing in cosmopolitan as opposed to nationalistic sentiments—while acknowledging that these developments can be explained through a nationalistic lens as well. In assessing the level of support for shared responsibilities for global health, one can look to recent political pledges such as the much-hailed MDGs, which include three health-related goals. The attention devoted to these political pledges suggests that political leaders may be moving towards an acceptance of shared responsibility for global health. Evidence suggests that MDG 6 (to combat HIV, malaria, and other diseases) is the health-related MDG that is most on target (Institute for Health Metrics and Evaluation 2010). This is so arguably because MDG 6 is the only goal that has managed to leverage international commitments into new institutions that embrace a concept of global justice beyond borders (see chapter 7). The discussion below outlining the history of the movement for global access to HIV treatment demonstrates how international commitments were leveraged to bring a degree of health justice beyond borders. However, others might argue that the encouraging progress on MDG 6 reflects the fact it is about communicable diseases, and that the willingness of the international community to provide open-ended assistance for achieving MDG 6 simply reflects the nationalist self-interest of richer countries to contain communicable diseases wherever they prevail. As shall be argued below, the UN Secretary-General's recently launched Global Strategy for Women's and Children's Health will hopefully show that the world can extend the progress made on some communicable diseases and not just commit but act on delivering the rights of the world's women and children.

Increasing Global Access to HIV Treatment

It is worth recalling that since the 1980s, American AIDS activists have pushed pharmaceutical companies to ramp up research on treatment and prevention and have called for an end to repressive stigmatising responses to HIV. The research of Jonathan Mann supported the argument that respecting the human rights of all people would help slow the spread of HIV and affirm the human dignity of those living with the disease (Mann et al., 1999). The profound marginalisation and stigma that American activists experienced while campaigning for the right to treatment pushed them to extend their goals beyond national borders and advocate for universal access to HIV treatment globally.

In South Africa, the country with the largest number of people living with HIV, national and international activists have pressured the government and international pharmaceutical companies to remove trade and other legal barriers to universal access to HIV treatment (Treatment Action Campaign 2011; see chapter 9). At the 2001 UN General Assembly Special Session on HIV/AIDS, world leaders committed to establishing a fund that would offer global resources to fight HIV/AIDS, tuberculosis, and malaria instead of expecting countries to finance treatment from their national budgets.[17] The resulting Global Fund to Fight AIDS, Tuberculosis and Malaria has been a key actor in rolling out access to HIV treatment in countries that lack the means to fund such treatment. The Global Fund's executive director has made it clear that the Global Fund does not support a nationalist or state-centric view regarding access to treatment: "The Global Fund has helped to change the development paradigm by introducing a new concept of sustainability. One that is not based solely on achieving domestic self-reliance but on sustained international support as well" (Kazatchkine 2008). Furthermore, the Global Fund's governance platforms can be considered platforms where "consent of the governed"—among all citizens of the world—can be (and has been) reached.[18]

This recognition of human solidarity beyond borders is arguably an example of a cosmopolitan view of the right to health. Yet we cannot exclude the possibility that governments of richer countries largely ignore the values espoused by AIDS activists and are simply acting out of nationalist self-interest. It remains a matter of fact that similar human solidarity beyond borders does not yet exist for non-communicable health issues, and it is unclear whether this is due to a lack of broader health-related activism (e.g., related to maternal health and health systems strengthening) or the (mistaken) belief that broader health issues do not have cross-border implications.

In recent years, advocacy around maternal mortality has spread beyond the health community. The engagement of the international community is evidenced in MDG 5 and that of the human rights community in Amnesty International's Demand Dignity campaign.[19] However, in contrast to HIV and other communicable diseases, combating maternal mortality requires both long-term investment in health systems and strategies for addressing the complex issue of gender-based discrimination, making it harder to achieve measurable results in the short term (see chapter 6).

The recently announced Global Strategy is arguably a cosmopolitan approach to addressing maternal and child health with a rights-based focus, for it concentrates the world's attention and resources on the most vulnerable individuals. Interestingly, it mirrors some of the key elements of the Global Fund's approach: country-led health plans with predictable and sustainable investment, innovative approaches to financing, and monitoring and accountability mechanisms. Importantly, it also focuses on the strengthening of health systems, staffing, and the integrated delivery of care. The Global Strategy is the product of a multiple-stakeholder process engaging more than 170 countries and organisations, including governments, non-governmental organisations (NGOs), community advocates, multinational corporations, and faith-based groups (UN Secretary-General 2010). This broad-based support suggests that it is an example of the consent of the governed. However, as with many excellent initiatives, it is critical that both donors (including countries and international NGOs) and implementers (including countries and national and international NGOs) are held accountable for their commitments (Partnership for Maternal, Newborn and Child Health 2011).

Health Systems

Health systems strengthening has recently attracted attention from donors, implementing countries, implementing agencies, and the human rights community. The importance of health systems strengthening on the global health stage is evidenced by the weighty players involved in the newly formed Health Systems Funding Platform.[20]

First, it is important to review some definitions from WHO, a Platform member charged with norm setting and providing leadership on global health matters (WHO 2011). According to WHO, "A health system consists of all organizations, people and actions whose *primary intent* is to promote, restore or maintain health" (2007, p. 2). WHO takes an instrumentalist approach in its definition, noting that health systems are a means to achieving better health outcomes (WHO 2007, p. 2). Health systems strengthening is defined as building capacity in critical components ("the six building blocks"[21]) of health systems to achieve more equitable and sustained improvements across health services and health outcomes (WHO 2007, p. 4; see chapter 4).

The international community's focus on health systems is a welcome development because an effective and integrated health system accessible to all is fundamental to achieving the right to health for all.[22] However, as WHO research (2007) shows, health systems in low-income countries are failing. A recent study by Gunilla Backman et al. (2008) provides extensive guidance on how a human rights framework can be used to develop and implement policies, thus enabling countries to comply with their international legal obligation to guarantee the right to health for all. Their study stresses the importance of international cooperation and assistance in achieving the right to health, noting that such cooperation is a legal duty incumbent on both low- and high-income countries: low-income countries should seek, and high-income countries should provide. Such an approach seems to be consistent with a cosmopolitan approach to realising the right to health, as it recognises the importance of international solidarity in achieving health for all. The issue of self-sufficiency is not mentioned in the study because it is irrelevant to defining international legal obligations to cooperate and provide assistance.

As noted above, the Global Fund approach embodied a paradigmatic change from nationalist to cosmopolitan. What about the efforts of the

Platform? At present, this remains unclear. However, if WHO acts as the Platform's normative guide, the assessment is mixed. WHO's *World Health Report 2010* recognises the important role of the international community in achieving health for all, encouraging it to increase the predictability of donor funding, support the development of national health plans, avoid fragmentation in the way in which funding is delivered, and strengthen domestic capacity and systems (pp. 99–101). The report does not discuss how long-term international financing can help low-income countries achieve health for all, though it does recommend that donors move away from annual commitments and towards three- to five-year cycles. In an earlier *World Health Report*, WHO notes that "external funds [for low-income countries] need to be progressively re-channelled in ways that help build institutional capacity towards a longer-term goal of self-sustaining, universal coverage" (2008, p. 106). If this is the guidance that WHO is providing to the Platform, it is unlikely that the Platform will embrace a cosmopolitan approach to financing health systems strengthening because the aforementioned longer-term goal of self-sustaining universal coverage and a more cosmopolitan vision of long-term global health solidarity are at odds. As Backman et al. note, "The international dimension of health systems is reflected in countries' human-rights responsibilities of international assistance and cooperation that can be traced through the Charter of the UN, the Universal Declaration of Human Rights, and some more-recent international human-rights declarations and binding treaties" (2008, p. 2052). WHO should therefore be looking to the international human rights obligations of WHO members to guide its advice. These obligations are not time bound.

Balancing the demands of state autonomy and interdependence are fundamental to achieving the right to health for all. Backman et al. claim that "of all the important human rights that bear upon health systems, the right to the highest attainable standard of health is the cornerstone of … an effective health system" (2008, p. 2048). It could be argued that the success of the health-systems-strengthening agenda requires a cosmopolitan approach to ensure that the interaction of national and global produces positive outcomes for all.

PHILOSOPHICAL UNDERPINNINGS

International human rights instruments lean towards a cosmopolitan view of the right to health. There is also evidence that recent international assistance efforts for health lean towards a cosmopolitan view, too. This chapter argues that elements of the global AIDS response have broken down some of the nationalist barriers that exist both in people's minds and in practice, leading to a new paradigm for addressing global health. Shared responsibility has moved to the forefront at the same time that full national responsibility has moved to the back burner. The paradigm shift from "international health" to "global health"—i.e., from the idea that health is a concern limited by national borders to an idea that health is a global concern—reflects a cosmopolitan rather than a nationalist view. Thomas Quinn and David Serwadda echo this view, arguing that

> African nations should transition to a model of longterm sustainability in which the responsibility for the HIV/AIDS response is more effectively shared between African partner states and the broader international community. This model must compel African countries to take a lead role in this fight, eventually to assume the responsibility entirely. (2010, pp. 1133–1134)

Such a shift in thinking needs to be expanded to all health-related issues if the aim is to achieve the right to health for all. However, supposing that none of these arguments are strong enough to convince the international community to embrace the cosmopolitan view beyond communicable diseases, can the philosophical underpinnings of the right to health provide guidance?

First, it is important to note that some human rights scholars fiercely resist any attempt to clarify the philosophical underpinnings of human rights. Jack Donnelly, for example, argues that "the common complaint that non-foundational theories leave human rights 'vulnerable' is probably true but certainly irrelevant" (2003, p. 20) and that "while recognizing that human rights are at their root conventional and controversial, we should not place more weight on this fact than it deserves" (Donnelly 2003, pp. 20–21). For Donnelly, human rights are what they are because they have been included in a convention referring to human rights, and any attempt to clarify their content through reference to philosophical underpinnings will only weaken them—because there is no agreement on these underpinnings.

Donnelly's position flies in the face of Ruger's assessment that legal scholars and health activists have mistakenly ignored the philosophical underpinnings of the right to health; according to Donnelly, these underpinnings deserved to be ignored, even rejected.

However, Donnelly's position is unhelpful when we are faced with a dichotomy between cosmopolitan and nationalist views of the right to health. If human rights are what they are because they have been included in a convention referring to human rights, recent practice in the area of international assistance might suggest a "silent convention" that rejects the existence of international responsibility and legal obligations.[23]

A "foundational" explanation of what human rights are is fleshed out by Ooms (2010), who argues that the natural evolution of human beings, who originally lived in small hunter-gatherer tribes, endowed humans with a natural sense of justice that entails an expectation of reciprocal support as a condition for cooperation. While this natural sense of justice is not easily adapted to a global society of seven billion humans, a global society divided into some two hundred countries that reject mutual responsibility for something essential to survival is unlikely to become a functional global society. In our increasingly interconnected world, there is a need to further explore the logic underpinning the treatment of only some, but not all, health issues as matter of global responsibility. Both human rights law and international development practice must evolve to address the issue of delineating national and international obligations in achieving health for all.

This position cannot be explored in depth here. However, it is worth highlighting the preamble of the Universal Declaration of Human Rights: "Whereas it is essential to promote the development of friendly relations between nations." Can any view of relations between countries that rejects mutual responsibility for human survival, for the sake of a "consent of the governed" principle, be considered "friendly"? Can we expect to achieve a functional (and friendly) global society that is based on the idea that countries bear no responsibility for the survival of humans living in different countries? How would that translate to enhancing cooperation on cross-border problems, such as climate change, terrorism, and international organised crime? This chapter argues that recognising a shared responsibility for the realisation of human rights as a precondition for a functional and friendly global society can help. As a starting point, this shared responsibility would apply to all health efforts that are reasonably understood as essential by communities around the world (from a legal perspective, this would be defined as the core obligations outlined in General Comment 14; see discussion above). Only then can we expect communities around the world to engage in efforts to develop a functional and friendly global society.

CONCLUSION

Why should wealthy countries care about the health of the world's poorest people? As outlined above, such concern in recent history may have been motivated largely by nationalist self-interest—namely, stopping the spread of communicable diseases—and/or a cosmopolitan view of the right to health held by activists.

This chapter started from the premise that the global health lottery seems fundamentally unjust. As a truly universal right, the right to health entails both national and international obligations. The worldwide movement for access to HIV treatment has successfully used a concept of solidarity to expand the health debate from a national level to a global level—from national obligations to international obligations. This chapter has tried to challenge the reader by asking, if we accept the premise that a theory of global health justice is needed to underpin global and national responses to health inequalities, what might such a theory look like?

This chapter has asserted that such a theory would be underpinned by the universal norms enshrined in international human rights agreements and that responsibility for ensuring all people's enjoyment of the core content of the right to health has both international and national dimensions. From a theoretical perspective, intense work on reconceptualising the human rights framework is necessary in order to delineate what obligations different actors owe to whom. Pharmaceutical companies and new global health actors such as the Bill and Melinda Gates Foundation are examples of highly influential players whose activities affect the health rights of millions, in both negative and positive ways.[24] Determining how to define such actors' human rights obligations and how to confront other important issues, such as accountability mechanisms, are rich areas for research and action. As the world becomes increasingly interconnected, such an examination is increasingly important. From a practical perspective, several elements of the Global Fund's approach—specifically, civil society's role in project design and implementation, the pooling of donor resources, and accountability mechanisms—can serve as an example for a new international model based on shared responsibilities (Ooms and Hammonds 2010). Given the massive scale of ongoing human rights violations, it is a matter of extreme urgency that the international community fulfil its obligations, starting with small steps, such as providing the long-promised 0.7% of gross domestic product to international assistance and implementing structural reforms, that help the world achieve health for all.

REFERENCES

Alston, P. 2005. "Ships Passing in the Night: The Current State of the Human Rights and Development Debate Seen through the Lens of the Millennium Development Goals." *Human Rights Quarterly* 27 (3): 755–829.

Backman, G., P. Hunt, R. Khosla, et al. 2008. "Health Systems and the Right to Health an Assessment of 194 Countries." *The Lancet* 372 (9655): 2047–2085.

Baker, B. 2010. *CTT-for-Health/FTT-with-Health: Resource-Needs Estimates and an Assessment of Funding Modalities.* Action for Global Health and International Civil Society Support. http://www.actionforglobalhealth. eu/fileadmin/AfGH_Intranet/AFGH/Publications/CTL-HSS_Funding_ Mechanisms_Final.pdf.

Beitz, C. 1999. *Political Theory and International Relations.* Princeton, NJ: Princeton Univ. Press.

Business and Human Rights Resource Centre. 2011. "UN Secretary-General's Special Representative on Business and Human Rights: UN 'Protect, Respect and Remedy' Framework." Accessed 11 June 2011. http://www.business- humanrights.org/SpecialRepPortal/Home/Protect-Respect-Remedy- Framework.

Carrin, G., D. Evans, and D. Xu. 2007. "Designing Health Financing Policy Towards Universal Coverage." *WHO Bulletin* 85 (9): 652.

Donnelly, J. 2003. *Universal Human Rights in Theory and Practice.* 2nd edition. Ithaca, NY: Cornell Univ. Press.

GAVI Alliance (Global Alliance for Vaccines and Immunisation). 2010. *Health Systems Funding Platform: Frequently Asked Questions.* http://www.gavialliance.org/resources/FAQ_ HealthSystemsFundingPlatform.pdf

Institute for Health Metrics and Evaluation. 2010. *Building Momentum: Global Progress Toward Reducing Maternal and Child Mortality*. Seattle, WA: Institute for Health Metrics and Evaluation.

Kazatchkine, M. 2008. "Dr. Kazatchkine's Closing Speech at the XVII International AIDS Conference in Mexico" (speech). August 11. http://www.theglobalfund.org.en/pressreleases/?pr=pr_080811.

Mann, J. M., S. Gruskin, M. A. Grodin, et al., eds. 1999. *Health and Human Rights: A Reader*. New York: Routledge.

Ooms, G. 2010. "Why the West Is Perceived as Being Unworthy of Cooperation." *The Journal of Law, Medicine and Ethics* 38 (3): 594–613.

Ooms, G., and R. Hammonds. 2010. "Taking Up Daniels' Challenge: The Case for Global Health Justice." *Health and Human Rights* 12 (1): 29–46.

Partnership for Maternal, Newborn and Child Health. 2011. *A Review of Global Accountability Mechanisms for Women's and Children's Health*. Geneva: Partnership for Maternal, Newborn and Child Health.

Quinn, T., and D. Serwadda. 2010. "The Future of HIV/AIDS in Africa: A Shared Responsibility." *The Lancet* 377 (9772): 1133–1134.

Rawls, J. 1971. *A Theory of Justice*. Cambridge, MA: Harvard Univ. Press.

—. 1999. *The Law of Peoples*. Cambridge, MA: Harvard Univ. Press.

Ruger, J. P. 2006. "Toward a Theory of a Right to Health: Capability and Incompletely Theorized Agreements." *Yale Journal of Law and the Humanities* 18:273–326.

—. 2009. "Global Health Justice." *Public Health Ethics* 2 (3): 261–275.

Tan, K-C. 2004. *Justice Without Borders: Cosmopolitanism, Nationalism and Patriotism*. Cambridge: Cambridge Univ. Press.

Treatment Action Campaign. 2011. "About the Treatment Action Campaign." Accessed 11 June 2011. http://www.tac.org.za/community/about.

UNICEF (UN Children's Fund). 2008a. *Progress for Children: A Report Card on Maternal Mortality*. No. 7. New York: UNICEF.

—. 2008b. *Tracking Progress in Maternal, Newborn and Child Survival*. New York: UNICEF.

UN Secretary-General. 2010. *Global Strategy for Women's and Children's Health*. Geneva: Partnership for Maternal, Newborn and Child Health.

WHO (World Health Organization). 2007. *Everybody's Business: Strengthening Health Systems to Improve Health Outcomes; WHO's Framework for Action*. Geneva: WHO.

—. 2008. *The World Health Report: Primary Health Care; Now More Than Ever*. Geneva: WHO.

—. 2010. *The World Health Report: Health Systems Financing; The Path to Universal Coverage.* Geneva: WHO.

—. 2011. "About WHO." Accessed 11 June 2011. http://www.who.int/about/en.

NOTES

1 Declaration of Alma-Ata, International Conference on Primary Health Care, Alma-Ata, USSR, 6–12 September 1978.

2 We define this term very broadly to include nation states, international organisations (such as the UN and the World Bank), the European Union, international non-governmental organisations, and multinational corporations.

3 MDG 4 focuses on reducing child mortality, MDG 5 on improving maternal health, and MDG 6 on combating HIV/AIDS, malaria, and other diseases. The MDGs are political commitments, not legally binding goals, to address a selected number of human rights issues. As such, the MDG framework does not engage directly with a human rights accountability framework. However, the MDGs cannot escape the indivisibility and interdependence of all human rights. This means that the health MDGs cannot be achieved without progress in the other MDGs, including, for example, MDG 2 focusing on achieving universal primary education and MDG 7 focusing on environment sustainability.

4 Universal Declaration of Human Rights, G.A. Res. 217A (III), U.N. Doc A/810 at 71 (1948).

5 Charter of the United Nations, 26 June 1945, 59 Stat. 1031, entered into force 24 October 1945.

6 International Covenant on Civil and Political Rights, G.A. Res. 2200A (XXI), 21 U.N. GAOR Supp. (No. 16) at 52, U.N. Doc. A/6316 (1966), 999 U.N.T.S. 171, entered into force 23 March 1976; International Covenant on Economic, Social and Cultural Rights, G.A. Res. 2200A (XXI), 21 U.N. GAOR Supp. (No. 16) at 49, U.N. Doc. A/6316 (1966), 993 U.N.T.S. 3, entered into force 3 January 1976. The division of these rights into two separate Covenants was a by-product of the Cold War ideological battle. The indivisibility and interdependence of human rights has been affirmed in numerous UN Declarations, including the Vienna Declaration and Programme of Action, World Conference on Human Rights, 25 June 1993, U.N. Doc A/Conf.157/23 (1993), para. 5.

7 Committee on Economic, Social and Cultural Rights, General Comment 14, U.N. Doc. E/C.12/2000/4 (2000).

8 "The States Parties to the present Covenant agree that international action for the achievement of the rights recognized in the present Covenant includes such methods as the conclusion of conventions, the adoption of recommendations, the furnishing of technical assistance and the holding of regional meetings and technical meetings

for the purpose of consultation and study organized in conjunction with the Governments concerned."

9   Convention on the Rights of the Child, G.A. Res. 44/25, Annex, 44 U.N. GAOR Supp. (No. 49) at 167, U.N. Doc. A/44/49 (1989), entered into force 2 September 1990.

10 Article 24(4) of the Convention on the Rights of the Child recognises that, as with other economic and social rights, the rights enshrined in the Convention will be achieved progressively and not immediately.

11 Committee on Economic, Social and Cultural Rights, General Comment 3, U.N. Doc. E/C.12/1991/23 (1990), para. 9.

12 General Comment 14, *supra* note 7, paras. 43–45.

13 An example of the importance of the core obligation in developing a national health plan is evidenced in the work of major global health actors; for example, the Health Systems Funding Platform (which brings together the GAVI Alliance, the Global Fund, and the World Bank, and is coordinated by WHO) requires that a national health plan (assessed and refined through a joint assessment process) serve as the basis for all health-related funding that the Health Systems Funding Platform coordinates. Details are available at http://www.gavialliance.org/resources/HSF_Platform_FAQ_15.01.2010.pdf.

14 While the contents and cost of a basic package are disputed, even a low estimate far exceeds what low-income countries can afford. For a recent examination of the costing issue, see Baker (2010).

15 Committee on Economic, Social and Cultural Rights, Summary Record of the 10th Meeting: Portugal, U.N. Doc. E/C.12/2000/SR.10 (2000), para. 27.

16 The distinction between unwillingness and inability to realise rights is of immense importance. A government that chooses to devote domestic financing to military rather than social goals would, for example, be "unwilling." In such cases, international development assistance organisations should look beyond the state to help fulfil human rights obligations (e.g., by partnering with civil society organisations).

17 Declaration of Commitment on HIV/AIDS, General Resolution of the United Nations General Assembly, U.N. Doc. A/RES/S-26/2 (2001), arts. 90–91.

18 The Global Fund is not an implementing agency but a financial enabler that pools resources from donor countries and distributes them to recipient countries. Funding decisions are made by the Global Fund Board, which includes representatives of donor and recipient governments, NGOs, the private sector, and communities affected by the diseases. The decision process works as follows: the board issues a call for proposals, and interested countries apply for funds through a national-level Country Coordinating Mechanism (CCM) comprised of various stakeholders. The proposals are then reviewed by the independent Technical Review Panel, which makes recommendations to the board. Once a proposal is approved, a grant is signed with a Principal Recipient, proposed by the CCM. A Local Fund Agent oversees implementation, acts as an independent auditor of expenditure and activities, and

liaises with the Global Fund's Secretariat. Details are available at
http://www.theglobalfund.org/en/how/?lang=en.

19 See the campaign's website, http://www.amnesty.org/en/demand-dignity.

20 The Platform brings together the Global Fund, the World Bank, and the GAVI
Alliance, with facilitation from WHO, to allow countries to use new and existing funds
more effectively for health systems development and to help them access donor funds
in a manner that is aligned to their own national processes (GAVI Alliance 2010).

21 The six building blocks include service delivery; health workforce; information;
medical products, vaccines, and technology; leadership and governance; and
financing (WHO 2007, p. 14).

22 Paul Hunt, Report of the Special Rapporteur on the right of everyone to the enjoyment
of the highest attainable standard of physical and mental health, Human Rights
Council, U.N. Doc. A/HRC/7/11 (2008), para. 15.

23 Paul Hunt, Report of the Special Rapporteur on the right of everyone to the enjoyment
of the highest attainable standard of physical and mental health, Mission to Sweden,
Human Rights Council, U.N. Doc. A/HRC/4/28/Add.2 (2007).

24 Given the increasing effect that pharmaceutical companies and international
NGOs are having on right-to-health issues, particularly in low-income countries,
innovative thinking on defining these actors' responsibilities is needed. With respect
to pharmaceutical companies, the soon-to-be finalised UN Guiding Principles on
Business and Human Rights (implementation of the respect, protect, and remedy
framework) should be a useful contribution (Business and Human Rights Resource
Centre 2011). Similar work is needed with respect to other non-state actors, including
international NGOs.

CHAPTER 3

Public Health, Primary Health Care, and the Right to Health

HELEN POTTS

INTRODUCTION

This chapter discusses primary health care (PHC) and its relationship to the right to health. It begins by clarifying the differences between public health and medicine, followed by a brief explanation of the history of public health. The chapter then turns to the 1978 Alma-Ata Declaration, which positioned PHC on the world stage as a way of dealing with increasing health inequalities within and between countries and the rising costs of health care.[1] Unfortunately, the implementation of PHC faced substantial barriers, such as vague concepts and definitions, and over the years the original intent of the PHC approach has been narrowed to the provision of health services and first contact with the health sector. The chapter then briefly revisits the content of the right to health in order to highlight the similarities between this right and PHC and to identify two essential elements present in the right to health but lacking in PHC: accountability and legal obligations. It is precisely these two elements that offer the potential to overcome barriers to PHC's implementation. The chapter concludes by suggesting that adoption of the right to health as a means of implementing PHC offers one way of ensuring that, this time around, PHC will have a greater chance of success.

DEFINING PUBLIC HEALTH

In thinking about public health, it is important to understand what this term means and how it differs from medicine. As Jonathan Mann notes, medicine and public health, both important components of health systems, are not the same. Medicine focuses on individuals—assessment, diagnosis, treatment, and prevention at an individual level (Mann 1997, p. 6). It adopts a biomedical approach, using the absence of disease as its model, which does not consider how social, economic, and other external factors affect health. Public health, on the other hand, is collective in nature. In the words of Robert Beaglehole and Ruth Bonita, it is "collective action for sustained population-wide health improvement" (2004, p. 174). The authors point out that public health is defined in terms of its aims rather than in terms of a theoretical foundation (2004, p. 173). To achieve better health for the population at large, public health entails a principal role for the state, an emphasis on prevention, concern for the underlying socio-economic determinants of health, a multidisciplinary approach, partnership with the populations served, and a focus on populations rather than individuals (Beaglehole and Bonita 2004, p. 175).

Despite the general recognition that public health programmes should include participation of the populations served, adopt intersectoral or collaborative approaches, and be comprehensive to ensure that external factors are addressed, many countries have adopted approaches that focus on "risk factors" at the individual level, depend too heavily on personal responsibility and individual behavioural change, and continue to rely on the development and enforcement of public health legislation.

A BRIEF HISTORY OF PUBLIC HEALTH

Knowledge that a multitude of external factors influence health is not new (Link and Phelan 2002, p. 730). The evidence of an association between external factors and inequalities in health status dates back to ancient China, India, Greece, and Egypt (Porter 1999, pp. 12–14). The rise of the bureaucratic Roman Empire favoured the direct effect of sanitary improvement on health and facilitated the development of technology in water provision and sanitary reform. It also established infirmaries, although they were reserved principally for sick slaves and the military (Porter 1999, pp. 19–22). These initiatives stand in contrast to the contemporary understanding of "public health," as they were designed largely by and for the benefit of the elite and did not seek to improve the health conditions of the general population.

Public health measures from the fourteenth century—implemented in response to plague outbreaks—represent the earliest direct involvement of civil governments in the control and prevention of epidemic disease. Though these measures introduced the concept of quarantine, control of travelling between towns, and sanitation reforms, they were largely motivated by concerns over trade, maintenance of the social status quo, and control of the poor. For those who could afford it, the response was flight, resulting in the need for protection of the property of the rich. Fearing revolt among the poor who were unable to leave, elaborate regulations were created to control the behaviour of the urban poor who were viewed as an increasing risk to social stability (Porter 1999, pp. 31–36).

From the sixteenth to eighteenth centuries, colonial, trade, and urban expansion created new patterns of disease that often threatened national economies. Governments developed various responses, many of which remain current: statistics, vaccinations, isolation, and individual behaviour modification. However, these responses showed little concern for the underlying socio-economic determinants of disease (Porter 1999, p. 49). A country's strength was assessed by the state of its population's health, promoting interest in the social scientific analysis of health. Statistical inquiries into population (e.g., regarding births, deaths, causes of death, levels of literacy, and levels of ill health), economic activity, and epidemic diseases were undertaken in Britain, France, Germany, Italy, Spain, Sweden, and their associated colonies. These statistical inquiries represented a growing science of biopolitics at the end of the eighteenth century and facilitated increasingly disciplinary interventions upon individuals and society as a whole. This growing science was used to justify the creation of "medical police" to regulate intimate individual behaviour that might spread or engender disease. Implemented in France, Germany, and Sweden, the conceptual theory was outlined by the Austrian physician Johann Peter Frank, who proposed regulating public behaviour, implementing public hygiene measures (e.g., drainage, pure water supply, street cleaning, and control of vice and overcrowding), and sanitary reform for hospitals (Porter 1999, pp. 50–52).

The nineteenth century heralded an era of rigorous and sustained investigation of health and disease. Through the work of social investigators such as Louis-René Villermé and Rudolph Virchow, premature mortality was definitively identified as an economic, social, and political disease. However, this identification did not translate into reform of the social and economic structures that caused ill health (Oppenheimer, Bayer, and Colgrove 2002,

p. 526; Porter 1999, pp. 66–69). Rather, it was the belief in miasma as the cause of disease that resulted in the consideration of certain external factors in public health delivery. This theory proposed a single cause of disease: poisons in the atmosphere (Hamlin 1994, p. 97; Oppenheimer, Bayer, and Colgrove 2002, p. 525; Porter 1999, pp. 86–87). In Britain, Edwin Chadwick, through his *Report on the Sanitary Conditions of the Labouring Population of Great Britain* (published in 1842), advanced the idea that disease did not result from poverty but from one cause alone—environmental filth—and that the appropriate response was sanitation: closed sewers, eradication of cesspools, and waste removal (Oppenheimer, Bayer, and Colgrove 2002, p. 525; Porter 1999, p. 68). At the same time, others stood in outright opposition to Chadwick. Friedrich Engels drew on Chadwick's 1842 report to reverse the causal pathway from "disease to poverty" to "poverty to disease" (Oppenheimer, Bayer, and Colgrove 2002, p. 526; Susser 1993, p. 419). Engels and others, in contrast to Chadwick, saw health as a social and political value. Nonetheless, public health policies adopted during this time did not reflect the belief that socio-economic conditions affected the morbidity and mortality of populations, and hence overlooked the underlying socio-economic determinants of poor health.

A shift in focus occurred at the beginning of the twentieth century as a result of "germ theory" and the rise of bacteriology. With the identification of bacteria as the cause of disease, germ theory provided a sound scientific basis for a focus on disease and curative care and came to dominate the public health agenda in Britain and its colonies, continental Europe, and the United States (Fidler 2000, p. 92). Individuals were categorised into "risk populations" (Porter 1999, pp. 139–140). Science, rather than social and sanitary measures, was seen as the answer to achieving population health. Through the provision of health care, diseases would be eradicated. Although important social reforms during this period (e.g., school meals, regulation of working conditions, baby clinics, baby bonuses, and antenatal and postnatal care) had a positive impact on the health of these countries' populations, the motivation behind these reforms was largely for a "purer" population and not out of concern for the political, economic, and social factors that affected health (Hamlin 1994, p. 153; Porter 1999, p. 175). While governments acknowledged the squalid conditions in which people lived and worked, their responses were firmly focused on the individual. Through health education, it was believed, the public would be educated in domestic hygiene and made conscious of the social impact of individual behaviour on the community's health (Bryder 1994, p. 319; Porter 1999, pp. 178–179).

By the end of World War II, confidence in the belief that the decline of infectious diseases owed much to medical science and health care was high. The discoveries of sulphonamides, antibiotics, and new vaccines promised to protect entire populations against certain diseases. These new forms of health care, appealing to governments, were considered both affordable and effective. In addition, universally available medical care was seen as essential, and many countries took steps to ensure that health care was widely available (Blane, Brunner, and Wilkinson 1996, pp. 1–2). A public health-care system guided by scientific rationality became the primary vehicle for improving health.

The period following the 1950s represented a tumultuous time for both high- and low-income countries. In the former, new political and social movements emerged, including the women's, disability, black, environmental, and gay and lesbian movements. These new social movements demanded political and social equality, justice, and a genuine, participatory democracy (Croft and Beresford 1996, p. 177). Low-income countries, in turn, witnessed demands for a greater share of the world's resources. The political and intellectual centres of these countries became increasingly aware that their countries' poverty resulted from a pattern of worldwide relations in which a few countries controlled a lot and many countries controlled very little. Structural change was required, demanding a new economic order and a redistribution of worldwide resources (Navarro 1984, p. 162).

These movements influenced activity in the public health sector. There was general dissatisfaction with the paternalistic nature of the health sector and the fact that health care was "owned" by special groups and imposed on populations (Newell 1988, p. 903). Public health research conducted during this period began to reveal that the reduction in infectious disease, at least in the West, was due not only to the provision of chemotherapy but also to improvements in economic and social conditions (Colgrove 2002, pp. 725–728; Szreter 1988, p. 1). New "diseases of affluence" were also emerging, which were related to lifestyle factors and which required an approach beyond mere access to drugs. Influential studies argued that the appropriate response to such diseases was one that was comprehensive, collaborative, and participatory (Lalonde 1974; Lee 1997, p. 24; Newell 1975); these studies were, in part, a return to the responses advocated by the social reformers of the nineteenth century.

During the same period, the Western medical model of health that had been exported to low-income countries during the colonial period was failing to meet the basic health needs of their populations. Developed along centralised lines, this model tended to create sophisticated health-care services centred largely in cities and towns and accessible only to small and elite sections of the population (Cueto 2004, p. 1864; WHO 1975, p. 7; Navarro 1984, pp. 160–163). In fact, approximately 80% of these countries' populations lacked access to health services. The time had come to take a fresh look at an alternative approach to health, one that sought to distinguish health as a separate, though related, entity from health care (Segall 1983, p. 27). The following section reviews this alternative approach.

PRIMARY HEALTH CARE

This section reviews the alternative approach to global and national health policy proposed in PHC and as expressed in the Alma-Ata Declaration. PHC and the "Health for All" campaign developed to implement PHC have been described as providing a detailed programme for the implementation of article 12 of the International Covenant on Economic, Social and Cultural Rights (ICESCR) (Trubek 1984, p. 244).[2] When drafting its General Comment 14, the UN Committee on Economic, Social and Cultural Rights relied on the Declaration for its compelling guidance on the core obligations of the right to health.[3] Despite this endorsement, PHC has faced a rocky road since its inception: after its public rollout in the Alma-Ata Declaration, its implementation was complicated by a variety of barriers, including confusion over its very definition. These barriers continue to be particularly relevant in view of WHO's renewed call for implementation of PHC (WHO 2008).

THE ALMA-ATA DECLARATION

Halfdan Mahler, Director-General of WHO from 1973 to 1988, instigated the *Alternative Approaches to Meeting Basic Health Needs in Developing Countries* study (WHO 1975), which launched PHC onto the world stage.[4] This report followed WHO's Executive Board organisational study in 1973, *Methods of*

Promoting the Development of Basic Health Services (Newell 1988, p. 903). Hence, by the mid-1970s, member countries of the World Health Assembly, WHO's decision-making body, appeared to be convinced that the research conducted by WHO provided sufficient evidence of there being a better approach to protecting the health of the world's population. This approach in part returned to the environmental issues of the nineteenth century—but this time, it also acknowledged the need for equity in health development and curative care and for public participation in health-care decision making. An ideological shift within WHO was responsible for this dramatic change in health policy, which culminated in the landmark Alma-Ata Declaration declaring PHC as the key to achieving "Health for All" by the year 2000.[5]

THE PHC APPROACH

The Declaration contains ten paragraphs. Health as a human right is reaffirmed, as is the definition of health contained in the WHO Constitution (para. I). Inequalities in health are considered unacceptable (para. II). The importance of economic and social development to reducing inequalities in health is recognised (para. III). Emphasis is placed on people's right to participate in planning and implementing their health care (para. IV). The Declaration confirms that governments have a responsibility for the health of their people, which can be achieved only through the provision of adequate health and social measures (para. V). PHC is seen to be critical in order for people to attain a level of health that enables them to live socially and economically productive lives. Paragraph VI describes PHC as

> essential care based on practical, *scientifically sound* and *socially acceptable* methods and technology made *universally accessible* to individuals and families in the community through their full participation and at a cost that the community and country can *afford* to maintain at every stage in their development in the spirit of self-reliance and self-determination. It forms an integral part both of the country's health system, of which it is the central function and main focus, and of the overall social and economic development of the community. It is the first level of contact of individuals, the family and community with the national health system bringing health care as close as possible to where people live and work, and constitutes the first element of a continuing health care process.

PHC is to be accessible and appropriate (Mahler 1988, p. 76; WHO 1978, p. 59). Accessibility has four overlapping components:

- geographical accessibility: accessible in terms of distance, travel time, and means of transportation
- financial accessibility: affordable by the community and the country
- cultural accessibility: culturally accessible technical and managerial methods
- functional accessibility: appropriate care delivered by trained health professionals

Appropriateness refers to both the scientific and cultural acceptability of any technology used and its adaptability to local circumstances.

Read in isolation, paragraph VI appears to refer to the provision of health services at the local level only. However, when read with the whole of the Declaration, it indicates that the approach is based on a broad understanding of health (social, cultural, and biomedical) and public health experience, reflects the socio-economic and political conditions of a country and the health concerns of the community, and emphasises effective community participation in health-care planning.

Under the Declaration, the PHC approach was to include, at a minimum, health-related education, food and nutrition, an adequate supply of safe water and basic sanitation, maternal and child health care (including family planning), immunisation, prevention and control of locally endemic diseases, appropriate treatment of common diseases and injuries, and provision of essential drugs (para. VII(3)). To ensure that PHC did not develop as an isolated project at the edge of the health sector, coordination with other social and economic sectors (including education, environment, agriculture, public works, communications, and industry) at the national, intermediate, and community levels was obligatory (para. VII(4)). PHC was to prioritise those most in need and to provide appropriately trained health workers to respond to community health needs as expressed by the community (para. VII(7)).

Recognising that political will would be required to implement the approach, the Declaration called on governments to develop national strategies and plans of action for implementation (para. VIII). The national strategies and plans of action were to have well-defined goals, which were to be subject to a review process that would ensure their appropriate adaptation to the national context and their prioritisation of under-served groups and areas (WHO 1978, Recommendation 19). Governments were also encouraged to express their political will by committing to implementing PHC as part of an overall social and economic development strategy, with the involvement of all relevant sectors and the adoption of enabling legislation where necessary (WHO 1978, Recommendation 18).[6] Despite this recommendation, few countries, if any, adopted enabling legislation to support implementation of the approach.

In summary, the Declaration adopted a broad understanding of health and required a "whole-of-government" approach to the development and implementation of health programmes. Health services were to be accessible, appropriate, affordable, and available. By emphasising public participation in health-related decision making, the PHC approach placed people at the centre of the health system. The Declaration was ground-breaking in the sense that it represented a paradigm shift in approaches to population health and health care: it effectively demanded a shift from an exclusively biomedical model of health (focused on disease and access to health care) to a more holistic model that considered external factors that affect people's health. Unfortunately, it did not take long for this comprehensive approach to be undermined for a variety of reasons, including selective primary health care (discussed below), confusion over what the term "primary health care" actually meant, health professional barriers, and the neo-conservative environment of the late 1970s and 1980s. The following section explores the adoption of selective PHC and the dual use of the term "primary health care"—two barriers in particular that continue to influence public health practice and programming, as well as health system reform.

BARRIERS TO IMPLEMENTATION

Selective PHC is considered to have arisen out of a joint Ford-Rockefeller Foundation symposium on health and population development, held in Bellagio, Italy, in April 1979. At the symposium, Julia Walsh and Kenneth Warren presented a paper entitled "Selective Primary Health Care: An Interim Strategy for Disease Control in Developing Countries." First published in the *New England Journal of Medicine* (1979) and subsequently reprinted in *Social Science and Medicine* (1980), the article led to a famous and lively debate within the international health literature on selective health care as an alternative to the PHC approach adopted only seven months earlier.[7]

The selective PHC approach consisted of classifying major infectious diseases according to their prevalence, morbidity, and mortality, and subsequently placing them into priority groups of high, medium, and low. Feasibility of control was considered in terms of the effectiveness and cost of available technology. Selective PHC was intended not to supplant PHC but rather to serve as an initial step towards it, whereby limited resources would be directed to the most effective means of improving the health of the greatest number of people (Warren 1988, p. 891). In the conservative political climate of the late 1970s and 1980s, the selective PHC approach proved attractive to governments and multilateral and bilateral donors alike (Unger and Killingsworth 1986, p. 1010). The approach resulted in a continuation of selected and targeted strategies to treat disease. As vertical programmes, these strategies relied heavily on specific and focused activities, representing a major departure from the original intent of PHC.

Additional barriers to PHC's implementation included confusion over the meaning of the term "primary health care" (Vuori 1984, p. 221) and its dual use as access to health care at the local level and an approach to reorganising health systems. As a result of its dual use, the term PHC became confused with "primary care." As Helen Keleher notes, primary care is drawn from a biomedical model of health and refers to a person's first point of entry into the health system (2001, pp. 57–58). It is delivered by health professionals: general practitioners, nurses, and allied health workers. Primary care is not intended to deliver social programmes, as it is oriented towards disease prevention and is concerned with health risks. While it may include some forms of opportunistic health education on an individual level to encourage the adoption of better health behaviours, this health education targets individual behavioural change rather than the underlying social or environmental conditions that have caused an illness or disease. This interchangeable use of "PHC" and "primary care" continues today.

GLOBAL AND NATIONAL HEALTH POLICY POST-ALMA-ATA

PHC was a controversial political issue from the beginning. This was acknowledged in both the Alma-Ata Declaration (para. VIII) and the Alma-Ata conference report (WHO 1978, p. 19). Despite the PHC approach being in line with WHO's definition of health, the World Health Assembly failed to marshal the necessary political commitment to utilise WHO's international lawmaking powers and to develop international law to promote implementation of PHC at a country level, despite many of its members being signatories to the ICESCR. Instead, WHO continued with its technical orientation (e.g., quarantine and epidemic intelligence, nomenclature, international standardisation, statistics, and public health administration), this time directed towards the implementation of PHC via the "Health for All" campaign, and did not move beyond exhortations to implement PHC.

By the mid-1980s, it was clear that high-income countries were paying scant attention to the implementation of PHC and that another approach was needed. A series of international conferences on health and health promotion commenced, with the first held in Ottawa, Canada.[8] Health as a basic human right and the PHC approach were recognised and endorsed in the Ottawa Charter and subsequent health promotion charters and declarations.[9] These charters and declarations also confirmed that strategies for health promotion required "healthy" public policy that was intersectoral (i.e., involving sectors such as non-health governmental sectors, private sectors, and non-governmental organisations), coordinated in action, and participatory (WHO 1997).

Some changes were implemented as a result of these health promotion charters and declarations. For example, the "Healthy Cities Project," launched in 1986, became a major instrument for the implementation of the Ottawa Charter (Baum 2002, pp. 474–508) and continues today in countries such as Australia, Canada, and Scotland. Some projects have been sustained while others have struggled. Additionally, by focusing on individual cities and their communities, such projects ignore wider political, social, and economic factors (Beaglehole and Bonita 2004, p. 255). Despite all of the conferences and meetings, PHC has remained largely elusive in low-income countries, and the comprehensive approach originally intended has received scant attention in high-income countries.

By 1993, it was becoming obvious that with no binding rules in place, governments were not implementing the major demands embodied within PHC. Indicators often pointed to regression rather than progression, and it was growing clear that a re-launch of the "Health for All" campaign in the twenty-first century would be required. WHO called for the campaign's renewal in 1995 in response to accelerated global change and in order to "ensure that individuals, countries and organisations are prepared to meet the challenges of the 21st Century."[10]

Nearly three and a half decades after the Alma-Ata Declaration, many critics have concluded that the PHC approach was a failed experiment. Others argue that the approach has actually never been tried in its true form. Over the years, its original intent has been lost, and PHC has instead become associated primarily with the provision of health services and first contact with the health sector. This is revealed in how the term is now used: interchangeably with primary care. As originally intended, however, the PHC approach is inextricably connected with comprehensive, collaborative, and partici-patory programming. WHO (2008) has renewed its call for implementation of PHC, and the Commission on Social Determinants of Health (2008) has highlighted the importance of, among other things, incorporating social determinants into health policy and tackling inequitable distributions of power, money, and resources.[11] Perhaps the time has come for those who fought to implement PHC in the first place, together with new actors in the public health realm, to consider adopting an approach that is strikingly similar to the "old" PHC, with one critical difference: an approach that is also based on international human rights law.

THE RIGHT TO HEALTH AND PHC

This section revisits the right to health with two aims in mind. First, it seeks to draw attention to the similarities between the right to health (as established by the ICESCR) and PHC (as established by the Alma-Ata Declaration). Once these similarities are identified, the barriers to the implementation of PHC become very important, particularly in light of WHO's renewed calls for its implementation. Second, it aims to identify two elements of the right to health that are absent in the PHC approach: an international human rights legal obligation and accountability. These two elements have the potential to overcome existing barriers to PHC's implementation.

Other authors have noted that PHC provides a framework for implementing the right to health (Trubek 1984, p. 244; Yamin 1996, p. 417). This is not surprising, given the similarities between PHC and the right to health. Just as PHC contains its own analytical framework, so too does the right to health, though with minor differences. The PHC analytical framework addresses the accessibility, acceptability, affordability, and appropriateness of health services, whereas the right-to-health framework addresses the availability, accessibility, acceptability, and quality (AAAQ) of the health services. Within the latter framework, this means that services are to be available in sufficient quantity, accessible (encompassing the elements of non-discrimination, physical accessibility, affordability, and information accessibility), culturally appropriate and gender sensitive, and of good quality (scientifically and medically appropriate).[12] Unlike the "4 As" of PHC, "quality" under the right-to-health approach separates medical and scientific appropriateness from cultural appropriateness, each of which are included under "acceptability" in the PHC approach.

The right to health, as established by the ICESCR, is concerned with non-discrimination and equality in order to address issues of vulnerability and marginalisation. The Alma-Ata Declaration is concerned with equity in order to give priority to those most in need. Both the Declaration and the ICESCR consider public participation in health-related decision making to be an essential component. Indeed, participation, along with non-discrimination, is contained in the minimum core obligations of the right to health.[13] They both also view health as more than absence of disease and require governments to incorporate the social determinants of health into health reform programmes. States are encouraged under both the Declaration and the ICESCR to develop national plans to implement the respective approaches. In essence, both PHC and the right to health call for a "whole-of-government" approach: one that incorporates other governmental sectors in addition to the obvious health-related bodies and one that is collaborative, coordinated, and participatory.

A POINT OF DEPARTURE

Two important elements absent from the PHC approach but included in the right to health approach—a legal obligation and accountability—have the potential to overcome the obstacles faced by those attempting to implement PHC.

All state parties that have ratified the ICESCR have an international legal obligation to implement the right to health. This legal obligation is either immediate or progressive in nature. Whereas the Alma-Ata Declaration calls on states to develop national plans, the ICESCR obliges them to immediately undertake the development and implementation of a national public health strategy and plan of action.[14] This strategy should be based on a broad understanding of epidemiology (inclusive of social epidemiology at a minimum), address the health concerns of the whole population, be devised and reviewed through a participatory and transparent process, include right-to-health indicators and benchmarks for monitoring, and pay particular attention to vulnerable and marginalised groups (Potts 2008b, p. 730; see chapter 4).[15]

The right to health also includes the essential element of accountability. Accountability is a process that entitles individuals and groups to monitor their governments' activities and to demand that governments explain how they have discharged their right-to-health obligations (Potts 2008a). Where there have been violations, accountability requires remedies in one or more of the following forms: restitution, rehabilitation, compensation, satisfaction, and guarantees of non-repetition.[16]

By relying on international human rights law, monitoring governmental activity, and ensuring governmental accountability via various accountability mechanisms—judicial, quasi-judicial, political, administrative, and social— communities across the globe have managed to advance implementation of the right to health (Potts 2008a). In the presence of renewed calls for the implementation of PHC, public health programmers might consider utilising the right to health as a facilitating framework (see chapter 1).

CONCLUSION

This chapter has attempted to show that the public's health has frequently been viewed in terms of its instrumental rather than intrinsic value. When a global movement emerged to incorporate political, economic, and social determinants into public health policy and programmes, it was quickly undermined. Beaglehole and Bonita note that public health has always been drawn in two directions (2004, p. 251). In one direction is a broad path that adopts a holistic approach to health and relies on comprehensive, collaborative, and participatory approaches to address political, economic, and social determinants and health status. In the other direction is reliance on a narrow path concerned with medical care, risk factors, and cost containment. Implementation of the right to health, an approach extremely similar to that of PHC, has the potential to ensure that the health sector adopts the broad path when responding to WHO's call for a renewal of PHC—and, in the process, overcome the barriers to its implementation.

REFERENCES

Baum, F. 2002. *The New Public Health*. 2nd ed. Melbourne: Oxford Univ. Press.

Beaglehole, R., and R. Bonita. 2004. *Public Health at the Crossroads: Achievements and Prospects*. 2nd ed. Cambridge: Cambridge Univ. Press.

Berman, P. 1982. "Selective Primary Health Care: Is Efficient Sufficient?" *Social Science and Medicine* 16 (10): 1054–1059.

Blane, D., E. Brunner, and R. Wilkinson. 1996. "The Evolution of Public Health Policy: An Anglocentric View of the Last Fifty Years." In *Health and Social Organization: Towards a Health Policy for the Twenty-First Century*, ed. D. Blane, E. Brunner, and R. Wilkinson, 1–15. London: Routledge.

Bryder, L. 1994. "A New World? Two Hundred Years of Public Health in Australia and New Zealand." In *The History of Public Health and the Modern State*, ed. D. Porter, 313–334. Amsterdam: Editions Rodopi B. V.

Colgrove, J. 2002. "The McKeown Thesis: A Historical Controversy and Its Enduring Influence." *American Journal of Public Health* 92 (5): 725–729.

Commission on Social Determinants of Health. 2008. *Closing the Gap in a Generation: Health Equity through Action on the Social Determinants of Health; Final Report of the Commission on Social Determinants of Health*. Geneva: WHO.

Croft, S., and P. Beresford. 1996. "The Politics of Participation." In *Critical Social Policy A Reader: Social Policy and Social Relations*, ed. D. Taylor. London: Sage Publications.

Cueto, M. 2004. "The Origins of Primary Health Care and Selective Primary Health Care." *American Journal of Public Health* 94 (11): 1864–1874.

Fidler, D. 2000. *International Law and Public Health: Materials on and Analysis of Global Health Jurisprudence*. New York: Transnational Publishers.

Gish, O. 1982. "Selective Primary Health Care: Old Wine in New Bottles." *Social Science and Medicine* 16 (19): 1049–1054.

Hamlin, C. 1994. "State Medicine in Great Britain." In *The History of Public Health and the Modern State*, ed. D. Porter, 132–164. Amsterdam: Editions Rodopi B. V.

Keleher, H. 2001. "Why Primary Health Care Offers a More Comprehensive Approach for Tackling Health Inequalities than Primary Care." *Australian Journal of Primary Health* 7 (2): 57–61.

Lalonde, M. 1974. *A New Perspective on the Health of Canadians*. Ottawa: Canadian Department of National Health and Welfare. http://www.phac-aspc.gc.ca/ph-sp/pdf/perspect-eng.pdf.

Lee, S. 1997. "WHO and the Developing World." In *Western Medicine as Contested Knowledge*, ed. A. Cunningham and B. Andrews, 24–45. Manchester: Manchester Univ. Press.

Link, B., and J. Phelan. 2002. "McKeown and the Idea That Social Conditions Are Fundamental Causes of Disease." *American Journal of Public Health* 92 (5): 730–732.

Lipkin, M. 1982. "Commentary of Mack Lipkin." *Social Science and Medicine* 16 (10): 1062–1063.

Mahler, H. 1988. "Present Status of WHO's Initiative, 'Health for All by the Year 2000.'" *Annual Review of Public Health* 9:71–97.

Mann, J. 1997. "Medicine and Public Health, Ethics and Human Rights." *The Hastings Center Report* 27 (3): 6–13.

Navarro, V. 1984. "A Critique of the Ideological and Political Position of The Brandt Report and The Alma Ata Declaration." *International Journal of Health Services* 14 (2): 159–172.

Newell, K. 1975. *Health by the People*. Geneva: WHO.

—. 1988. "Selective Primary Health Care: The Counter Revolution." *Social Science and Medicine* 26 (9): 903–906.

Oppenheimer, G., R. Bayer, and J. Colgrove. 2002. "Health and Human Rights: Old Wine in New Bottles?" *Journal of Law, Medicine and Ethics* 30 (4): 522–532.

Porter, D. 1999. *Health, Civilization and the State: A History of Public Health from Ancient to Modern Times.* London: Routledge.

Potts, H. 2008a. *Accountability and the Right to the Highest Attainable Standard of Health.* Colchester: Univ. of Essex. http://www.essex.ac.uk/human_rights_centre/research/rth/docs/HRC_Accountability_Mar08.pdf.

—. 2008b. "The Right to Health in Public Health: Is This a New Approach?" *Journal of Law and Medicine* 15 (5): 725–741.

Rifkin, S., and G. Walt. 1986. "Why Health Improves: Defining The Issues Concerning 'Comprehensive Primary Health Care' and 'Selective Primary Health Care.'" *Social Science and Medicine* 23 (6): 559–566.

Segall, M. 1983. "The Politics of Primary Health Care." *IDS Bulletin* 14 (4): 27–37.

Susser, M. 1993. "Health as a Human Right: An Epidemiologist's Perspective on the Public Health." *American Journal of Public Health* 83 (3): 418–426.

Szreter, S. 1988. "The Importance of Social Intervention in Britain's Mortality Decline c. 1850–1914: A Re-interpretation of the Role of Public Health." *Social History of Medicine* 1 (1): 1–38.

Trubek, D. 1984. "Economic, Social and Cultural Rights in the Third World: Human Rights Law and Human Needs Program." In *Human Rights in International Law*, ed. T. Merton. Oxford: Clarendon Press.

Unger, J. P., and J. Killingsworth. 1986. "Selective Primary Health Care: A Critical Review of Methods and Results." *Social Science and Medicine* 22 (10): 1001–1013.

Vuori, H. 1984. "Primary Health Care in Europe: Problems and Solutions." *Community Medicine* 6 (3): 221–231.

Walsh, J. 1982. "Comments of Julia A. Walsh." *Social Science and Medicine* 16 (10): 1060–1061.

—. 1988. "Selectivity within Primary Health Care." *Social Science and Medicine* 26 (9): 899–902.

Walsh, J., and K. Warren. 1979. "Selective Primary Health Care: An Interim Strategy for Disease Control in Developing Countries." *New England Journal of Medicine* 301 (18): 967–974.

—. 1980. "Selective Primary Health Care: An Interim Strategy for Disease Control in Developing Countries." *Social Science and Medicine – Part C: Medical Economics* 14 (2): 145–163.

Warren, K. 1982. "Comments of Kenneth S. Warren." *Social Science and Medicine* 16 (10): 1059–1060.

—. 1988. "The Evolution of Selective Primary Health Care." *Social Science and Medicine* 26 (9): 891–898.

WHO (World Health Organization). 1975. *Alternative Approaches to Meeting Basic Health Needs in Developing Countries.* Geneva: WHO

—. 1978. *Primary Health Care: Report of the International Conference on Primary Health Care, Alma-Ata, USSR, 6–12 September 1978.* Geneva: WHO.

—. 1997. *Intersectoral Action for Health: A Cornerstone for Health-for-All in the Twenty-First Century; Report of the International Conference, 20–23 April 1997, Halifax, Nova Scotia, Canada.* Geneva: WHO.

—. 2008. *The World Health Report: Primary Health Care; Now More Than Ever.* Geneva: WHO.

Yamin, A. 1996. "Defining Questions: Situating Issues of Power in the Formulation of a Right to Health under International Law." *Human Rights Quarterly* 18 (2): 398–438.

NOTES

1 Declaration of Alma-Ata, International Conference on Primary Health Care, Alma-Ata, USSR, 6–12 September 1978.

2 International Covenant on Economic, Social and Cultural Rights, G.A. Res. 2200A (XXI), 21 U.N. GAOR Supp. (No. 16) at 49, U.N. Doc. A/6316 (1966), 993 U.N.T.S. 3, entered into force 3 January 1976.

3 Committee on Economic, Social and Cultural Rights, General Comment 14, U.N. Doc. E/C.12/2000/4 (2000), para. 43.

4 The study examined "successful or promising" national programmes for delivering primary health care in several countries, including Bangladesh, Cuba, India, Niger, Tanzania, Venezuela, and Yugoslavia. All of the programmes studied featured a common political strategy, which saw health, as well as strong community involvement, as integral to a country's overall social and economic development. Although some of the programmes were implemented in capitalist countries, often involving non-governmental organisations, the most notable demonstrations of successful alternative approaches came from developing socialist countries.

5 Alma-Ata Declaration, *supra* note 1, para. V. See also WHO (1978). The Alma-Ata conference report expands on the content of the Declaration and provides the context for understanding the primary health care approach. It contains a summary of discussions from the conference and twenty-two recommendations for implementing the primary health care approach.

6 Alma-Ata Declaration, *supra* note 1, para. VIII.

7 In addition to the Walsh and Warren article, other key articles from the debate include the following: Berman (1982); Gish (1982); Lipkin (1982); Newell (1988); Rifkin and Walt (1986); Unger and Killingsworth (1986); Walsh (1982, 1988); Warren (1982, 1988).

8 Ottawa Charter for Health Promotion, First International Conference on Health Promotion, 21 November 1986, Ottawa, Canada, WHO/HPR/HEP/95.1.

9 Adelaide Recommendations on Healthy Public Policy, Second International Conference on Health Promotion, 5–9 April 1988, Adelaide, South Australia; Sundsvall Statement on Supportive Environments for Health, Third International Conference on Health Promotion, 9–15 June 1991, Sundsvall, Sweden; Jakarta Declaration on Leading Health Promotion into the 21st Century, Fourth International Conference on Health Promotion, 21–25 July 1997, Jakarta, Indonesia; Mexico Ministerial Statement for the Promotion of Health, Fifth Global Conference on Health Promotion, 5 June 2000, Mexico City, Mexico; Bangkok Charter for Health Promotion in a Globalized World, Sixth Global Conference on Health Promotion, 7–11 August 2005, Bangkok, Thailand. These charters, declarations, and recommendations are available at WHO's website, http://www.who.int/healthpromotion/conferences/en.

10 WHO Response to Global Change: Renewing the Health-for-All Strategy, Resolution adopted by the World Health Assembly, WHA Res. 48.16 (1995).

11 WHO established the Commission on Social Determinants of Health in 2005, with the aim of identifying actions to promote health equity between and within countries and fostering a global movement around the issue. The Commission, which presented its final report in 2008, was a global collaboration between policy makers, researchers, and civil society.

12 General Comment 14, *supra* note 3, para. 12.

13 Ibid., para. 43.

14 Ibid., para. 43.

15 Ibid., para. 43(f).

16 Ibid., para. 59.

CHAPTER 4

Health Systems and the Right to Health

GUNILLA BACKMAN

INTRODUCTION

A health system that is effective, responsive, integrated, of good quality, and accessible to all without discrimination is a requirement of the right to health (Hunt and Backman 2008).

Strong health systems are critical for improving health outcomes, such as addressing mental disability, reducing the spread of HIV, and reaching the Millennium Development Goals, which include reducing maternal and child mortality. At a time of economic crises, new pandemics, globalisation, and climate change, strong health systems are needed more than ever (WHO 2009). Yet, according to the World Health Organization (WHO), many health systems are collapsing and failing, and a large number are inequitable, regressive, and unsafe (2007a).

This chapter provides a brief introduction to a large number of highly complex and wide-ranging issues regarding health systems and the right to health that demand much closer scrutiny than the chapter will be able to provide. The aim of this chapter is to introduce health systems and their relationship with the right to health, and to explore the features that health systems should have in order to be respectful of the right to health. It starts by defining health systems, their building blocks, and their overall goal, followed by a brief history of health systems. The chapter then focuses on why a right-to-health approach to health systems should be adopted and on the features that a health system should have in order to be respectful of the right

This chapter draws to a great extent on Paul Hunt, Report of the Special Rapporteur on the right of everyone to the enjoyment of the highest attainable standard of physical and mental health, Human Rights Council, U.N. Doc. A/HRC/7/11 (2008); Backman et al. (2008); Hunt and Backman (2008).

to health. Due to space constraints, this chapter neither describes the different structures and constructs of health systems nor provides a specific analysis of concerns related to health systems in different settings. The analysis of the right-to-health features of health systems will be left to the reader to consider when reading section II of this book.

DEFINITION, STRUCTURE, AND VITALITY OF HEALTH SYSTEMS

DEFINITION OF HEALTH SYSTEMS

There are various definitions of health systems. WHO's definition of a health system, which will be used in this chapter and throughout this book, is "all organizations, people and actions whose *primary intent* is to promote, restore or maintain health" (WHO 2007a, p. 2). This definition encompasses health care and efforts to influence the determinants of health. The health system includes public and private providers; the mother who takes care of her sick child; public health programmes; insurance organisations; occupational health and safety legislation; and intersectoral collaboration (for example, working with and encouraging the Ministry of Education to include health education in schools that encompasses sexual and reproductive health and discusses contraceptives, including condoms).

THE STRUCTURE AND OVERALL GOAL OF HEALTH SYSTEMS

Health systems are socio-historic constructs reflecting various political, historical, and economic influences. As a result, they are very contextual (Fryatt, Mills, and Nordström 2010); just like disease patterns, concerns and needs of health systems vary between and within countries.

Irrespective of the national structure, certain features are required of a country's health system. WHO (2007a, 2009) has identified six essential building blocks that make up a health system:

- health information system
- leadership, governance, and stewardship
- financing
- health workforce

- vaccines, technologies, and medicines
- health services (medical and public health)

These building blocks alone do not constitute a health system; it is the interrelationship and interactions between them, with the patient at the centre, that make up a health system. How well these building blocks are interrelated and affect one another will determine how well the system is able to realise the objectives that it is designed to meet (WHO 2009; see figure 4.1).

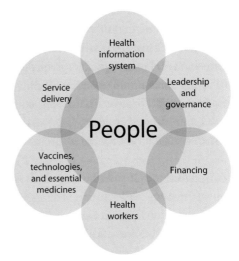

FIGURE 4.1 The interrelationship of the WHO building blocks.

Adapted from WHO (2009, figure 1.2).

The overall goal of a health system is to "improve health and health equity in ways that are responsive, financially fair, and make the best or most efficient use of available resources" (WHO 2007a, p. 2).

How the Six Building Blocks Contribute to a "Good" Health System

A *health information system* is the base for how the other building blocks need to be structured and what services should be provided. It answers such questions as the following: Should there be a greater emphasis on HIV and sexual reproductive health services? Should the oncology department be expanded? What is the structure of the population (age, sex, rural/urban, ethnicity, socio-economic group) using the services? A well-functioning health information system ensures the production, analysis, dissemination, and use of reliable and timely information on health determinants, health system performance, and health status. *Leadership and governance*, a component of health systems that is often underestimated or overlooked, is fundamental. It involves ensuring that strategic policy frameworks exist and that they are combined with effective oversight, regulation, attention to system design, and accountability. An *appropriate health financing system* raises adequate funds for health in order to ensure that people can access needed services and are protected from financial ruin and impoverishment associated with having to pay for them out of pocket. It provides incentives for providers and users to be efficient. A well-functioning *health workforce* is one that utilises responsive, fair, and efficient methods for achieving the best health outcomes possible, given available resources and circumstances (i.e., there must be sufficient staff—fairly distributed—who are competent, responsive, and productive). *Access to essential medical products, vaccines, and technologies* of assured quality, safety, efficacy, and cost-effectiveness, is also required for a properly functioning health system. These products, vaccines, and technologies should also be equitable, as well scientifically sound and cost-effective to use. Finally, *health services* should efficiently deliver effective, safe, and good-quality personal and non-personal health interventions to those in need, in a timely and appropriate manner (WHO, 2007a, p. 3; see figure 4.2).

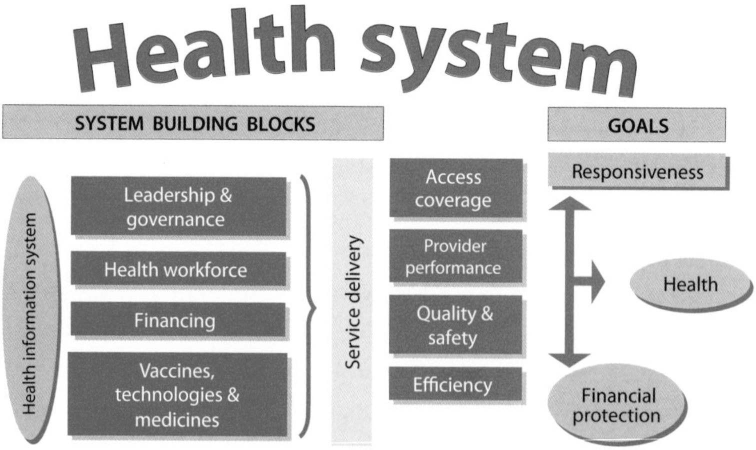

FIGURE 4.2 Health system with its building blocks.
Adapted from WHO (2007a).

THE IMPORTANCE OF HEALTH SYSTEMS

Recognition that a strong health system is an essential element of a healthy and equitable society is growing, and there is a general global consensus on the need to strengthen health systems (WHO 2007a).[1] However, health systems are not new to the health sector. While they have existed for as long as people have endeavoured to protect their health, organised health systems are only about one hundred years old (WHO 2007a). Moreover, the importance placed on health systems has varied through history. At one time or another, all countries have introduced structural changes to their health systems, shaped by national and international values and goals. The 1978 Alma-Ata Declaration, with its focus on primary health care, was the international community's first attempt to bring different values and ideas about health into one policy framework (WHO 2007a; see box 4.1; for more on the Alma-Ata Declaration and primary health care, see chapter 3).[2]

BOX 4.1

ALMA-ATA DECLARATION (1978)

Principal themes

> The importance of equity
> The need for community participation
> The need for a multisectoral approach to health problems
> The need for effective planning
> The importance of integrated referral systems
> An emphasis on health-promotional activities
> The crucial role of suitably trained human resources
> The importance of international cooperation

Essential health interventions

> Education concerning prevailing health problems
> Promotion of food supply and proper nutrition
> Adequate supply of safe water and basic sanitation
> Maternal and child health care, including family planning
> Immunisation against major infectious diseases
> Prevention and control of locally endemic diseases
> Appropriate treatment of common diseases and injuries
> Provision of essential drugs

The Alma-Ata Declaration was developed at a time when the world economy was generally doing well. However, in the 1990s, many countries experienced an economic downturn and were advised to focus public spending on interventions that were cost-effective and to introduce user fees. The importance of health systems was lost, and vertical programmes came to dominate, pushing health systems to "the point of collapse" (WHO 2007a, p. 9). As the world economic crisis deepened, countries undertook health-sector reform in which efficiency (i.e., "doing more for less") became a key focus. As WHO has observed, "the results were predictable" (WHO 2007a, p. 9): the poor, vulnerable, and marginalised were dissuaded from receiving treatment, and user fees yielded limited income. Despite the increased inequality among both people and countries, the international community did not intervene or speak out openly about these problems. It was not until the end of the 1990s that the international community, assisted by the work of the WHO Commission on Macroeconomics and Health, began an open discussion about how health systems could not be not viably run on US $10 per person or less, as had been the advice during the "efficiency" phase (WHO 2007a, p. 9). Thereafter, there was again a focus on health systems and on the importance of protecting people from catastrophic health expenditure (WHO 2007a). For example, WHO's *World Health Report 2000* on health systems emphasised social security, as well as issues of leadership and governance. Further, its *World Health Report 2003* stressed the importance of an integrated approach based on the core principles outlined in the Alma-Ata Declaration.

The global health agenda—shaped by donors; global disease-specific initiatives, such as the Global Alliance for Vaccines and Immunisation (GAVI Alliance) and the Global Fund to Fight AIDS, Tuberculosis and Malaria; and policy makers—also highlights the importance of health systems and directly or indirectly funds health systems strengthening (Reich and Takemi 2009; Travis et al. 2004).

Despite the re-focus and agreement on the importance of health systems and health systems strengthening, national health systems are still faced with many pressures, such as increasing ageing populations and changes in disease patterns from communicable to non-communicable diseases. Many health systems still lack basic capacity in governance, health financing, human resources, health information, and procurement (vaccines, medicines, and technologies)—weaknesses that effectively hamper service delivery. Too many health systems also remain inequitable, regressive, and unsafe (WHO 2007a). In addition, many health and human rights workers and policy makers, including donors, do not have a clear understanding that "every intervention, from the simplest to the most complex, has an effect on the overall [health] system, and the overall [health] system on every intervention" (WHO 2009, p. 19). Furthermore, health systems themselves often lack methods for measuring their own weaknesses and constraints and for evaluating whether they should adopt a vertical or integrated approach. This latter issue has led to the coining of "diagonal intervention" (i.e., combination of vertical and integrated approaches) and has added an additional dimension to the discussion. Thus, it is difficult for policy makers to understand what needs to be done, given the lack of scientifically sound ideas and consensus on what can strengthen or improve a health system (WHO 2009). And with the increased recognition of the importance of health systems strengthening, "the world now confronts a proliferation of models, strategies and approaches" (Reich and Takemi 2009, p. 510), leading to fragmentation.

HEALTH SYSTEMS AND THE RIGHT TO HEALTH

In 2006, the UN Human Rights Council asked the then UN Special Rapporteur on the Right to Health to identify the features that health systems should have in order to be respectful of the right to health. The Special Rapporteur undertook this assignment, presenting his final report to the Council in 2008.[3] In December of the same year, building on the Special Rapporteur's report, the *Lancet* published the results of an assessment of health systems and the right to health in 194 countries (Backman et al. 2008; see chapter 1). This section highlights some reasons for applying a right-to-health approach to health systems and then clarifies what features a health system should possess in order to be respectful of the right to health.

THE REASONS FOR A RIGHT-TO-HEALTH APPROACH TO HEALTH SYSTEMS

In any society, an effective health system is a core institution, no less than a fair justice system or a democratic political system (Hunt and Backman

2008). Weak or collapsed health systems give rise to grave and widespread human rights violations. At the heart of the right to health lies an effective and integrated health system that encompasses preventive, curative, and palliative care and the underlying determinants of health; is responsive to local and national priorities; and is accessible to all without discrimination. Without such a system, the right to health can never be realised. It is only by having functioning health systems that "it will be possible to secure sustainable development, poverty reduction, economic prosperity, [and] improved health" for the population (Hunt and Backman 2008, p. 82).

WHO's six building blocks provide a useful way of looking at health systems; the blocks can be thought of as building blocks for the realisation of the right to health. However, it is possible for a health system to have all of these building blocks yet still not serve human rights. For example, the system might include both medical care and public health, while leaving out mental health services or palliative care; it might provide poor-quality reproductive health services; or though it might have an information system, key data might not be suitably disaggregated. The services need to have properly trained staff available in adequate numbers throughout the country. Of course, expectations are subject to resource availability: more and better facilities are required of Sweden and the UK than of Peru, for example.

The right to health can help identify and expose problem areas, such as health services that are absent or groups that cannot access health services. Also, direct discrimination, marginalisation, and inequity can be detected and, if recognised and acted upon, avoided (Rubenstein 2011). In addition, a rights-based approach can improve the planning and organisation of the health system so that it works towards its goals and ensures that health services are available, accessible, acceptable, and of good quality (AAAQ).

Moreover, General Comment 14 of the UN Committee on Economic, Social and Cultural Rights (ESCR Committee) provides a common right-to-health language for all actors and sets out a road map for realising the right to health, making it easier for practitioners and policy makers to understand and apply the right, including in relation to designing a health system.[4] However, a major challenge for human rights is to apply or integrate the right to health across the six building blocks of a health system. The right-to-health analysis provided by General Comment 14 must be systematically and consistently applied to these building blocks. Box 4.2 identifies some of the issues that arise when a right-to-health analysis is applied to the second WHO building block: the health workforce.

BOX 4.2

APPLICATION OF THE RIGHT TO HEALTH TO THE "HEALTH WORKFORCE" BUILDING BLOCK

- General Comment 14 requires a comprehensive national health plan encompassing human resources (paras. 43(6), 55). Is there an up-to-date plan for human resources in preventive, curative, and palliative care that encompasses both physical and mental health?
- Is there a role for mid-level providers who can increase access to health care, such as assistant medical officers and surgical technicians, and for public-health professionals?
- Are there outreach programmes for the recruitment of health workers from marginalised communities and populations, such as indigenous peoples, in order to reduce non-discrimination and improve respect for cultural differences?
- Are effective measures in place to achieve a gender balance among health workers in all fields in order to ensure equality, non-discrimination, and respect for cultural differences?
- Because health-related services must be available in sufficient quantity (subject to resource availability), are effective measures in place to ensure that the number of domestically trained health workers is commensurate with the health needs of the population?
- Is health information about the number of health workers by category (e.g., nurses and public health professionals) collected, centralised, and made publicly available on a regular basis?
- Are human rights, including respect for cultural diversity, as well as the importance of treating patients and others with courtesy, a compulsory part of the training for all health workers?
- General Comment 14 requires appropriate training for health personnel (para. 44(5)). Are opportunities for further professional training in place for all health workers, without discrimination? Is training in place to realise the goals set out in the national health plan?

- A lack of reasonable terms and conditions of employment, one of the causes of the "skills drain," is likely to undermine a health system. Are health workers receiving domestically competitive salaries, as well as other reasonable terms and conditions of employment?
- Are incentives in place to encourage the appointment and retention of health workers in underserved areas in order to improve access, especially for marginalised communities and populations?

Source: Backman et al. (2008, p. 2051)

Without the right to health, health systems run the risk of being impersonal, top-down, and dominated by experts; with the right to health, the well-being of individuals, communities, and populations is placed at the centre (WHO 2007b).

RIGHT-TO-HEALTH FEATURES OF HEALTH SYSTEMS

The right-to-health features of health systems are based on General Comment 14, including core obligations,[5] and reflect many of the themes outlined in the Alma-Ata Declaration and WHO's six building blocks. The Convention on the Rights of the Child, General Comments 3 and 4 of the UN Committee on the Rights of the Child, and General Recommendation 24 of the UN Committee on the Elimination of All Forms of Discrimination against Women also assist in the identification of these features.[6] While the features highlighted below do not include the essential services and facilities that are needed for a well-functioning health system, they encompass other important features that are often neglected. These right-to-health features are informed by good practices and are required of all health systems. Furthermore, they are underpinned by legal obligations (see figure 4.3).

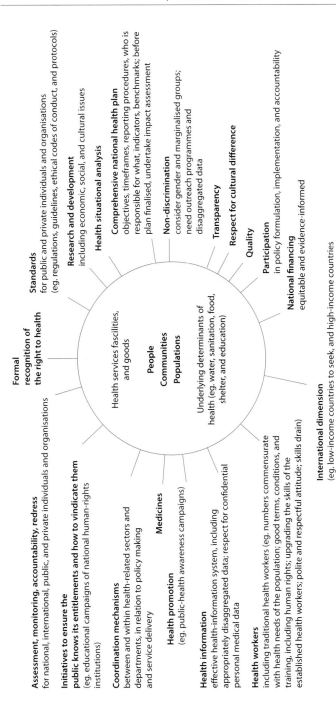

FIGURE 4.3 Right-to-health features of health systems.

Legal Recognition

Countries should recognise the right to health in national law. After a country has ratified an international treaty, the treaty should be recognised by and incorporated into the national constitution or other relevant statute. However, a study published in the *Lancet* in 2008 revealed that of the 158 countries that had ratified the International Covenant on Economic, Social and Cultural Rights (ICESCR), only 56 had included the right to health in their national constitutions or other statutes (Backman et al. 2008, p. 2059). Recognition of the right to health is more common at the international level than at the national level. One reason for this might be that international accountability is weaker than national accountability. Once a country has ratified an international human rights treaty, it has a legal obligation to respect, protect, and fulfil its obligations at least at the international level (see chapters 1, 6, and 10). Dedicated national legislation can legally reinforce health goals, plans, and polices, and help ensure that they are in line with international human rights and internationally approved standards and guidelines (WHO 2011).

In some countries, legal provisions on the right to health are generating significant case law (Singh, Govender, and Mills 2007; Yamin and Gloppen 2011). One concrete example is the study by Hans Hogerzeil and colleagues, who analysed seventy-one court cases from twelve countries and concluded that in fifty-nine cases, access to essential medicines was enforced through the courts as part of the right to health (Hogerzeil et al. 2006; see chapter 9). Legal recognition is just one of the first steps to realising the right to health—if not followed up by implementation and monitoring, such recognition is likely to be an empty promise.

Standards

Legal recognition of the right to health, while important, is usually confined to a general formulation that does not set out in any detail what is required of those with responsibilities for health. Consequently, countries must also ensure that their laws and policies contain detailed provisions clarifying what society can expect by way of health-related services and facilities. Clarification is important for health providers, so that they know what is expected of them; it is also important for health-system users, so that they know what they can legitimately expect. For example, provisions are needed for the quality and quantity of drinking water, blood safety, essential medicines, and the quality of medical care. Such provisions may be included in a country's laws, regulations, protocols, guidelines, and codes of conduct. WHO has published important standards on various health issues, which are meant to serve as a guide for health service providers and governments, among others (WHO 2008a, 2008b).

Equity, Equality, and Non-Discrimination

Health systems must be accessible to all, including those living in poverty, minority groups, indigenous people, women, children, people living in rural areas, people with disabilities, and other disadvantaged individuals and groups.[7] Additionally, health systems must be responsive to the particular health needs of groups such as women, children, adolescents, and elderly people.[8]

The right to health encompasses physical and mental health. Mental health, however, is grossly neglected. Of all the world's low-income countries, only 36% have mental health legislation (WHO 2011, p. 10). Few countries have sufficient mental health facilities properly serviced by trained staff (Hunt and Mesquita 2006), and few countries allocate sufficient funds to mental health services. Globally, mental health spending is less than US$2 per person; in low-income countries, it is less than US$0.25 (WHO 2011, p. 10; see chapter 8).

The human rights principles of equality and non-discrimination are akin to the concept of equity in health. All three concepts have a social justice component. In some respects, equality and non-discrimination, being reinforced by law, are more powerful than equity (Braveman and Gruskin 2003). For example, if a government or other body does not take effective steps to tackle discrimination, it can be held to account and required to take remedial measures.[9] Although the right to health provides for progressive realisation, some of its components are of immediate effect—and one of these is non-discrimination.

Participation

The right to health is also interested in process. Community participation is a key principle of the Alma-Ata Declaration (see chapters 3 and 6). WHO has stressed that "the role of the people is highlighted, not just as the centre of the system as mediators and beneficiaries but as actors in driving the [health] system itself" (WHO 2008a, 2009, p. 32). Health systems must include institutional arrangements for the active and informed participation in strategy development, policy making, implementation, and account-ability by all relevant stakeholders, including disadvantaged individuals, communities, and populations.[10] In New Zealand, for example, there is a legislative requirement of Maori participation in the country's district health boards. Participation improves the effectiveness and quality of health services, which, in turn, improve health outcomes (WHO 2008a). Despite legal obligations regarding participation, as well as scientific evidence of improved health outcomes arising from participation (Mandahar et al. 2004), there is a significant gap between rhetoric and practice. A review of countries' implementation of the Alma-Ata Declaration shows that participation has been especially neglected (Lawn 2008, p. 924; see chapter 3). If communities participate and set priorities, the process might be slower, but it will also be more sustainable (Lawn 2008, p. 924; see chapter 11). Preconditions for meaningful participation include having access to information, being free to speak openly without intimidation, and being free to organise without restriction. Yet, in 2008, only 73 out of 194 countries had laws protecting the right to information (Backman et al. 2008, p. 2071). These safeguards are also vital for carrying out health promotion. Additional examples of the critical importance of participation, and the consequences when overlooked or ignored, are presented in section II of this book.

Transparency

Tempered by the confidentiality of personal data, this requirement applies to all those working in health-related sectors, including national governments, international organisations, public-private partnerships, business enterprises, and civil-society organisations.[11] Transparency demands that health plans, including the accompanying budgets, be made publicly available (see chapters 6, 7, and 11). In many countries, however, this is not the case; Sweden and Ecuador, for example, were not transparent in their budget allocations for mental health. Sweden remarked that this was partly a consequence of the objective not to stigmatise people with mental disabilities. Not being transparent can mean perpetuating the marginalisation and neglect experienced by many people with mental health issues (Backman et al. 2008, p. 2060).

Respect for Cultural Differences

Health systems must be respectful of cultural differences (Hunt 2006).[12] In particular, health workers must be sensitive to issues of culture, ethnicity, and sex. Participation helps ensure that cultural aspects are taken into account (for more on the consequences of not respecting cultural differences, see chapter 6).

Quality

All health-related services and facilities must be of good quality.[13] Quality is also related to the competence of the staff (see chapters 3, 6, 8, and 10). A study in Uganda showed that one of the main reasons for people leaving public providers and seeking care with private providers was patients' lack of confidence in the competence of staff at public health facilities (Lindfors, Sundevall, and Forsberg 2008). The good-quality requirement also extends to the manner in which patients and others are treated: health workers must treat patients and others politely and with respect. In addition, due to the problem of counterfeit medicines, governments must establish appropriate regulatory systems for drugs (Hunt and Khosla 2008). Further, water-quality regulations and standards consistent with WHO's guidelines (2010) on this issue should be in place.

Planning

Some important implications arise from the right to health being subject to progressive realisation and resource availability. The crucial importance of planning is recognised in the Alma-Ata Declaration, General Comment 14, and elsewhere (Green 2007). A health plan is a core obligation of immediate effect. States must have comprehensive national health plans, encompassing both the public and private sectors, for the development of health systems; because the plans have to be evidence based, a situational analysis or rapid assessment needs to be carried out, with disaggregated data, before the plan is drafted. Health research and development should also inform the planning process (Allotey et al. 2008; Hunt et al. 2007).

According to General Comment 14, a country's health plan must include certain features, such as clear objectives (and how these are to be achieved), time frames, effective coordination mechanisms, reporting procedures, a detailed budget, financing arrangements (national and international), assessment arrangements, indicators and benchmarks to measure achievement, and one or more accountability devices. The national health plan should also be gender mainstreamed. Indicators and benchmarks are already commonplace features of many health systems, but they rarely have all the elements that are important from a human rights perspective, such as appropriate disaggregation.

The identification of indicators and benchmarks to measure the progressive realisation of the right to health is a national and international process that involves countries, international organisations, the ESCR Committee, and others (see chapter 1).

The process of crafting a national health plan also requires a fair, transparent, participatory, and inclusive process for prioritising competing health needs—one that takes into account explicit criteria, such as the well-being of those living in poverty, and not just the claims of powerful groups with vested interests (Hunt 2007). The process of prioritisation should give particular attention to the core obligations identified in General Comment 14, as such obligations are required of all countries, whatever their stage of economic development. It is important to note that the list of core obligations is illustrative rather than exhaustive (Chapman and Russell 2002). One of the core obligations is to adopt and implement a national public health strategy and plan of action, on the basis of epidemiological evidence, that addresses the health concerns of the whole population (see chapters 6, 7, 8, and 11).[14]

Before the finalisation of the plan, key elements must undergo impact assessment to ensure that they are consistent with national and international legal obligations, including those relating to the right to health (Hunt and MacNaughton 2006; see chapter 1). In addition, the present realisation of the right to health must be maintained, although this might be waived in exceptional circumstances.[15] Progressive realisation does not mean that a government is free to choose whatever measures it wishes to take, so long as they reflect some degree of progress. General Comment 14 requires that governments take deliberate, concrete, and targeted steps to ensure progressive realisation as quickly and effectively as possible.

Progressive realisation, maximum available resources, and core obligations need closer conceptual and operational attention. Some courts have rejected the idea of core obligations, requiring instead that governmental policies be "reasonable."[16] Other courts have taken the same position as the ESCR Committee in its General Comment 14, finding that some health-related responsibilities are so fundamental that they are subject to neither progressive realisation nor resource availability.[17] This position most closely matches the right to health: progressive realisation is an important concept with a crucial role, but only up to the boundaries of core obligations.

Referral Systems

Health systems should have a mix of primary (community-based), secondary (district-based), and tertiary (specialised) facilities and services that provide a continuum of prevention, curative, and palliative care (WHO 2000; see chapter 11).[18] They also need to establish an effective process by which health workers assess whether patients will benefit from additional services and by which patients are referred from one facility or department to another. Such a procedure should also include referrals between alternative health systems (e.g., traditional health practitioners) and mainstream health systems. The absence of an effective referral system is inconsistent with the right to health, as well as WHO's recommendations for improving primary health care and the overall health system (WHO 2008a).

Coordination

Health systems and the right to health depend on effective coordination across a range of public and private stakeholders (including non-govern-mental organisations) at the national and international levels. Effective coordination between various sectors and departments—such as health, environment, water, sanitation, education, food, shelter, finance, and transport—is important for health systems. The need for coordination extends to policy making and delivery of services, as well as to actors other than the state (WHO 2000; see chapters 3, 6, 10, and 11).[19]

International Cooperation

Health systems have international dimensions, including the control of infectious diseases, the dissemination of health research, and regulatory initiatives, such as the International Health Regulations (WHO 2008b) and the WHO Framework Convention on Tobacco Control.[20] The international dimension of health systems is reflected in countries' human rights responsibilities of international assistance and cooperation, which can be traced through the UN Charter, the Universal Declaration of Human Rights, and some more recent international human rights declarations and binding treaties (Skogly 2006; see chapters 1 and 2).[21]

Monitoring, Accountability, and Redress

Individuals and communities should have the opportunity to understand how those with responsibilities have discharged their duties. They should also provide these actors the opportunity to explain what they have done and why (Potts 2008). Where mistakes have been made, accountability requires redress. Accountability is not a matter of blame and punishment but a fair and reasonable process to identify what works, so it can be repeated, and what does not, so it can be revised (Potts 2008).

Something as complex and important as a health system needs several effective, transparent, accessible, and independent accountability mechanisms—health commissioners, national human rights institutions, democratically elected local health councils, public hearings, patients' committees, impact assessments, and judicial proceedings. Civil society organisations and the media also have crucial roles (Potts 2008).

Unfortunately, accountability mechanisms in many health systems are extremely weak. In many cases, accountability is often little more than a device to check that health funds were spent as they should have been. Also, in some countries, the body that provides and regulates health services is the same body charged with holding those responsible to account. Furthermore, the private health sector is often largely unregulated.

Human rights accountability helps remedy these problems. It is concerned not just with monitoring health funds but also with ensuring that health systems are improving and that the right to health is being progressively realised for all, including disadvantaged individuals, communities, and populations. The requirement of human rights accountability extends to both the public and private health-related sectors and to international bodies working on health-related issues (Clapham 2006).

Accountability mechanisms are urgently needed for all bodies—public, private, national, and international—working on health-related issues. However, for monitoring and accountability to take place, the people, as users and providers, need to be able to obtain information, be aware of their rights, and understand the right to health. The last decade has witnessed a growing understanding of the right to health; as a result, people are increasingly monitoring, questioning, and holding governments to account. To take one example, in a landmark 2008 decision, the Colombian Constitutional Court, on the basis of a detailed understanding of the right to health, effectively ordered a phased restructuring of the country's health system by way of a participatory and transparent process based on current epidemiological information (Baderin and McCorquodale 2006; Gauri and Brinks 2008; Ghai and Cotrell 2004; Inter-American Commission on Human Rights 2007; Yamin and Gloppen 2011).[22]

Striking the Balance

Human rights are not unrealistic. Few are absolute. Human rights are aware that health systems face pressure to respond to multiple needs within finite budgets and that this gives rise to difficult policy choices (such as whether to prioritise more trained health workers, better community-based health services, improved mental health facilities, enhanced access to antiretrovirals, or subsidies for effective but expensive cancer drugs). However these priorities are made, human rights do not provide neat answers any more than ethics or economics do (Hunt and Backman 2008, p. 86). Crucially, the features presented above are not optional but rather legally binding requirements. As such, if a government decides not to respect these features, or decides to make a trade-off between one human right and another, human rights require that the reasons be reviewed in a "fair, transparent, participatory process, taking into account explicit criteria, such as the well being of those living in poverty and [marginalised] men and women, and not just the claims of powerful interest groups" (Hunt and Backman 2008, p. 86).

CONCLUSION

Health system are core social institutions. Because of their importance, they are reinforced and protected by the right to health and other human rights. Health systems should have certain right-to-health features, as highlighted in this chapter. These features are not new "add-ons" but qualities that many health sectors have highlighted as critically important. The international community has agreed on the importance of human rights, and numerous stakeholders—civil society, governments, donors, and international bodies— are increasingly advocating for the systematic integration of all human rights, including economic, social, and cultural rights, into health systems. Despite this, the features presented above are often overlooked. These features are legally binding requirements, not optional extras. Governments should be monitored to ensure that health systems have, in practice, the features required by international human rights law; and if such features are not present, governments should be held to account and forced to explain why not. In addition, states providing international assistance should be monitored to see if they are assisting towards the realisation of the right to health. This chapter does not demonstrate how these features are applied in practice—that is the task of the second part of this book, which uses case studies to demonstrate what happens when these features are not respected and what the consequences are.

REFERENCES

Allotey, P., D. Reidpath, H. Ghalib et al. 2008. "Efficacious, Effective, and Embedded Interventions: Implementation Research in Infectious Disease Control." *BMC Public Health* 8. doi:10.1186/1471-2458-8-343.

Backman, G., P. Hunt, R. Khosla, et al. 2008. "Health Systems and the Right to Health an Assessment of 194 Countries." *The Lancet* 372 (9655): 2047–2085.

Baderin, M. A., and R. McCorquodale, eds. 2006. *Economic, Social, and Cultural Rights in Action.* Oxford: Oxford Univ. Press.

Braveman, P., and S. Gruskin. 2003. "Defining Equity in Health." *Journal of Epidemiology Community Health* 57:254–258.

Chapman, A., and S. Russell, eds. 2002. *Core Obligations: Building a Framework for Economic, Social and Cultural Rights.* Antwerp: Intersentia.

Clapham, A. 2006. *Human Rights Obligations of Non-State Actors.* Oxford: Oxford Univ. Press.

Fryatt, R., A. Mills, and A. Nordstrom. 2010. "Financing of Health Systems to Achieve the Health Millennium Development Goals in Low-Income Countries." *The Lancet* 375 (9712): 419–426.

Gauri, V., and D. M. Brinks, eds. 2008. *Courting Social Justice: Judicial Enforcement of Social and Economic Rights in the Developing World.* Cambridge: Cambridge Univ. Press.

Ghai, Y., and J. Cottrell, eds. 2004. *Economic, Social and Cultural Rights in Practice: The Role of Judges in Implementing Economic, Social and Cultural Rights.* London: Interights.

Green, A. 2007. *An Introduction to Health Planning for Developing Health Systems.* Oxford: Oxford Univ. Press.

Hogerzeil, H. V., M. Samson, J. V. Casanovas, et al. 2006. "Is Access to Essential Medicines as Part of the Fulfilment of the Right to Health Enforceable through the Courts?" *The Lancet* 368 (9532): 305–311.

Hunt, P., 2006. "The Human Right to the Highest Attainable Standard of Health: New Opportunities and Challenges." *Transactions of the Royal Society of Tropical Medicine and Hygiene* 100: 603–607.

Hunt, P., and G. Backman. 2008. "Health Systems and the Right to the Highest Attainable Standard of Health." *Health and Human Rights* 10 (1): 40–59.

Hunt, P., and R. Khosla. 2008. "The Human Right to Medicine." *SUR* 5:99–116.

Hunt, P., and G. MacNaughton. 2006. "Impact Assessments, Poverty and Human Rights: A Case Study Using the Right to the Highest Attainable Standard of Health." Health and Human Rights Working Paper Series No. 6, World Health Organization and UNESCO.

Hunt, P., R. Stewart, J. Mesquita, et al. 2007. *Neglected Diseases: A Human Rights Analysis.* Geneva: Special Programme for Research and Training in Tropical Diseases.

Inter-American Commission on Human Rights. 2007. *Access to Justice as a Guarantee of Economic, Social and Cultural Rights: A Review of the Standards Adopted by the Inter-American Commission on Human Rights.* Washington, DC: IACHR.

Kjellström, T., C. Håkansta, and C. Hogstedt. 2007. "Globalisation and Public Health: Overview and a Swedish Perspective." *Scandinavian Journal of Public Health* 35 (5): 2–68.

Koivusalo, M. 2006. "The Impact of Economic Globalisation on Health." *Theoretical Medicine and Bioethics* 27 (1): 13–34.

Labonte, R., and R. Torgerson. 2002. *Frameworks for Analyzing the Links between Globalization and Health.* Geneva: WHO.

Lawn, E. J. 2008. "Alma-Ata 30 Years On: Revolutionary, Relevant, and Time to Revitalise." *The Lancet* 372 (9642): 917–926.

Lindfors, A., J. Sundevall, and B. Forsberg. 2008. "Sjukvard i laginkomstlander ofta privat. For god vard pa lika villkor kravs nya systemlosningar." *Lakartidningen* 105 (4): 215–219.

Mandahar, D. S., D. Osrin, B. P. Shrestha, et al. 2004. "Effect of a Participatory Intervention with Women's Groups on Birth Outcomes in Nepal: Cluster-Randomised Controlled Trial." *The Lancet* 364 (9438): 970–979.

Potts, H. 2008. *Accountability and the Right to the Highest Attainable Standard of Health.* Colchester: Univ. of Essex. http://www.essex.ac.uk/human_rights_centre/research/rth/docs/HRC_Accountability_Mar08.pdf.

Raviola, G., A. E. Becker, and P. Farmer. 2011. "A Global Scope for Global Health: Including Mental Health." *The Lancet.* doi:10.1016/S0140-6736(11)60941-0.

Reich, M. R., and K. Takemi. 2009. "G8 and Strengthening of Health Systems: Follow-Up to the Tokyo Summit." *The Lancet* 373 (9662): 508–515.

Rubestenin, L. 2011. "Post-Conflict Health Reconstruction: Search for a Policy." *Disaster* 35 (4): 680–700.

Singh, A. J., M. Govender, and E. Mills. 2007. "Do Human Rights Matter to Health?" *The Lancet* 370 (4): 521–527.

Skogly, S. 2006. *Beyond National Borders: States' Human Rights Obligations in International Cooperation.* London: Intersentia.

Travis, P., S. Bennett, A. Haines, et al. 2004. "Overcoming Health Systems Constraints to Achieve the Millennium Development Goals." *The Lancet* 364 (9437): 900–906.

WHO (World Health Organization). 2000. *World Health Report: Health Systems; Improving Performance.* Geneva: WHO.

—. 2003. *World Health Report 2003: Shaping the Future.* Geneva: WHO.

—. 2007a. *Everybody's Business: Strengthening Health Systems to Improve Health Outcomes; WHO's Framework for Action.* Geneva: WHO.

—. 2007b. *People at the Centre of Health Care: Harmonizing Mind and Body, People and Systems.* Geneva: WHO.

—. 2008a. *Framework and Standards for Country Health Information Systems.* 2nd ed. Geneva: WHO.

—. 2008b. *International Health Regulations (2005).* 2nd ed. Geneva: WHO.

—. 2009. *Systems Thinking for Health Systems Strengthening.* Geneva: WHO.

—. 2010. "Water for Health: WHO Guidelines for Drinking-Water Quality." Accessed 10 September 2011. http://www.who.int/water_sanitation_health/ WHS_WWD2010_guidelines_2010_6_en.pdf.

—. 2011. *Mental Health Atlas 2011.* Geneva: WHO.

Yamin, A. E., and S. Gloppen, eds. 2011. *Litigating Health Rights: Can Courts Bring More Justice to Health?* Boston: Human Rights Program, Harvard Law School.

NOTES

1 Rio Political Declaration on Social Determinants of Health, World Conference on Social Determinants of Health, 19–21 October 2011, Rio de Janeiro, Brazil, para. 13(2)(ii).

2 Declaration of Alma-Ata, International Conference on Primary Health Care, Alma-Ata, USSR, 6–12 September 1978.

3 Paul Hunt, Report of the Special Rapporteur on the right of everyone to the enjoyment of the highest attainable standard of physical and mental health, Human Rights Council, U.N. Doc. A/HRC/7/11 (2008) [hereinafter Hunt Report].

4 Paul Hunt, Report of the Special Rapporteur on the right of everyone to the enjoyment of the highest attainable standard of physical and mental health, Commission on Human Rights, U.N. Doc. E/CN.4/2005/51 (2005).

5 Committee on Economic, Social and Cultural Rights, General Comment 14, U.N. Doc. E/C.12/2000/4 (2000), para. 43.

6 Convention on the Rights of the Child, G.A. Res. 44/25, Annex, 44 U.N. GAOR Supp. (No. 49) at 167, U.N. Doc. A/44/49 (1989), entered into force 2 September 1990; Committee on the Rights of the Child, General Comment 3, U.N. Doc. CRC/ GC/2003/3 (2003); Committee on the Rights of the Child, General Comment 4, U.N. Doc. CRC/GC/2003/4 (2003); CEDAW Committee, General Recommendation 24, U.N. Doc. CEDAW/C/1999/I/WG.II/WP.2/Rev.1 (1999). For details of the methodology of identifying the features of health systems, see Hunt Report, *supra* note 3; Backman et al. (2008).

7 General Comment 14, *supra* note 5, paras. 18–19.

8 Ibid., paras. 24–27.

9 *Hoffmann v. South African Airways*, Constitutional Court of South Africa, Case CCT 17/00 2000, 29 September 2000; *Eldridge v. British Columbia*, Supreme Court of Canada, [1997] 3 S.C.R. 624.

10 General Comment 14, *supra* note 5, para. 43(f).

11 Ibid.

12 Ibid., para. 12(c).

13 Ibid., para. 12(d).

14 Ibid., para. 43(f).

15 Ibid., paras. 28–29.

16 *Minister of Health and Others v. Treatment Action Campaign and Others,* Constitutional Court of South Africa, 2002 (5) SA 721 (CC).

17 Sentencia T-760/2008, Colombian Constitutional Court, 31 July 2008; *Paschim Banga Khet Mazdoor Samity v. State of West Bengal,* Supreme Court of India, 1996 AIR SC 2426/(1996) 4 SCC 37.

18 General Comment 14, *supra* note 5, para. 17.

19 Ibid., para. 64.

20 WHO Framework Convention on Tobacco Control, adopted by the 56th World Health Assembly, 31 May 2003.

21 Charter of the United Nations, 26 June 1945, 59 Stat. 1031, entered into force 24 October 1945; Universal Declaration of Human Rights, G.A. Res. 217A (III), U.N. Doc A/810 at 71 (1948); Paris Declaration on Aid Effectiveness, 2005; Maastricht Principles on Extraterritorial Obligations of States in the area of Economic, Social and Cultural Rights, 28 September 2011; General Comment 14, *supra* note 5, para. 38.

22 Sentencia T-760/2008, *supra* note 17.

CHAPTER 5

Ethics and the Right to Health

JOHN PORTER AND SRIDHAR VENKATAPURAM

"When enacted with conscience, public health work includes a moral or ethical aspect to one's conduct together with the urge to prefer right over wrong."

— Milstein (2008)

INTRODUCTION

The Universal Declaration of Human Rights, along with the many legally binding international and national instruments that enshrine its vision, helps uphold the intention behind "the right to health" (Brownlie 2006; Marks 2006).[1] These legal instruments are meant to regulate actions. And the rights articulated in national laws have been created through a historical, ethical process of reasoning that links individuals to their communities, governments, and the international structures of the UN. In turn, human rights law also reflects an enduring ethical global consensus regarding the rights or moral[2] claims of human beings, wherever we find them.

In all aspects of health care (research, planning, service provision, and evaluation) and at all levels (individual, local, national, and international), reflecting on our actions is an ethical process. This is because "doing ethics" involves reflecting on and reasoning about what the right, good, or obligatory thing to do is in a particular situation. All actions—whether performed by ourselves, another person, our community, our government, or international organisations and corporations—have ethical dimensions and consequences. We can ask a variety of questions: Was this the right or wrong action to take?

This chapter is based on the course Ethics, Public Health and Human Rights, which has been taught for over ten years at the London School of Hygiene and Tropical Medicine.

Is this how we or they ought to be acting in this situation? Are these the values that we want to uphold in our health-care system? Through ethically evaluating what is happening (or, indeed, not happening) around us at all levels (self, other, community, world, and whole), we are able to examine ourselves, our roles in health, the goodness of our health-care system, and societies more broadly.

Within this process of evaluating what are good, right, or obligatory actions in health care, the right to health serves as a reference point; it is both an ethical principle to guide our actions and a legal obligation with varying levels of enforcement. The relationship between ethics and the right to health is mutually reinforcing, clear, and broad.

This chapter expands on the relationship between ethics and the right to health. It provides a brief understanding of ethics and its role in relation to the right to health and health systems. Throughout the chapter, a framework of five broad perspectives is highlighted (see figure 5.1): the self, the other, the community, the world, and the whole.[3] Such a framework is meant to emphasise the need to be conscious of ethical issues at all levels, from the individual to the population, and of our duties at each of these levels.

The chapter begins by introducing this framework. It then explores ethics and rights (rights in general as well as human rights) and presents some of the ethical categories and theories that are useful to consider when thinking about rights and health systems (virtue, deontology, consequentialism, justice and political philosophy, and religious ethics). This is followed by a brief history of ethics in health systems and a discussion of its role in current health systems and policy research.

ETHICAL FRAMEWORK: FOCUS ON SELF

WHO AM I? WHAT ROLE AM I PLAYING, AND HOW CAN ETHICS HELP?

It has been said that the best way to understand human behaviour is to examine individuals in their social, cultural, and historical contexts (Mooney 1998). But philosophy often tends to move us towards abstractions and away from context. "Even when philosophy focuses on the individual it tends to do so in abstract terms: the 'unsituated self' divorced from constitutive attachments to family, friends, community and history" (Sandel 1982). While there is good reason to abstract away from context in order to focus on the primary moral issue, there is a fine balance to such reasoning. We must be careful to ensure that abstracting, in order to do ethical reasoning, does not go so far as to be irrelevant or make us lose sight of the fact it is human beings that are the centre of attention. It seems to be important to ensure that individuals working in the field of health care understand this aspect of philosophy. It is crucial to ensure that when using philosophy and philosophical principles and applying them to health care and the right to health, we are "situated" appropriately in context. This is where a process of self-reflection is important (see figure 5.1).[4]

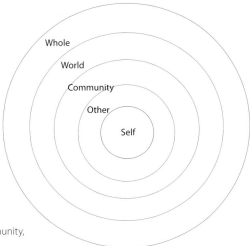

FIGURE 5.1 The self, the other, community, world, and the whole.

In figure 5.1, the first level is the self; the second is the other, meaning relationships with other people; the third is the community; the fourth is the world; and the fifth is the whole.[5] The definition of each of these words is important in deciding what each level means for you. When facing an ethical dilemma, we begin with a reflection on ourselves (Who am I? Why am I here? What is my role? How should I act?). At each level, we remain rooted in ourselves while at the same time trying to put ourselves in the shoes of others as we find ways to determine how we "ought" to act in particular situations and relate to others. Perspectives of community, world, and whole allow us to link our individual role in the day-to-day running of the health system with the management, power, politics, and policy that control the overall health system (see chapter 6). By linking the bottom with the top, we can get an idea of top-down and bottom-up health policy processes and how they affect us in our work (Porter, Ogden, and Pronyk 1999). Some of these top-down policies will be declarations, while others, such as the Universal Declaration of Human Rights, will be codes and laws that direct how we "ought" to act.

ETHICS AND RIGHTS AND THE PHILOSOPHIES FOR THE RIGHT TO HEALTH

ETHICS AND RIGHTS

The academic discipline of philosophy has some commonly recognised areas of intellectual inquiry. These include metaphysics (nature and structure of reality), epistemology (what is knowledge and how do we know?), logic (logical consequences, validity, and argument), aesthetics, political philosophy, and ethics. Within ethics, there are three basic types of ethical inquiry: normative ethics, meta-ethics, and descriptive ethics (Frankena 1973).

Normative ethics sets out to give answers to questions such as, what ought to be done? and what ought not to be done? Meta-ethics investigates the meaning of ethical terms—such as good, bad, wrong, and right—and the linguistics of ethical reasoning, making it the most abstract type of ethical inquiry. Lastly, descriptive ethics asks empirical questions, such as how people act or think when faced with situations where ethical values are vague or in conflict (Sugarman and Sulmasy 2001). All three types of ethical inquiry are relevant to health ethics, including the ethics of the right to health.

For example, the meaning of words, which is central to meta-ethics, is also a pressing concern for those working in health care (see chapter 11). The word "health" has profound implications for rights, duties, and social support, depending on how it is defined and used. Precisely because of this, the broad definition of health articulated in the World Health Organization's Constitution as "a state of complete physical, mental and social well-being and not merely the absence of disease or infirmity" has been controversial from the outset (see chapter 1). It is currently being questioned because of the absoluteness of the word "complete"; the changing demography of populations, which now include high numbers of individuals living for a long time with chronic impairments; and the difficulty in making the definition operational (Huber et al. 2011). The right to health, then, immediately raises meta-ethical questions, including, what is good and bad health? and what is a right? Other words—such as health care, illness, disease, well-being, ethics, equity, and justice—are crucial to evaluating actions in the health system. How they are defined and used can unite diverse perspectives or be a source of much disagreement.

Rights: Legal, Social, or Ethical

Rights can be legal, social, or ethical principles of entitlement. They are intimately linked to the law. One way in which we express our "common morality" is through rights, both ethical and legal. A country's legal system is the means through which a society orders and assigns these rights and responsibilities among the competing and conflicting interests of its citizens. Our laws represent the collection of enforceable rights and duties through which individuals relate to each other and their community (Capron 1979), and they are greatly influenced by ethical consensus and morality (Gaare 1989). The law helps replace or clarify morality where ethical principles fail to sufficiently guide human conduct. Therefore, "the law and ethics are similar in that they both prescribe human behaviour according to a set of rights and duties" (Capron 1979, p. 403).

The relationship between legal and ethical rights shows differences that help us distinguish these fields. Where ethical rights are grounded purely in a moral tradition, legal rights and corresponding duties exist as part of our social structure—our "social contract"[6] or sphere of security and welfare (Pence 1998; Walzer 1983). Thus, according to this perspective, "laws do not appear from a moral foundation, but are expressed by a political majority (through legislation), elected or appointed governmental officials (through administrative law) or members of the judiciary (through case law)" (Hodge and Gostin 2001, p. 89).

One of the common misunderstandings between philosophers and human rights advocates concerns the foundations of human rights. Human rights advocates often see rights as an a priori list of entitlements; everything begins from the list or legal document of rights. Philosophers see moral and legal rights as the "moral fruits" harvested from foundational reasoning, such as theories of justice (Daniels 1985). They see the necessity for background theoretical architecture because of the need for justification: why are these human rights? Background theories also provide principles to guide conflicts between rights and to locate rights in relation to other social values and goals.

Indeed, most countries have a constitution that identifies a list of basic rights. Such basic constitutional rights are often based on some background reasoning about the good society or ethical social contracts. Because the human interests within each legal human right are seen to be so important, many non-philosophers express impatience and exasperation with the need for clarity, coherence, and justification. Philosophers and human rights advocates often come to blows because philosophers seek to build a solid foundation for human rights by questioning the coherence and justification of rights, while human rights professionals see such questions as undermining vital protections for the most vulnerable people in the world. In these often difficult conversations between philosophers and human rights advocates, ethics is relevant not just to the foundations of the right to health but also to the actions of the participants in the debates; ethics applies to the self, other, community, world, and whole.

PHILOSOPHIES FOR THE RIGHT TO HEALTH

Some moral and political philosophers try to create a theory or an approach that will provide principles of morality, their ambition being to offer an adequate normative framework for addressing problems in moral life (De Grazia and Beauchamp 2001). Usually, these frameworks take the form of a theory of right action, but they may also take the form of a theory of good character. The types of ethical theories important in the health sector include *virtue ethics*, *deontology*, and *consequentialism*.[7] Because health is often not just a personal matter between individuals, *political and religious philosophies* are also relevant, especially when considering the relationship between the individual and the state and when reflecting on pain and suffering.

Virtue Ethics

Virtue theory focuses on the individual and asks how one ought to shape one's own character (Pence 1997). Who am I? How am I going to behave? Am I courageous? What is courage? Questions about personal character are clearly central in ethics—what a good person would do in a particular situation, how such a person would interact with others, and how this person would perform his or her duties in society. Virtue theory has a long history, believed to emanate from the ancient Greek philosophers. In particular, Aristotle specified the virtues of courage, temperance, wisdom, and justice. Virtue theorists feel that there has been too much focus on actions in ethics and not enough attention paid to the people carrying out these actions and to their virtues as human beings.[8] **A focus of this theory is on "the self."**

Deontology

Deontologists highlight concepts such as duty and relationships. Deontological theories are often referred to as Kantian because duty or absolute actions were central to Immanuel Kant's philosophy. Kant argued that morality provides a rational framework of universal principles and rules that constrain and guide everyone. He focused on the concept of reason and on the connection between morality and reason, constructing principles of ethics according to rational or reasoned procedures. What makes an action right or wrong? What ought I to do? (O'Neill 1997) In answering such questions, Kant proposed asking, can I, as a rational moral agent, consistently will that everyone should act as I am now proposing to act? The principle "Always act in such a way that you can will that everyone should act in the same manner in similar situations" comes from Kant and is known as the categorical imperative (Kant 1959). Another important Kantian idea is that persons are ends in themselves; every individual must be respected for being a rational agent with values and independent goals. Respect for the equality and dignity of human beings prohibits using one individual for another's ends or purposes. The principle of individuals as ends in themselves requires us to treat persons as having their own autonomously established goals. **A focus of this theory is on "the other," on relationships.**

Consequentialism

In contrast to the deontological approach, which identifies particular universal duties, consequentialism looks towards the end result. Deontology requires that come what may, a certain action must always be taken. In contrast, consequentialism is focused on—as implied by its label—consequences. It has most often been associated with the philosophy of utilitarianism, an approach that looks towards producing "happiness" and "utility." Utilitarianism was formulated in the nineteenth century by Jeremy Bentham and John Stuart Mill, although it builds on ideas that go back at least as far as the ancient Greeks (Beauchamp and Steinbock 1999). The core of utilitarianism is the "greatest happiness principle," which holds that actions are right insofar as they tend to promote the greatest happiness or "greatest good." The theory can be applied to actions, motives, and policies, and can be judged to be right or wrong, depending on the consequences that are produced or expected to be produced. **A focus of this theory is on "community"** (see chapters 1 and 3).

Political Philosophy

"Political philosophy can be defined as philosophical reflection on how best to arrange and run our collective life—our political institutions and our social practices, such as our economic system and our pattern of family life" (Miller 1998). Moral philosophies, such as Kantian categorical imperatives and utilitarianism, are important perspectives within political philosophies.

Currently, the dominant philosophy in health systems is utilitarianism. Whether out of concerns to reduce prevalence levels, maximise cases averted, or increase cost-efficiency in health care, the notion of pursuing the greatest good is readily apparent. But if governments treat all individuals as "an end in themselves," as suggested by Kant, and at the same time utilitarianism aims to maximise the good in a population, then we have a conflict of ethical principles. The philosopher Bernard Williams (1995) has stated that one of the problems with utilitarianism is that it "ignores the separateness of persons, and is prepared illegitimately to sacrifice the interest of any given person with the aim, not just of protecting, but even of increasing the aggregate welfare." This is a problem with regard to access to health care because the poorest, most vulnerable, and most marginalised groups ("the outliers")[9] often have limited access to the health-care system and can be very difficult to reach and treat (Pradhan et al. 2010; Singh et al. 2002; see chapters 4, 6, 7, 8, and 10).

To address this sort of problem, John Rawls (1999) developed his theory of social justice, which has important applications in health care. Starting from absolute equality, the theory suggests that social and economic inequalities are acceptable insofar as they work to the benefit of the least advantaged. That is, socio-economic inequality is acceptable, while other conditions of equality remain, as long as they also improve the lot of the least advantaged. As a result, societies and their health systems are encouraged to pay attention to the most vulnerable members and to ensure that they benefit. In his book *Just Health Care*, Norman Daniels (2001) builds on the work of Rawls. He draws attention to the ethical importance of the process of health-care resource allocation, as well as the outcome of health-care resource decisions. Daniels argues that the allocation of health-care resources should, insofar as it is a causal factor, offer equal opportunity to all to flourish and carry out their projects in life. He calls this "accountability for reasonableness" (Daniels 1985, 2000).

While many of the principal theories of justice (like that of John Rawls) concentrate overwhelmingly on how to establish just institutions and institutional systems, Amartya Sen, is his book *The Idea of Justice* (2009), looks at how we can proceed to enhance justice and remove injustice rather than try to identify perfect or ideal institutions. He indicates that justice is ultimately connected with the way people's lives go and not merely with the nature of the institutions surrounding them. Therefore, to help create justice in our societies, we must pay attention both to institutions and to the behaviour of ourselves, our communities, and groups. **A focus of these theories is on "the world."**

Religious Ethics

There are many distinct ethical traditions in our globalised world whose wisdom can be drawn upon to help with our ethics and rights dilemmas. These traditions are major contributors to perspectives that have shaped our current norms and practices. These traditions include Indian ethics, Buddhist ethics, Chinese ethics, Jewish ethics, Christian ethics, and Islamic ethics (Singer 1997). These traditions seek to interpret the "unknown," along with pain and suffering. They quest to understand the major philosophical questions: Who am I? Why was I born? What it the purpose of my being here? Who made me? (Viveka Shadami 1975)

Thomas Aquinas said, "The Human will is subject to three orders. Firstly, to the order of its own reason, secondly to the orders of human government, be it spiritual or temporal, and thirdly it is subject to the universal order" (Aquinas 1963–1975). Aquinas links the reason of the individual human being with spirit, with governments, and with the universal order, or "the whole." **A focus of these theories is on "the whole."**

HEALTH SYSTEMS AND ETHICS

HISTORY OF HEALTH-CARE ETHICS AND LINKS TO PHILOSOPHIES

Ethics in health systems, or at least in relation to taking care of people's health, dates back to the Greeks and before. In the nineteenth and twentieth centuries, the ethics of health care was principally expressed through oaths, codes, declarations, and principles.[10] In 1803, Thomas Percival published a manual of ethics entitled *Medical Ethics; or, a Code of Institutes and Precepts, Adapted to the Professional Conduct of Physicians and Surgeons.* This title represents the birth of the term "medical ethics" in the literature on the morality of physicians. Percival indicated that jurisprudence and ethics are similar but distinct, citing Justinian's definition of jurisprudence as "the precepts of law are: live morally, hurt no one, and give each his due" (Percival 1803, pp. 61–114).

By 1847, the newly formed American Medical Association had adopted a Percivalian code of ethics, which was the first code of ethics adopted by a national professional society and the first to be termed as such. By the beginning of the twentieth century, codes became the dominant form of embodying professional ethics. The word "code" derives from the Latin term for an authoritative system of laws, which Emperor Justinian called "dige-code" (Pojman 2002).

The end of World War II produced codes of ethics for medical research and health-care practice, starting with the 1947 Nuremberg Code and the World Medical Association's 1964 Declaration of Helsinki.[11] The Nuremberg Code's historical narrative shows how the plight of individuals (namely, the medical and research abuse of prisoners) and their relationships with other people (including camp guards and other prisoners who were able to recount the stories of abuse) led to a global event of accountability (the Nuremberg Trials). From these trials emerged a code of conduct for medical research and practice.

These codes then informed the identification of certain ethical principles, or moral rules, that could be applied to bioethical[12] problems. The Belmont Report of 1979 established three main ethical principles for clinical research: (1) *respect for person*, which meant recognising a person's right to exercise autonomy; (2) *beneficence*, which meant minimising risk and maximising benefits; and (3) *justice*, which meant ensuring that investigations would not unduly involve persons from groups unlikely to benefit from subsequent applications of the research. The group that wrote the report derived these basic ethical principles from the concept that we, as individuals, should treat others as we wish to be treated ourselves. A society in which this principle would be realised is one that protects the autonomy of each person and that is eminently fair and just (National Commission for the Protection of Human Subjects of Biomedical and Behavioral Research 1979). These principles have been further developed by Tom Beauchamp and James Childress into "the principles approach," which has been a mainstay of medical ethics since the 1980s. The approach argues that common morality[13] can be summarised in the form of generally accepted principles. The principles are autonomy, beneficence, non-maleficence, and justice (Beauchamp and Childress 1983).

Much has happened in the world and regarding health ethics since the development of bioethical principles. Contemporary medical ethics and bioethics has developed through four distinct stages (Wikler 1997). In the first phase, bioethics represented a code of professional conduct for health-care professionals, as demonstrated by the work of Thomas Percival and the Nuremberg Code. Bioethics reached its second phase beginning in the 1960s, when the debate was extended to doctors who entered into dialogue with society on such issues as euthanasia, confidentiality, and transparency (see chapter 11). By the 1980s, in the third phase, the societal debate had been expanded to encompass discussions over health-care reform and the role of ethics in health policy. In the 1990s, a fourth phase evolved, which concentrated on the bioethics of population health. Through the work of Jonathan Mann and colleagues (Mann et al. 1999), the human rights framework began to be linked with health, and the term "public health ethics" began to be used.

There was also an interest in expanding health matters beyond health care to encompass the social determinants of health and in crossing over into other sectors, including education, agriculture, and the environment (Lerer et al. 1998; Porter, Ogden, and Pronyk 1999; see chapters 3, 4, 6, and 7).

HEALTH SYSTEMS AND ETHICS TODAY

Bioethics has evolved from a primarily individual domain, with a focus on the patient-provider relationship, to a field that focuses on community and, more recently, on societies and the "whole" globalised world. The fifth phase, which has been evolving since 2000, attempts to integrate human rights into public health (Gostin 2001) and to link the individual with the population through a focus on health systems and global justice. Today, there is an abundance of codes and declarations for health professionals and researchers; what is now needed are health systems that support and follow ethical processes linked to the right to health.

This phase is occurring in a time of unprecedented growth in health technologies, with findings from stem cell research and the Human Genome Project leading to major ethical questions. At the same time, there are exciting innovations in systems thinking, in modelling and social navigation (Milstein 2008), as well as in social technologies that seek to address how organisations work and learn (Scharmer 2009; Senge 1990). The speed and complexity of these changes is challenging us at all levels, from the individual to the family to the community to nation-states. Integration of these different ways of thinking and being is demanding that we become more "aware" and more "conscious"[14] by transcending our current modes of thinking about health (e.g., by altering the definition of health) and the systems that deliver health. Perhaps we are being given the opportunity to look at health through a different lens in order to create policies and systems that respect the individual and at the same time provide equitable health services, particularly for poor and vulnerable groups.

HEALTH SYSTEMS: SOFTWARE AND HARDWARE

How do ethics and human rights relate to health systems[15] and to research on health systems and policy? Currently, national and international discussions

on health systems and research are defined by the World Health Organization's structural (building-block) approach to health systems. This approach
conceptualises health systems in the functional or instrumental terms of
their constituents—finance, medical products, information systems, levels
and types of human resources, forms of service delivery, and governance—
understood as organisational structures and legislation (WHO 2007; see
chapter 4).

The health system is a "complex whole." However, sometimes the human
behavioural aspect is missing from discussions on health systems, with
human beings and their behaviour being given a subsidiary role in health
systems analysis, while structures and institutions are seen as the most critical
aspects. While it is important to create and conceptualise the structural,
functional, and instrumental aspects of a system, we also need to include
the human component. The "health" in health systems emerges through
the relationships and actions of the individuals at all levels within them, in a
sense through the ethics and the "essence"[16] of what we are working within.

One way of helping raise consciousness of the human behavioural aspects
of health systems is to divide the complex health system into its hardware
and software components (Sheikh et al. 2011; see figure 5.2). The hardware
contains the building blocks (i.e., WHO's six building blocks) while the
software contains the ideas and interests, values and norms, and affinities
and power that guide actions and underpin the relationships between system
actors and elements. The hardware constituents come alive through the
people and through the ethics of individual members of different parts of the
system. Who these individuals are, how they think, what they say, what values
they hold, and how they act is crucial to understanding why a system works
and why it does not—why one system is "healthy" and why another is not.

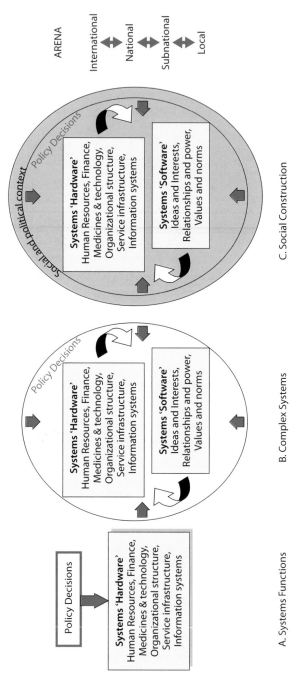

FIGURE 5.2 Health policy and systems research.

Reproduced by permission from Sheikh et al. (2011).

CONCLUSION

Across the myriad practices, professions, organisations, and individuals in the health system, ethics links actions with values and highlights the importance of respect for individuals at all levels. In health systems, we may create effective structural, organisational, financial, governmental, and legislative domains—but if we fail to understand and engage with human behaviour and the ethics of what it means to be a human being, we will fail in our vision of a "right to health." Through our own individual ethical reflection, we have the opportunity to place ourselves more consciously within the centre of our communities to ensure the creation of "healthy" systems for health that benefit ourselves, our friends, our families, our countries, and the international community as a whole.

REFERENCES

Aquinas, S. T. 1963–1975. "Summa Theologiae." In *Aquinas Thomas: Summa Theologias*, ed. T. Gilby. London: Blackfriars and Eyre and Spottiswoode.

Beauchamp, D., and B. Steinbock. 1999. *New Ethics for Public Health*. Oxford: Oxford Univ. Press.

Beauchamp, T. L., and J. F. Childress. 1983. *Principles of Biomedical Ethics*. Oxford: Oxford Univ. Press.

Brownlie, I. 2006. *Basic Documents of International Law*. Oxford: Oxford Univ. Press.

Capron, A. M. 1979. "Legal Rights and Moral Rights." In *Biomedical Ethics and the Law*, ed. J. M. Humber and R. F. Almeder, 400–405. New York: Plenum Press.

Daniels, N. 1985. *Just Health Care*. Cambridge: Cambridge Univ. Press.

—. 2000. "Accountability for Reasonableness." *British Medical Journal* 321: 1300–1301.

—. 2001. "Health Care Needs and Distributive Justice." In *Bioethics*, ed. J. Harris. Oxford: Oxford Univ. Press.

De Grazia, D., and T. L. Beauchamp. 2001. "Philosophy." In *Methods in Medical Ethics*, ed. J. Sugarman and D. L. Sulmasy, 31–46. Washington, DC: Georgetown Univ. Press.

Frankena, W. 1973. *Ethics*. Englewood Cliffs, NJ: Prentice Hall.

Gaare, R. D. 1989. "Introduction to the Legal System." In *Biolaw*, ed. J. E. Childress, P. A. King, K. H. Rothenburg, et al. Bethesda, MD: Univ. Publication of America.

Gostin, L. O. 2001. "Public Health, Ethics, and Human Rights: A Tribute to the Late Jonathan Mann." *Journal of Law, Medicine and Ethics* 29:121–130.

—. 2002. *Public Health Law and Ethics*. Berkeley: Univ. of California Press.

Hodge, J. G., and L. O. Gostin. 2001. "Legal Methods." In *Methods in Medical Ethics*, ed. J. Sugarman and D. L. Sulmasy, 88–103. Washington, DC: Georgetown Univ. Press.

Huber, M., J. A. Knottnerus, L. Green, et al. 2011. "How Should We Define Health?" *British Medical Journal* 343:d4163.

Kant, I. 1959. *Foundations of the Metaphysics of Morals*. Indianapolis: Boobs Merrill.

Lerer, L. B., A. Lopez, T. Kjellstrom, et al. 1998. "Health for All: Vision to Strategy; The Role of Health Status and Determinants." *World Health Statistics Quarterly* 51:7–20.

Macintyre, A. 2007. *After Virtue*. 3rd ed. London: Bristol Classical Press.

Mann, J., S. Gruskin, M. A. Grodin, et al., eds. 1999. *Health and Human Rights: A Reader*. New York: Routledge.

Marks, S. 2006. *Health and Human Rights: Basic International Documents*. Cambridge, MA: Francois-Xavier Bagnoud Center for Health and Human Rights, Harvard School of Public Health.

Miller, D. 1998. "Political Philosophy." In *Routledge Encyclopedia of Philosophy*, ed. E. Craig. London: Routledge. http://www.rep.routledge.com/article/S099.

Milstein, B. 2008. *Hygeia's Constellation: Navigating Futures in a Synamic and Democratic World*. Atlanta, GA: Centers for Disease Control and Prevention.

Mooney, G. 1998. "Economics, Communities and Health Care." In *Health, Health Care and Health Economics Perspectives on Distribution*, ed. M. L. Barer, T. E. Getzen, and G. L. Stoddart. Chichester, Sussex: John Wiley and Sons.

National Commission for the Protection of Human Subjects of Biomedical and Behavioral Research. 1979. *The Belmont Report: Ethical Principles and Guidelines for the Protection of Human Subjects of Research*. Washington, DC: U.S. Government Printing Office.

O'Neill, O. 1997. "Kantian Ethics." In *Companion to Ethics*, ed. P. Singer, 175–185. Oxford: Blackwell.

Pence, G. E. 1997. "Virtue Theory." In *Companion to Ethics*, ed. P. Singer, 249–258. Oxford: Blackwell.

—. 1998. "Ethical Theories and Medical Ethics." In *Classic Works in Medical Ethics*, ed. G. E. Pence. Boston: McGraw Hill.

Percival, T. 1803. *Medical Ethics; or, a Code of Institutes and Precepts, Adapted to the Professional Conduct of Physicians and Surgeons*. Manchester: S. Russell.

Pojman, L. P. 2002. *Discovering Right and Wrong*. Montreal: Wadsworth.

Porter, J., J. Ogden, and P. Pronyk. 1999. "Infectious Disease Policy: Towards the Production of Health." *Health Policy Plan* 14 (4): 322–328.

Pradhan, A., K. Kielmann, H. Gupte, et al. 2010. "What 'Outliers' Tell Us about Missed Opportunities for Tuberculosis Control: A Cross-Sectional Study of Patients in Mumbai, India." *BMC Public Health* 10:263–271.

Rawls, J. 1999. *A Theory of Justice*. Oxford: Oxford Univ. Press.

Roth, G. 2004. *Connections: The Five Threads of Intuitive Wisdom*. New York: Jeremy Tarcher/Penguin.

Sandel, M. 1982. *Liberalism and the Limits of Justice*. Cambridge: Cambridge Univ. Press.

Scharmer, O. 2009. *Theory U: Leading from the Future as It Emerges*. San Francisco: Berrett Koehler.

Seedhouse, D. 1998. *Ethics: The Heart of Health Care*. Chichester, Sussex: John Wiley and Sons.

Sen, A. 2009. *The Idea of Justice*. Cambridge, MA: Belknap Press, Harvard Univ.

Senge, P. 1990. *The Fifth Discipline: The Art and Practice of the Learning Organisation*. New York: Doubleday.

Sheikh, K., L. Gilson, I. A. Agyepong, et al. 2011. "Building the Field of Health Policy and Systems Research: Framing the Questions." *PLoS Medicine* 8:e1001073.

Singer, P., ed. 1997. *A Companion to Ethics*. Oxford: Blackwell.

Singh, V., A. Jaiswal, J. D. Porter, et al. 2002. "TB Control, Poverty, and Vulnerability in Delhi, India." *Tropical Medicine and International Health* 7:693–700.

Sugarman, J., and D. L. Sulmasy, eds. 2001. *Methods in Medical Ethics*. Washington, DC: Georgetown Univ. Press.

Viveka Shadami, S. 1975. *Shankara's Crest Jewel of Discrimination*. Hollywood, CA: Vedanta Press.

Walzer, M. 1983. *Spheres of Justice: A Defence of Pluralism and Equality*. New York: Basic Books Inc.

WHO (World Health Organization). 2007. *Everybody's Business: Strengthening Health Systems to Improve Health Outcomes; WHO's Framework for Action*. Geneva: WHO.

Wikler, D. 1997. "Bioethics, Human Rights and the Renewal of Health for All: An Overview." In *Ethics, Equity and Health for All*, ed. Z. Bankowski, J.H. Bryant, and J. Gallagher, 23–24. Geneva: Council for International Organisations of Medical Sciences.

Wilber, K. 2001. *A Theory of Everything*. Boston: Shambala.

Williams, B. 1995. "Ethics." In *Philosophy: A Guide through the Subject*, ed. A. Grayling, 545–582. Oxford: Oxford Univ. Press.

NOTES

1 Universal Declaration of Human Rights, G.A. Res. 217A (III), U.N. Doc A/810 at 71 (1948).

2 Moral: pertaining to right and wrong conduct. Ethical: relating to morals (Oxford Dictionary). These terms are used interchangeably in this chapter.

3 This framework has evolved from the course Ethics, Public Health and Human Rights at the London School of Hygiene and Tropical Medicine. Each week of the course concentrates on a particular perspective: week one focuses on philosophy; week two on research ethics and health-care priorities; week three on human rights; week four on environment and development; and the final week on completion and the process of linking ethics, public health, and human rights. Each of the weeks is connected to the framework, beginning in week one with "self" and ending in week five with "the whole." Viewing ethical issues through these different lenses may help students understand more about themselves and their own perspectives on ethics and rights, as well as more about local, national, and international health systems, policy and public health. See Wilber (2001, Great Holarchy); Seedhouse (1998, ethical grid); Roth (2004, five rhythms).

4 See Seedhouse's ethical grid (1998) for a way of helping with self-reflection.

5 Self: one's own person or individuality. Other: other person, not this, not the same, alternative, different. Community: body of people with something in common. World: sphere of existence, mankind, people generally, society, the planet earth, the universe. Whole: complete, containing all parts of elements, entire (Oxford Dictionary).

6 Social contract theory posits that a person's moral and political obligations are dependent on an agreement or contract among themselves to form the society in which they live. See Thomas Hobbes, John Locke, and Jean-Jacques Rousseau for examples.

7 For other ethical theories in public health, see Gostin (2002).

8 In his book *After Virtue*, first published in 1981, Alisdair MacIntyre (2007) argues that modern moral philosophy is essentially misplaced and flawed. The preoccupation with analytical work and normative theory has accompanied historical developments, during which a key component has been lost—a common conception of the good.

9 Outlier: a person whose residence and place of business are at a distance; something (as a geological feature) that is situated away from or classed differently from a main or related body; a statistical observation that is markedly different in value from the others of the sample (Merriam-Webster Dictionary).

10 Oath: confirmation of truth of statement by naming something sacred; curse. Code: systems of letters, symbols, and rules for their association to transmit messages secretly or briefly; scheme of conduct; collection of laws. Declaration: a formal announcement. Principle: moral rule, settled reason of action, uprightness, fundamental truth or element (Collins Gem Dictionary).

11 *Trials of War Criminals before the Nuremberg Military Tribunals under Control Council Law No. 10*, vol. 2, pp. 181–182, Washington, D.C., U.S. Government Printing Office, 1949; World Medical Association Declaration of Helsinki: Ethical Principles for Medical Research Involving Human Subjects, adopted by the 18th World Medical Assembly, Helsinki, Finland, June 1964 (6th revision in 2008).

12 Bioethics: bios, life; ethos, behaviour.

13 Common morality can be understood as morality shared by morally serious persons throughout the world (De Grazia and Beauchamp 2001).

14 "When enacted with conscience, public health work includes 'a moral or ethical aspect to one's conduct together with the urge to prefer right over wrong'" (Milstein 2008).

15 A system is defined as "a complex whole, organisation, method, classification" (Collins Gem Dictionary).

16 Essence: all that makes a thing what it is, existence, being, entity, reality (Oxford Dictionary).

PRACTICAL APPLICATION OF THE RIGHT TO HEALTH: FROM THEORY TO PRACTICE

CHAPTER 6

Maternal Mortality

ALICIA ELY YAMIN

CASE STUDY: EVARISTA, A PREGNANT WOMAN IN PERU

At the time of Evarista's death in late 2006, she and her common-law husband, Alejandro, were living in the small village of Cieneguilla, in the department of Huancavelica, in the southern Peruvian Andes. Evarista's other four children were all born at home without any problems, although one later died in infancy. Evarista went for prenatal checkups during all of her pregnancies. She was insured through the SIS (*Seguro Integral de Salud*), Peru's social insurance scheme and, according to her medical records, had three prenatal visits in her fifth and last pregnancy.

Evarista gave birth at home at approximately 3 a.m. When the placenta did not come out, Alejandro knew that something was wrong. He went to get his brother, Odilón, who lived next door. Upon seeing the situation, Odilón recommended that they immediately notify the health post. But since there was no phone or radio in the community, at around 3:30 a.m., Alejandro dispatched his son from a previous union, Godifredo, who lived in the same family compound, to the health post to communicate the emergency.

It had rained most of the night, and Godifredo, without so much as a flashlight, walked all the way down the steep mountainside to reach the health post, as there was no other means of transportation available.

Much of this chapter is based on Yamin (2007), as well as Yamin (2010). The author is grateful to Physicians for Human Rights for granting permission to use material from *Deadly Delays*. A short documentary film accompanies the *Deadly Delays* report and can be obtained from Physicians for Human Rights, http://physiciansforhumanrights.org.

When Godifredo arrived at approximately 5 a.m., he woke up the night guard at the post, who in turn roused the doctor, midwife, and nurse's aide, all of whom lived next door to the health post. Despite the obvious emergency, the doctor dispatched only the nurse's aide, Isabel.

Although it should have taken Isabel twenty to thirty minutes to arrive at Evarista's house by car, there were additional delays. Since the health post had no transportation, Isabel and Godifredo had to find, wake up, and convince a local resident to take them in his car to the house. However, about halfway there, the car tyre was punctured and it took another twenty minutes to repair the tyre.

When Isabel arrived shortly after 6 a.m., she attempted to insert an IV tube into Evarista's veins, but they had already hardened. Evarista had already died. Isabel berated Alejandro, telling him that his wife had died because he had waited too long before seeking help at the health post.

The health post, in violation of Peruvian law, imposed a fine on Alejandro because the baby had been born at home instead of at the health post, and told him that obtaining the baby's birth certificate would cost 50 nuevos soles (approximately US$16). Without a birth certificate, the baby could not be registered in the social insurance scheme and thus be able to access vaccinations and governmental benefit programmes. As an adult, she would not be able to obtain a national identity document, and therefore would not be able to vote.

At the same time, Isabel, the nurse's aide who attended Evarista that morning, was relieved of her post immediately after Evarista's death, despite the fact that there was no indication that Isabel was responsible for Evarista's death.

INTRODUCTION

Evarista's death illustrates many of the issues that underpin maternal mortality, which relate to both gender inequalities and the functioning of health systems. Drawing on this case narrative, this chapter examines aspects of maternal mortality from a rights-based perspective.

Maternal health is only one narrow aspect of sexual and reproductive health (SRH). Moreover, sexual and reproductive rights—which are not synonymous with one another—extend far beyond health rights and the health sector. Both sexual and reproductive rights entail a wide array of civil and political rights, as well as economic, social, and cultural rights, such as health.

The definition of SRH under international law recognises the indivisibility and interdependence of SRH and these other aspects of sexual and reproductive rights. SRH was defined through two foundational international consensus documents, the International Conference on Population and Development Programme of Action in Cairo and the Fourth World Conference on Women Platform for Action in Beijing.[1] According to these consensus and other normative documents, reproductive health includes sexual health, "the purpose of which is the enhancement of life and personal relations, and not merely counselling and care related to reproduction and sexually transmitted disease;" it should address the reproductive processes, functions and system at all stages of life, in the context of "complete physical, mental and social well-being."[2] SRH is predicated on the ability of men and women to have a

> responsible, satisfying and safe sex life and that they have the capability to reproduce and the freedom to decide if, when and how often to do so. Implicit in this are the rights of men and women to be informed of and to have access to safe, effective, affordable and acceptable methods of fertility regulation of their choice, and the right of access to appropriate health care services that will enable women to go safely through pregnancy and childbirth and provide couples with the best chance of having a healthy infant.[3]

SRH also requires "equal relationships between men and women in matters of sexual relations and reproduction, including full respect for the integrity of the person, [and] mutual respect, consent, and shared responsibility for sexual behavior and its consequences"; it also requires that women "have control over and decide freely and responsibly on matters related to their sexuality, including SRH, free of coercion, discrimination and violence."[4]

Despite the many statements and rich jurisprudence regarding SRH rights in international law, the topic continues to be subject to both tremendous neglect and political manipulation at the national and international levels. In 2010, an estimated 215 million women had an unmet need for contraception (UNFPA 2010). A World Health Organization (WHO) study found that across all countries, up to 75% of women had experienced gender-based violence, including emotional violence, in the last twelve months (2005, p. 9). Around the world, criminalisation of certain services and practices, such as sex work and sex between same-sex partners, isolates and further stigmatises marginalised populations, with dramatic health effects. For example, draconian anti-abortion laws, enacted recently in a number of countries, are linked to higher rates of maternal mortality (Amnesty International 2009; Grimes et al. 2006; Okonofua et al. 2009).

Indeed, maternal health is no exception to the hypocrisy and neglect that have characterised SRH more broadly. The spread of disinformation on abortions and governments' refusal to acknowledge that access to safe and legal abortion is a determinant of the number and distribution of maternal deaths are but one example (Amnesty International 2009; Grimes et al. 2006; Okonofua et al. 2009). Historically, maternal health has been subject to such neglect in international health circles that women's obstetric needs have largely been treated as though they were a subset of children's health needs (Rosenfield and Maine 1985). Despite increasing awareness in recent years of the scale and epidemiology of maternal mortality, after ten years of the Millennium Development Goals (MDGs), MDG 5 relating to improvement in maternal health has been the most underfunded and, not surprisingly, has shown very uneven progress.[5]

Although two important 2010 studies showed some promising evidence of improvement, it remains clear that enormous increases in global health funding over the last decade have not translated into the necessary investments in basic health services and reproductive health (Hogan et al. 2010; World Bank 2009). An estimated 358,000 women still die every year due to maternal causes, which means that even the global maternal mortality ratio, which masks regional disparities, is far higher than that required to achieve the 75% overall reduction since 1990 levels called for under the MDGs (Hill et al. 2007; Hogan et al. 2010). Further, for every woman who dies, an estimated twenty others are left with debilitating complications, such as fistula (Miller et al. 2005). The story is bleaker still when disparities within countries are taken into account. Progress on expanding access and improving care in urban and peri-urban areas has often left the most excluded and marginalised women in rural areas behind.[6]

The reasons for such painfully slow progress on improving maternal health are varied and complex. However, persistently high levels of maternal mortality reveal much about the "pathologies of power," in Paul Farmer's terms, that determine the distribution of health and illness within societies and across the globe (2003). Women and girls are not continuing to die by the tens of thousands because we do not know what to do about maternal mortality. We do—and in most of the global North, maternal mortality no longer presents a major public health problem. Indeed, 99% of maternal mortality occurs in the global South; of all public health indicators, maternal mortality is the one that shows the greatest disparity between the global North and South, and these disparities are much greater than with respect to indicators such as infant mortality or HIV/AIDS. These enormous gaps are not solely attributable to income; nor are they solely due to the status of women and girls in given societies—although both of these are critical factors. As this chapter shows, maternal mortality is also a sensitive indicator of the functioning of a country's health system and of how a health system both reflects and communicates norms and values, including gender equality and women's rights to SRH (Freedman 2005; UN Millennium Project Task Force on Child Health and Maternal Health 2005; Yamin and Norheim 2011).

MEDICAL/PUBLIC HEALTH ASPECTS

From a biomedical perspective, Evarista died of a post-partum haemorrhage, the most common cause of maternal death in Peru and in the world. From a health systems perspective, she died because of the absence of a skilled birth attendant, accessible emergency obstetric care (EmOC), and a functioning referral network, which together with family planning are the four pillars of maternal mortality prevention (Freedman, Graham, and Brazier 2007; see chapter 4).

Intravenous fluid resuscitation, manual removal of the placenta, and medications that contract the uterus might have been life saving if Evarista had received them in time. These interventions could have bought her time to be transferred to a facility capable of providing more comprehensive EmOC, such as surgery and blood.

A public health response to maternal mortality requires prioritisation of these key programme interventions. Further, it requires the development of standards or guidelines for every level of facility, such as those jointly set out by WHO, the UN Population Fund, the UN Children's Fund, and Averting

Maternal Death and Disability (2009). Once such standards are set, a survey of facilities and communities needs to be done, together with costing of the standards for planning and implementation purposes. Costing needs to address supplies and medications, but also non-medical items associated with communications, transportation, and the like. Such costing would also include expenses associated with a rational allocation of health-care personnel in light of the needs of the population, with a recognition of the twin needs for availability of skilled birth attendance and EmOC, and for respecting the labour rights of health-care workers. For example, demanding that any one person provide care 24/7 is not a reasonable expectation. In turn, these plans should be budgeted and executed at the national and district levels, and protocols (ranging from managing normal deliveries to managing different kinds of complications) should be implemented at the facility level. Finally, systematic monitoring of service delivery is crucial to an effective public health response (Gill et al. 2005).

In this particular case, the local health post was well equipped to provide routine prenatal care and attend to uncomplicated vaginal deliveries, but it did not have the capacity to perform surgery or store blood. It is highly unusual to have a midwife, let alone a midwife and a doctor, at a health post, the lowest level of facility in Peru. However, in this case, either of the two could have performed some basic EmOC, including manual removal of the placenta. By contrast, even if Evarista had still been alive when Isabel (a nurse's aide) arrived, Isabel would not have had the skills to manually extract the placenta, and it is unclear how she would have communicated to the health post or the nearest health centre for more help.

A variety of factors conspired to result in Evarista being unable to receive the necessary care in time. There were delays in taking the decision to seek care, as well as delays in having care arrive. Underlying those delays were deficiencies in the health system relating to accessibility of care. Addressing the lack of accessibility of care would in turn require specific steps to broach the cultural distance between the health establishment and its users, as well as the absence of communication and transportation.

First, the Peruvian government—and governments generally—must conduct outreach within the community to ensure that couples are aware of and prepared for potential complications during pregnancy or delivery. In Peru and elsewhere, families are often unable to recognise and plan for obstetric emergencies, and they can even be afraid of visiting the health post. Especially given Evarista's grand multipara status (this was her fifth pregnancy), both she and her common-law husband should have been educated about the possibility of having a complicated delivery. It is unclear whether such a discussion occurred at the time of her prenatal visits, but it should have. Based on her prenatal record, there was no documented plan for her to give birth at the health post.

In many cases, even the mere fear of user fees poses a significant barrier to accessing EmOC in a timely way. However, this was not the principal barrier here. According to Alejandro, Evarista did not like going to the health post even for prenatal care, as she felt mistreated because she was indigenous and the health workers did not speak Quechua. Alejandro said that despite having social insurance coverage, he and Evarista never planned to give birth at the health post because they were afraid that Evarista would need a caesarean section and require an expensive transfer to the department's capital. Many *campesinos* associate delivering at a health facility with having a caesarean section; there is an enormous reluctance for a woman to be "cut," and a belief that after a caesarean she will be "useless" or unable to work, as life is extremely hard in the mountainous and inhospitable terrain, and couples need to have both partners working just to survive.

Systematic efforts must be made to bridge these cultural distances between the health system and its users and to allay such fears by providing accessible information that explains the narrow circumstances under which a caesarean section would be necessary, what the surgery entails, and what recovery would be like in the event that such a surgery were required. It is crucial for there to be a relationship of trust not only with the health providers at the nearest health facility but with the health system in general. Cultural and emotional distances between health system users and health establishments create significant barriers to access by delaying or precluding the decision to seek care when an emergency arises.

Second, this case highlights critical elements impeding access to and delivery of EmOC once a decision is made to seek care. First, there was no radio or mobile phone available in the village. Therefore, in cases of obstetric—or other—emergencies, residents could not immediately communicate with the health post. Had there been a means of communication available, Godifredo's treacherous hour-and-a-half walk down the steep muddy hillside would have been averted. With that savings of time, it is possible that Isabel would have arrived in time to stabilise Evarista with fluids just long enough for her to reach the health post and receive further treatment.

In this regard, Evarista's case is unfortunately all too typical. It is still quite rare for communities in Huancavelica and elsewhere in rural Peru to have access to a radio or other means of communication, such as a telephone or mobile phone. Radios or telephones are usually available at health posts, but there is a significant delay in communicating an emergency when, as in this case, the health post is located at some distance from the community itself. Lack of communications is a major obstacle in treating obstetric emergencies in a timely manner, both in Peru and around the world.

Increasing interest in "mhealth" (for "mobile health")—using mobile telephones for clinical protocols and communications with and between health facilities—is promising in this regard. A number of recent initiatives seek to provide mobile phones to community health workers and community members; however, these initiatives are largely untested as yet, and coverage varies greatly. Mobile telephone coverage appears to be higher in Africa than in many parts of Latin America (including the Sierra of Peru), and the use of mobile phones for mobile banking, which could have implications for paying transportation and care costs, is also on the rise in Eastern and Southern Africa (Aker and Mbiti 2010; Bhavnani et al. 2008; Rashid and Elder 2009).

In Evarista's case, the lack of communication was compounded by an equally serious lack of transportation, another major obstacle to accessing care in a timely way and preventing maternal mortality. There was no means to reach the health post other than simply walking, as Godifredo was forced to do in complete darkness. Nor did the health post have a ready means of transportation. Reliance on a local resident means being subject to his availability and willingness in the event of an emergency, and also poses delays.

It is unrealistic for every health post in Peru, or in the global South generally, to have an ambulance at its disposal. Every health post, however, should have a transportation contingency plan, which will necessarily be adapted to the local context. Such a plan may include multiple local residents with vehicles who give prior agreement to act as ambulance drivers so that willingness—and fares—need not be negotiated at the time of an emergency. Under different circumstances, a contingency plan for transportation could entail the use of a boat or even a helicopter, and sometimes it will involve police or military personnel.

Moreover, hospitals—and to the extent possible, health centres (facilities larger than health posts but smaller than hospitals)—should have vehicles at their disposal, which can be dispatched in the event of an emergency. This requires that a budget be in place for regular maintenance, parts, and fuel, and that the use of such vehicles be subject to strict oversight. The global South is far too littered with cemeteries of broken-down vehicles that governments have been forced to purchase under bilateral or multilateral loan agreements or that have been donated without consideration as to suitability for the local terrain, maintenance, or regulation of their use.

Finally, a third delay—the delay in receiving appropriate treatment—would likely have played a role had Evarista survived the first two delays. That is, the health post did not send its most trained personnel to manage her obstetric emergency. Neither the doctor nor the midwife went to attend the emergency. Instead, Isabel, a nurse's aide, was dispatched, despite the fact that given the training that nurses' aides receive in Peru, she would likely have been unable to manually extract the placenta or do anything but administer intravenous fluids. In this case, Evarista had died by the time the Isabel arrived. However, had Evarista lived for a few more minutes, she might well have died anyway because there would have been significant further delays in receiving appropriate care from the health system. A protocol should have been in place to direct a more skilled health worker to attend Evarista's case.

ETHICAL AND LEGAL PERSPECTIVES

ETHICAL DILEMMAS AND CONCERNS

The case study raises significant ethical issues relating to punitive attitudes and incentives within the health system, as well as gender inequality. Further, the treatment of both of these issues illustrates how the health system interacts with and often reflects values commonly held in Peruvian society—values that can be at odds with human rights (see chapter 5).

First, the case highlights a commonly held punitive attitude towards patients, especially indigenous patients, by Peru's Western-oriented health system (Amnesty International 2006). Health-care providers often describe indigenous customs as "backwards" or "ignorant," arguing that indigenous populations "need to be taught to behave" (Yamin 2007).

In this case, Isabel told Alejandro that it was his fault that Evarista had died, and the staff at the health post felt that he needed to be punished for failing to notify the health facility immediately after Evarista went into labour. Consequently, health-care personnel were withholding the baby's birth certificate until Alejandro paid a de facto fine. The imposition of de facto fines on women who have home births, as a means of coercing institutional births, is widespread in Peru. Indeed, the Human Rights Ombuds Office conducted a nationwide investigation into this practice in 2004–05 and issued a scathing report. The imposition of such fines violates the Peruvian Constitution, which provides for a right to nationality. Additionally, as a result of that report, a new norm outlawing the fines was enacted (Defensoría del Pueblo 2005). Unfortunately, implementation of this norm has been haphazard (Amnesty International 2006; Yamin 2007), highlighting the Ombuds Office's lack of enforcement powers.

At the same time that these coercive measures are applied to patients, the professionals working in the health system are themselves subject to punitive and arbitrary treatment. Indeed, the fines imposed on patients often emerge as a result of health workers' salaries being tied to "productivity" measures, which are also commonly known as pay-for-performance. Thus, a health worker's remuneration in Peru, as well as in many other countries, often depends on how many institutional deliveries she or he has attended. Not only can this lead to overtly coercive behaviour but in circumstances where facilities are not equipped to deal with obstetric emergencies, it is the height of cynicism to draw women in to deliver when their health and rights cannot be guaranteed (Basinga et al. 2011; Mannion and Davies 2008; Montagu and Yamey 2011).

The immediate removal of the nurse's aide who attended Evarista that morning, despite the fact that she was not responsible for Evarista's death, is all too typical of maternal death cases, where someone tends to be scapegoated. Throughout Peru and elsewhere, frontline health professionals are routinely subject to summary dismissal when they are associated with a maternal death (Yamin 2007). In this case for example, the higher-up health professionals appear to have eschewed their obligations—probably thinking that it would be too late to save Evarista. Such widespread dismissals tend to create perverse incentives for health professionals to avoid handling emergency cases for fear of being fired.

A second ethical factor in this case is the fact that male family members made all the necessary decisions. Alejandro consulted with his brother, Odilón, but never with females in the household or community. By all accounts, Evarista herself had no voice in the decision making process from the outset, even though it fatally affected her—a dynamic all too typical in Peru and elsewhere (Ministerio de Salud, Peru 1999). In times of crisis, such as during obstetric emergencies, husbands and other male family members tend to take control of all decisions. Although in some cases mothers-in-law play important roles as well, male decision making reflects a basic divide in gender roles, as well as the fact that the men of the family typically control its economic resources, which often become necessary in times of crisis.

The absence of a birth plan on file indicates that Evarista likely did not receive adequate information during her pregnancy about what to do in the event of an emergency, or even how to recognise such an emergency. Alejandro accompanied her on all prenatal visits and acted as an interpreter for her. By all accounts—both from Alejandro and the workers at the health post—health-care workers' communication with Evarista was extremely limited in those interactions.

Moreover, male domination of women's bodies and reproductive decisions begins long before pregnancy. In *campesino* communities in this region of Peru, as well as many places around the globe, decisions regarding sex, contraception, and the use of health care are generally made by men. In Evarista's case, despite being informed of family planning at the health post, Alejandro had not wanted to use any family planning method, and therefore the couple did not utilise contraception. It is often difficult to get women even to visit a health post to discuss family planning, as their husbands usually make these types of decisions for them.

If a health worker tacitly condones a husband's or male family member's decision making with respect to contraception, she countenances violations of women's SRH rights and violates the principle of autonomy in medical ethics; every woman has a right to make decisions that affect her own body. Further, as unwanted pregnancies are always high-risk pregnancies, lack of information and counselling regarding family planning may literally place these women's lives in danger. At the same time, women who use contraception can be subject to domestic violence. Further, health workers must be vigilant that they are not substituting their own judgments about the best interests of the patient for those expressed by their patients, as in Peru and elsewhere such decisions have also led to violations of informed consent in surgical contraception and other forms of family planning (CLADEM 1999). In sum, for frontline health workers, negotiating cultural norms that affect gender equality must be done with great care and sensitivity, especially, as stated above, when it is essential for ensuring open communication and trust between community members and health facilities.

LEGAL CONTEXT

The government of Peru has assumed obligations under both domestic and international law to address the different factors that lead to persistently high levels of maternal mortality. Obligations for reducing and preventing maternal mortality derive directly from the rights enumerated in international treaties to which a state is a party, which are then meant to be implemented through the constitution and domestic legislation.[7] Additionally, at the UN Millennium Summit in 2000, states—including Peru—adopted the Millennium Declaration. The Millennium Declaration and the MDGs, which are drawn from the Declaration, include a commitment to reduce maternal mortality by three quarters from 1990 levels by the year 2015 (MDG 5). The Millennium Project Task Force on Child Health and Maternal Health report (2005) forcefully recognises the crucial importance of human rights in both understanding the underlying elements of MDG 5 and achieving it.

As do all state parties to the International Covenant on Economic, Social and Cultural Rights (ICESCR) and the Convention on the Elimination of All Forms of Discrimination against Women (CEDAW), Peru has specific obligations to *respect* women's SRH rights by refraining from interfering with, for example, access to contraceptives and other means of maintaining SRH.[8] It also has obligations to *protect* the enjoyment of the right from interference by third parties and to *fulfil* the right to health through proactive measures that, among other things, provide available, accessible (physically, economically, on a non-discriminatory basis, and with respect to information), acceptable (culturally and ethically), and quality health care (AAAQ) (see chapters 1 and 4).[9]

The ICESCR asserts that state parties must take all appropriate steps or measures to assure the fulfilment of the right to health, including medical attention in the event of sickness (such as obstetric complications), to "the maximum of [their] available resources."[10] In addition, CEDAW notes that it is incumbent upon states to

> eliminate discrimination against women in the field of health care in order to ensure, on a basis of equality of men and women, access to health-care services, including those related to family planning [and] appropriate services in connection with pregnancy, confinement and the post-natal period, granting free services where necessary, as well as adequate nutrition during pregnancy and lactation.[11]

The reduction of maternal mortality is explicitly mentioned in both the UN Committee on the Elimination of Discrimination against Women's (CEDAW Committee) General Recommendation 24 on women and health and the UN Committee on Economic, Social and Cultural Rights' (ESCR Committee) General Comment 14 on the right to the highest attainable standard of health,[12] which are often considered authoritative interpretations of state parties' obligations. The ESCR Committee's General Comment 14 states that "a major goal should be reducing women's health risks, particularly lowering rates of maternal mortality."[13] For its part, the CEDAW Committee calls on states "to ensure women appropriate services in connection with pregnancy, confinement and the post-natal period."[14] Both human rights treaty bodies explicitly acknowledge that obstetric services must be provided and made accessible to women.[15] Of course, obstetric services cannot be provided in isolation from women's other reproductive and sexual health needs, including contraception. The first UN Special Rapporteur on the Right to Health, Paul Hunt, issued several reports on state obligations regarding maternal mortality, including the importance of EmOC.[16]

More recently, the UN Human Rights Council adopted ground-breaking resolutions on maternal mortality,[17] underscoring the need to address gender inequality and violations of women's rights more broadly, as well as provide for necessary technical health interventions.

From the health and development side, the UN Secretary-General's Global Strategy for Women's and Children's Health (2010), which was released at the

Millennium Development Summit in September 2010, also underscores the need for inclusion of human rights in accelerating efforts to reduce maternal mortality. Based on the Global Strategy, the UN Commission on Information and Accountability for Women's and Children's Health was created, and is led by WHO. In 2011, the Commission issued ten recommendations regarding measures to promote women's and children's health and again underscored the importance of approaches based on human rights and equity. Two of those recommendations called for the creation of accountability mechanisms at the national and international levels (and an independent Expert Review Group) and the tracking of financial commitments and budgetary allocations relating to maternal and child health. Both of these are potentially important aspects of fostering accountability, a critical dimension of a rights-based approach to maternal mortality.

The following section analyses in greater depth what adopting a rights-based approach to maternal mortality might mean in concrete terms in the case of Evarista and more generally for health systems.

APPLICATION OF THE RIGHT TO HEALTH IN PRACTICE

RIGHTS APPROACHES BEGIN WITH THE INITIAL PLAN OF ACTION AND BUDGET

A comprehensive approach to fulfilling the right to maternal health at the national level involves the initial design of policies and programmes to address maternal mortality, their implementation and evaluation, and the remedies provided in the event of violations (Yamin 2010).

Although the right to health is subject to progressive realisation and cannot be realised from one day to the next, state parties to relevant treaties do have some immediate obligations, including the development of a national strategy and plan of action concerning their public health goals.[18] The ESCR Committee requires that states establish such strategies and plans, which must be evidence-based and set out deliberate targets, as one of the core obligations that all states must undertake as parties to the ICESCR.[19] Addressing maternal and reproductive health is an obligation of comparable priority, and there is no country in the world where a national plan of action should not include attention to maternal health.[20]

A country's plan of action should be based on a robust situational analysis regarding sexual, reproductive, and maternal health in the country, as well as the best evidence of the interventions required to address maternal morbidity and mortality, which are now well understood.[21] The situational analysis should also consider legal and policy frameworks relating to SRH and institutional capacity.

Therefore, every national plan of action on maternal health must prioritise family planning, skilled birth attendance, EmOC, and a functioning referral network in the context of strengthening the overall health system as the "appropriate" measures to be adopted pursuant to international law, although legislative and programming measures will vary contextually based on the situational analysis (Yamin 2010; Yamin and Maine 1999).[22] In keeping with international law, a national plan of action should also include a broad range of services related to sexual and reproductive health that are aimed at enabling women to exercise agency with respect to their bodies and, in turn, their lives.[23] Further, it should give particular attention to marginalised and vulnerable groups.[24]

While plans of action can be suffused with rights-based principles, progress towards fulfilling the right to maternal health requires expenditure. Budgets often offer the best evidence of whether governments are actually making maternal health a priority (IIMMHR 2009; Kgamphe and Mahony 2004). Therefore, transparency and accountability in budgets is key to transforming health systems to meet women's needs (Commission on Information and Accountability for Women's and Children's Health 2011; Yamin 2010).

OPERATIONALISING KEY CONCEPTS IN RIGHTS-BASED APPROACHES

Rights-based approaches to maternal health—and to health more broadly—emphasise accountability, equality and non-discrimination, and meaningful participation, among other characteristics.

Accountability

Accountability refers to holding governments responsible for meeting certain standards that are drawn from international law (Yamin 2010). Human rights accountability in the context of maternal health requires effective and accessible mechanisms of legal redress. Increasingly, courts are playing important roles in assessing the adequacy of governmental programmes relating to maternal health.[25]

However, accountability cannot refer only to legal redress; it also requires systematic monitoring and oversight of governments' efforts to comply with their obligation to adopt appropriate measures to realise the right to maternal health to the maximum extent of their available resources (Yamin 2010). At the international level, human rights based accountability also requires accountability for donors' commitments (Commission on Information and Accountability for Women's and Children's Health 2011; Partnership for Maternal, Newborn and Child Health 2010; UN Secretary-General 2010).

With respect to monitoring the health system in particular, if empirical evidence from public health indicates that EmOC, skilled attendance, and referral networks (together with family planning) are the keys to preventing and reducing maternal mortality, human rights law requires that these aspects of care be made available, accessible, acceptable, and of adequate quality for the entire population on the basis of non-discrimination.[26]

Using human rights to advocate for specific policy changes that can reduce maternal mortality and advance maternal health requires understanding the contextually bound ways in which the availability, accessibility, acceptability, and quality of EmOC are at play in a person's decision to seek care, arrive at care, and receive adequate treatment. Health systems and social, cultural, and legal contexts vary enormously. The three delays are universal, but how they play out in women's lives differs from setting to setting. If we seek to make governments and other actors more responsive to women's health needs—that is, more accountable—these differences are critical to understand because they point to specific deficiencies in governmental policies and programming.

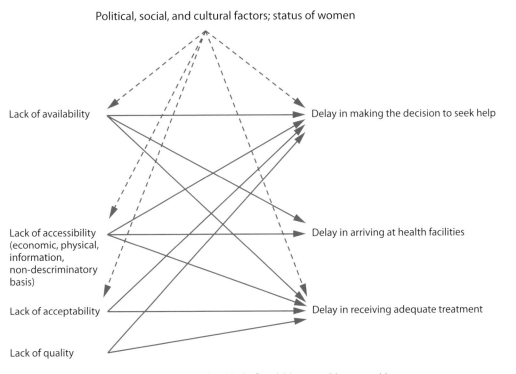

FIGURE 6.1 The three delays model and lack of available, accessible, acceptable, and quality EmOC.

Adapted from Maine (1991); Yamin (2007, p. 49).

As figure 6.1 shows, women's low social status factors into delays in the decision to seek care, largely because women rarely play a role in the decision-making process. It also undoubtedly factors into the political priority placed on making EmOC available, accessible, acceptable, and of adequate quality. Thus, as Paul Hunt stated in a report to the UN,

> Preventing maternal mortality and enhancing access to maternal health care is not simply about scaling up technical interventions or making the interventions affordable. It is also vital to address social, cultural, political and legal factors which influence women's decisions to seek maternal or other reproductive health-care services. This may require addressing discrimi-

natory laws, policies, practices and gender inequalities that prevent women and adolescents from seeking good quality services.[27]

However, in addition to undertaking such multipronged efforts to raise women's status and agency within both the household and the public sphere, providing concrete content to women's right to health requires making contextually specific assessments and recommendations with respect to the health system, which will reduce the three delays that lead to maternal deaths.

For example, in Evarista's case, a general lack of availability of communications and care in this rural region factored into all three delays. Second, a lack of accessibility played a determining role.[28] In this and many other cases, failure to recognise signs of obstetric emergencies can reflect lack of access to information, as discussed above, and lead to critical delays in seeking care. Overall distribution and location of health-care facilities can also reflect discrimination regarding access (Maine 1991; Yamin and Maine 1999).

Third, this case also demonstrates how a lack of cultural sensitivity and language barriers, as well as outright discrimination, can delay needed treatment. In understanding perceived cultural insensitivity of medical personnel, which can make women and their families hesitate to seek care, as a form of lack of acceptability under international law, a human rights approach places the obligation on the state rather than ascribing failures to the idiosyncrasies of individual families. Finally, a lack of quality was also an issue in this case because the most effective medical personnel were not deployed to the emergency.[29]

In short, by identifying the contextually specific causes of the three delays, it is possible to understand that maternal deaths are not random biological events but the foreseeable result of (in addition to social and cultural factors) systematic failures to adopt appropriate policy, programming, and budgeting decisions, for which governments and other actors can be held accountable. Obstacles to providing available, accessible, acceptable, and quality EmOC— and therefore to reducing maternal mortality—can be identified at the level of the household and community, the health centre, the regional government, the national government, and ultimately international actors, such as the World Bank and donor governments, which are playing a fundamental role in the restructuring health sectors around the world.

Equality and Non-Discrimination

The equal dignity of all human beings and non-discrimination are perhaps the most foundational principles of all human rights, including the right to health.[30] In addressing maternal mortality, these principles can be implemented at a variety of levels. First, there is of course individual discrimination by providers who are acting as agents of the state. Such instances abound; Evarista, for example, felt that the individual health providers at her health post had discriminated against her because of her indigenous status. Under international law, such instances of direct discrimination constitute per se violations, and their redress should be immediate, not subject to progressive realisation.

However, if we are to make human rights relevant to health systems planning and programme implementation, we must also be concerned with institutional and structural forms of exclusion that result in substantive inequality and discrimination. For example, at the institutional level, the health post, like many other facilities, did not permit traditional vertical birthing positions or other traditional practices, which in practice reduced accessibility of care and violates Peruvian law. Additionally, the lack of health personnel who speak the local language, coupled with the absence of any other form of accommodation, such as interpreters, constitutes a form of discrimination and a lack of acceptable care. Discrimination at the institutional level can often be indirect, but nonetheless violates international standards (see chapter 4).[31]

At a third level, structural inequality is pervasive in the Peruvian health system. The ESCR Committee has made it clear that "inappropriate health resource allocation can lead to discrimination that may not be overt."[32] The Committee has also stated that a core obligation of state parties includes ensuring "the equitable distribution of all health facilities, good and services."[33] In Peru, such structural factors result in de facto discrimination against ethnic minorities in a number of ways. Although many indicators are not disaggregated by ethnicity, which is itself a problem for tracking equity, there are greater health-related resources available on a per capita basis to Peruvians in areas with low indigenous populations, such as Moquegua and Tacna, as compared with areas such as Huancavelica that have high indigenous populations (Portocarrero Grados 2006).

This inequity translates into fewer health facilities, doctors, and specialists per capita—including anaesthesiologists, who are critical to caesarean sections—which has the "effect of nullifying or impairing the equal enjoyment or exercise" of the right to health for many women in Peru.[34] Such spending inequity results in measurably less availability and accessibility of care necessary to reduce maternal mortality, including skilled birth attendance, in regions such as Huancavelica, which have significant indigenous populations.

Peru is far from unique in this regard. The non-governmental organisation Fundar documented a similar pattern of inequities in Mexico's health system and linked the inequitable allocations to the fact that far more resources are spent on patients in the social security health system than on those in the public hospitals (Díaz et al. 2010). The Center for Economic and Social Rights documented a similar issue in Guatemala and linked the insufficient and inequitable allocations to poor fiscal policies (CESR and ICEFI 2009).

In Peru, this resource dichotomy—and the attendant implications for availability, accessibility, and quality of care—is replicated within the departments themselves, with significantly more resources devoted to health-care facilities in the more urbanised areas of these departments and fewer to rural areas, where the indigenous populations overwhelmingly reside. Although decentralisation of the health sector has given greater power to regional governments, many of the rural poor, who are largely indigenous, are not represented in regional decisions related to their own health. For example, the regional hospital in the capital city of Huancavelica has the capacity to perform laparoscopic surgeries with high-tech equipment, and women routinely receive three ultrasounds in every pregnancy, while indigenous *campesinas* in rural areas do not have ready access to even the most basic EmOC. This is particularly striking given that over two-thirds of the population in Huancavelica lives in rural areas; yet, the government is responsive not to their needs but to the needs of urban elites.

Peru's own progress reports on the MDGs acknowledge the continuing marginalisation of rural, disproportionately indigenous women: "the data reflect the persistence of enormous inequities that permeate the country" (República del Perú 2004, p. 64; 2008). Importantly, adopting a rights-based approach to health converts the issue of disparities into one of violations. However a comprehensive approach to remedies requires more than redress in the event of a documented abuse; it requires an entirely different chain of decision making from the government with respect to the financing, design, and management of health systems. Thus, the health systems can help ameliorate, rather than exacerbate, patterns of social exclusion that pervade overall society.

Finally, of course, it is impossible to address maternal mortality without considering how gender discrimination operates within a society. Gender inequality in Peru is inextricably linked to ethnic discrimination and rural poverty.[35] As in this case, women worldwide continue to remain disempowered as decision makers in their own right to seek health care. Evarista lacked control over decisions relating to her own bodily integrity and reproductive health. Even in cases of emergency, the men in the family make life-changing health decisions for their wives or other female relatives, as discussed above.

Gender discrimination in Peru and elsewhere is reflected in laws and policies that have a detrimental impact on women's health—and need to be changed. For example, under Peruvian law, abortion is illegal except when necessary to preserve the life or health of the mother. Both the woman who undergoes the procedure and the health professionals who perform it are subject to sanctions in all cases other than therapeutic abortions.[36] However, the definition of such "therapeutic abortions" has been interpreted narrowly to exclude situations where the woman's mental health is at risk. In the 2005 case *KL v. Peru*, which centred on a teenager who was forced to carry an anencephalic foetus to term and suffered grave psychological damage as a result, the UN Human Rights Committee found that the right to health includes both physical and mental health and that Peru's law was overly restrictive and violative of women's human rights.[37] As the Human Rights Committee held in its binding decision, the overly restrictive interpretation of therapeutic abortion not only presents a barrier to appropriate care but is directly damaging to women's health.[38]

The CEDAW Committee has stated that "laws that criminalize medical procedures only needed by women and punish women who undergo those procedures" constitute "barriers to women's access to appropriate health care" and are discriminatory.[39] In 2011, the CEDAW Committee issued a decision in *L.C. v. Peru*, a case that involved a thirteen-year-old girl who had become pregnant as a result of rape, calling for the government of Peru to modify its law to allow **abortion** in cases of rape and sexual assault, and to ensure the availability of and access to **abortion** services when abortion is in fact legal under the law.

Participation

Participation is recognised as critical to strengthening health systems in general, but in a rights-based approach to maternal mortality, participation goes beyond instrumental purposes (WHO 2007; Potts 2008).[40] Women are not the passive objects of policies or beneficiaries of programmes; rather, they are active agents entitled to have a voice in the decisions that affect their well-being. A rights-based approach to addressing maternal mortality in Peru calls for the democratisation of the entire health sector, with a transfer of planning and decision-making power to the individuals and communities the health system is supposed to serve, as well as to the health professionals who work within the system.[41]

Community participation, especially in indigenous communities. During his tenure as Special Rapporteur on the Right to Health, Paul Hunt called specifically for "the active and informed participation of indigenous people in the formulation, implementation and monitoring of health policies and programs."[42] In Peru, many indigenous communities perceive the health system as a westernizing, colonising force that does not respect indigenous cultural traditions and preferences.

Fortunately, there are examples of mechanisms that could facilitate greater community oversight and participation. For instance, the CLAS (*Comités Locales de Administración de Salud*) is a governmental programme in Peru in which staffing decisions and local priorities are determined with input from the local communities (Altobelli 2008). Other countries have adopted similar mechanisms, which require sustained funding.

Political participation, especially by rural women. The ESCR Committee has stated that "the right to health includes an entitlement to participate in health policy making at the local, national and international levels."[43]

However, numerous studies have found that many rural Peruvians, especially *campesina* women, do not possess the identity documents required to vote (Velázquez 2004). The Ombuds Office estimates that more than three million people lack these identity cards (Defensoría del Pueblo 2005), which are also needed to access certain social benefits and services, including the social insurance scheme (República del Perú 2004). Without the ability to vote, these rural residents—particularly women—are left invisible and uncounted when health policies and budget allocations are made.

Here, some positive examples of underwriting the creation and distribution of national identity documents can be found in experiences from the World Bank (2008) and the Inter-American Development Bank. Such funding, accompanied by meaningful efforts to increase voter participation among rural residents, especially women, can serve to increase the accountability of governments and improve monitoring efforts, ultimately leading to potential improvements in the health of marginalised women.

Participation by non-governmental organisations and civil society groups. Since the end of the Fujimori regime in 2000, Peru has seen a broad array of processes and institutions aimed at fostering civil society participation. Despite these efforts, civil society institutions have little actual power over policy or budgetary decisions (Cotlear 2006, p. 81). The World Bank has argued that the lack of clarity in roles and the great energy invested in these activities could even be producing "participation fatigue" and that such governmental efforts are often focused solely on civil society participation in the design of budgets and plans but not on the monitoring of implementation (Cotlear 2006, p. 82).

This is unfortunately all too common. Even when laws do not prohibit active monitoring and participation, non-governmental organisations are often underfunded and fragmented and cannot sustain monitoring efforts, as critical to rights-based accountability as these are. Furthermore, government-funded groups are often hamstrung by the governments on which they depend.

Participation within the health sector. As is often the case, Peru's health sector is highly autocratic and vertical. Health professionals who work in establishments have little control over how funds are spent or what policies their establishments follow. For example, many countries still impose quotas for institutional births and prenatal visits on frontline health workers in the name of promoting "productivity." In addition to the women in the population who bear the consequences of the perverse incentives created by such policies, the health professionals themselves—who are often on short-term contracts without benefits—suffer greatly from such quotas. WHO (2010) has raised questions with respect to pay-for-performance policies in health systems, which seem to undermine both patients' and health workers' rights.

Information. People must have access to adequate information, including budget numbers and health statistics, in order to participate in and evaluate programmes and policies to reduce maternal mortality—making it apparent that the right to health is interdependent on the right to information (Freedman 1995). Information regarding health at the individual, institutional, or systemic level is not widely accessible in Peru, and that is not uncommon.

An innovative example of attempting to collect information regarding budget priorities and use it for international advocacy is the "6 Question Campaign," whereby the International Budget Partnership (2010) partnered with civil society organisations in eighty-five countries in order to assess their governments' commitment to MDG 5, among other issues. Two of the six questions related to maternal health. The results of the campaign, which were released just before the Millennium Development Summit in 2010, showed that the overwhelming majority of countries did not have—or would not release to the public—such information.

CONCLUSION AND FUTURE CONSIDERATIONS

Adopting a rights-based approach to maternal mortality requires, first, recognising that maternal health—and SRH more broadly—is not merely a matter of "natural" biological causes or behavioural factors. On the contrary, patterns of maternal mortality (and SRH) are the products of social relations and social choices. In particular, maternal mortality is a telling indicator of the legal norms, policies, programmes, institutional arrangements, and practices concerning health systems that either promote not only formal but also substantive equality, as well as a wide array of rights—or, alternatively, do not (Freedman 2005; Hunt and Backman 2008).

However, human rights approaches must be operationalised and made relevant to health policy makers and programmers, as well as frontline service providers. Human rights should not be conceived as a separate topic relating only to laws and policies, or to the way in which individuals are treated at a facility. As evident from this chapter, human rights are relevant to health system decisions that run from the most macro-level of financing to the most micro-level of service delivery. A human rights framework can and should prove a highly useful tool in promoting accountability, equal treatment, and meaningful participation of women and health workers, for it transforms evidence-based public health policy into a legal obligation to meet certain standards under international law.[44]

There is no topic in SRH that more clearly demonstrates the centrality of health systems in ensuring women's rights and dignity. As in Evarista's case, women often face multiple burdens relating to exclusion based not only on gender but on other factors as well, such as race, ethnicity, and disability. If we are to make meaningful improvements to women's sexual and reproductive health, including maternal health, we must transform health systems to reflect and communicate respect for their rights and dignity.

REFERENCES

Aker, J. C., and I. M. Mbiti. 2010. "Mobile Phones and Economic Development in Africa." Center for Global Development Working Paper 211, June.

Altobelli, L. C. 2008. "Case Study of CLAS in Peru: Opportunity and Empowerment for Health Equity." Paper prepared for Case Studies of Programmes Addressing Social Determinants of Health and Equity, organised by the Priority Public Health Conditions–Knowledge Network of the WHO Commission on Social Determinants of Health. http://www.future.org/publications/case-study-clas-peru.

Amnesty International. 2006. *Peru: Poor and Excluded Women; Denial of the Right to Maternal and Child Health.* London: AI Publications.

—. 2009. *The Total Abortion Ban in Nicaragua: Women's Lives and Health Endangered, Medical Professionals Criminalized.* London: AI Publications.

Basinga, P., P. J. Gertler, A. Binagwaha, et al. 2011. "Effect on Maternal and Child Health Services in Rwanda of Payment to Primary Health-Care Providers for Performance: an Impact Evaluation." *The Lancet* 377 (9775): 1421–1428.

Bhavnani, A., R. Won-Wai Chiu, S. Janakiram, et al. 2008. *The Role of Mobile Phones in Sustainable Rural Poverty Reduction.* Washington, D.C.: World Bank.

Campbell, O. M. R., et al. 2006. "Strategies for Reducing Maternal Mortality: Getting On with What Works." *The Lancet* 368 (9543): 1284–1299.

CESR (Center for Economic and Social Rights) and ICEFI (Instituto Centroamericano de Estudios Fiscales). 2009. *Rights or Privileges? Fiscal Commitment to the Rights to Health, Education and Food in Guatemala.* Brooklyn, NY: CESR and ICEFI.

CLADEM. 1999. *Nada Personal: Reporte de Derechos Humanos sobre la Aplicación de la Anticoncepción Quirúrgica en el Perú, 1996–1998.* Lima: CLADEM.

Commission on Information and Accountability for Women's and Children's Health. 2011. *Keeping Promises, Measuring Results.* Geneva: WHO.

Cotlear, D., ed. 2006. *A New Social Contract: An Agenda for Improving Education, Health, and the Social Safety Net in Peru.* New York: World Bank.

Defensoría del Pueblo. 2005. *El Derecho a la Identidad y la Actuación de la Administración Estatal: Problemas Verificados en la Supervisión Defensorial.* Lima: Peru. http://www.ombudsman.gob.pe/modules/Downloads/informes/defensoriales/informe_100.pdf.

Díaz, D., M. A. Castaneda Pérez, and S. Meneses Navarro. 2010. *Implicaciones del Seguro Popular en la Reducción de la Muerte Maternal: Perspectivas a Nivel Nacional y en los Estados de Chiapas y Oaxaca.* Mexico: Fundar.

Farmer, P. 2003. *Pathologies of Power: Health, Human Rights, and the New War on the Poor.* Berkeley: Univ. of California Press.

Freedman, L. P. 1995. "Censorship and Manipulation of Reproductive Health Information." In *The Right to Know: Human Rights and Access to Reproductive Health Information*, ed. S. Coliver, 1– 37. Philadelphia: Univ. of Pennsylvania Press.

—. 2005. "Achieving the MDGs: Health Systems as Core Social Institutions." *Development* 48 (1): 19–24.

Freedman, L. P., W. J. Graham, E. Brazier, et al. 2007. "Practical Lessons from Global Safe Motherhood Initiatives: Time for a New Focus on Implementation." *The Lancet* 370 (9595): 1383–1391.

Gill, Z., P. Bailey, R. Waxman, et al. 2005. "A Tool for Assessing 'Readiness' in Emergency Obstetric Care: The Room-by-Room 'Walk-Through.'" *International Journal of Gynecology and Obstetrics* 89:191–199.

Grimes, D. A., J. Benson, S. Singh, et al. 2006. "Unsafe Abortion: the Preventable Pandemic." *The Lancet* 368 (9550): 1908–1919.

Hill, K., K. Thomas, C. AbouZahr, et al. 2007. "Estimates of Maternal Mortality Worldwide between 1990 and 2005: An Assessment of Available Data." *The Lancet* 370 (9595): 1311–1319.

Hogan, M. C., K. J. Foreman, M. Naghavi, et al. 2010. "Maternal Mortality for 181 Countries, 1980–2008: A Systematic Analysis of Progress towards Millennium Development Goal 5." *The Lancet* 375 (9726): 1609–1623.

Hunt, P., and G. Backman. 2008. "Health Systems and the Right to the Highest Attainable Standard of Health." *Health and Human Rights* 10 (1): 81–92.

IIMMHR (International Initiative on Maternal Mortality and Human Rights). 2009. *The Missing Link: Applied Budget Work as a Tool to Hold Governments Accountable for Maternal Mortality Reduction Commitments.* New York: IIMMHR.

International Budget Partnership. 2010. "Ask Your Government Initiative." Accessed 3 August 2011. http://www.internationalbudget.org/cms/index. cfm?fa=view&id=3653.

Kgamphe, L., and L. Mahony, eds. 2004. *Using Government Budgets as a Monitoring Tool: The Children's Budget Unit in South Africa.* Minneapolis: New Tactics.

Maine, D. 1991. *Safe Motherhood Programs: Options and Issues.* New York: Center for Population and Family Health.

Mannion, R., and H. T. O. Davies. 2008. "Payment for Performance in Health Care." *British Medical Journal* 336:306–308.

Miller, S., F. Lester, M. Webster, et al. 2005. "Obstetric Fistula: A Preventable Tragedy." *Journal of Midwifery and Women's Health* 50:286–294.

Ministerio de Salud, Peru. 1999. *Mujeres en Negro: La Muerte Maternal en Zonas Rurales del Perú.* Lima: Ministerio de Salud.

Montagu, D., and G. Yamey. 2011. "Pay-for-Performance and the Millennium Development Goals." *The Lancet* 377 (9775): 1383–1385.

Okonofua, F. E., A. Hammed, E. Nzeribe, et al. 2009. "Perceptions of Policymakers in Nigeria Toward Unsafe Abortion and Maternal Mortality." *International Perspectives on Sexual and Reproductive Health* 35 (4): 194–202.

Partnership for Maternal, Newborn and Child Health. 2010. "Delhi Declaration 2010: 'From Pledges to Action and Accountability' Outcome Document from the PMNCH Partners' Forum." Accessed 3 August 2011. http://www.who.int/ pmnch/media/press_materials/pr/2010/20101114_delhideclaration.pdf.

Portocarrero Grados, A. 2006. "La Equidad en la Asignación Regional del Financiamiento del Sector Público de Salud 2000–2005." Accessed 3 August 2011. http://www.forosalud.org.pe/Equidad_en_Asignacion_de_ financiamiento.pdf.

Potts, H. 2008. *Accountability and the Right to the Highest Attainable Standard of Health.* Colchester: Univ. of Essex. http://www.essex.ac.uk/human_rights_ centre/research/rth/docs/HRC_Accountability_Mar08.pdf.

Rashid, A. T., and L. Elder. 2009. "An Analysis of IDRC-Supported Projects." *Electronic Journal of Information Systems in Developing Countries* 36 (2): 1–16.

República del Perú. 2004. *Hacia el Cumplimiento de los Objetivos de Desarrollo del Milenio en el Perú: Un Compromiso del País para Acabar con la Pobreza, la Desigualdad y la Exclusió*. Accessed 3 August 2011. http://www.cepis.ops-oms.org/bvsair/e/repindex/repi83/milenio/informes/peru-odm.pdf.

—. 2008. *Objetivos de Desarrollo del Milenio: Informe de Cumplimiento Perú; 2008*. Accessed 3 August 2011. http://www.onu.org.pe/upload/documentos/IODM-Peru2008.pdf.

Rosenfield, A., and D. Maine. 1985. "Maternal Mortality: A Neglected Tragedy. Where's the M in MCH?" *The Lancet* 326 (8446): 83–85.

UN Millennium Project Task Force on Child Health and Maternal Health. 2005. *Who's Got the Power? Transforming Health Systems for Women and Children*. Accessed 3 August 2011. http://www.unmillenniumproject.org/documents/maternalchild-complete.pdf.

UNFPA (UN Population Fund). 2010. UNFPA Head Asks World Leaders to Put Women's Health at Heart of Development Priorities. Press release, 20 September. http://www.unfpa.org/public/home/news/pid/6664.

UN Secretary-General. 2010. *Global Strategy for Women's and Children's Health*. New York: Partnership for Maternal, Newborn and Child Health. http://www.who.int/pmnch/topics/maternal/20100914_gswch_en.pdf.

Velázquez, T. 2004. *Vivencias Diferentes: La Indocumentación entre las Mujeres Rurales del Perú*. Lima: DEMUS, DFID, and Oxfam.

WHO (World Health Organization). 2005. *WHO Multi-Country Study on Women's Health and Domestic Violence against Women: Initial Results on Prevalence, Health Outcomes, and Women's Responses*. Geneva: WHO.

—. 2007. *Everybody's Business: Strengthening Health Systems to Improve Health Outcomes; WHO's Framework for Action*. Geneva: WHO.

—. 2010. *The World Health Report: Health Systems Financing; The Path to Universal Coverage*. Geneva: WHO.

WHO, UNFPA (UN Population Fund), UNICEF (UN Children's Fund), and AMDD (Averting Maternal Death and Disability). 2009. *Monitoring Emergency Obstetric Care: A Handbook*. Geneva: WHO.

World Bank. 2008. "World Bank Donates 205 Vehicles to Support Identification, Civil Registry Modernization in Côte d'Ivoire." 24 November. http://go.worldbank.org/XHR9A8H9H0.

—. 2009. "World's Progress on Maternal Health and Family Planning is Insufficient." 9 July. http://go.worldbank.org/70P0CCPUF0.

Yamin, A. E. 2007. *Deadly Delays; Maternal Mortality in Peru.* Cambridge, MA: Physicians for Human Rights.

—. 2010. "Toward Transformative Accountability: A Proposal for Rights-Based Approaches to Maternal Health in the MDGs and Beyond." *Sur: International Journal on Human Rights* 7 (12): 95–122.

Yamin, A. E., and D. P. Maine. 1999. "Maternal Mortality as a Human Rights Issue: Measuring Compliance with International Treaty Obligations." *Human Rights Quarterly* 21 (3): 563–607.

Yamin, A. E., and O. F. Norheim. 2011. *Taking Equality Seriously: Priority Setting and the Right to Health.* Cambridge: Cambridge Univ. Press.

NOTES

1 Programme of Action, International Conference on Population and Development, 5–13 September 1994, U.N. Doc. A/CONF.171/13 (1995), para. 7.2; Beijing Declaration and Platform for Action, Fourth World Conference on Women, 4–15 September 1995, U.N. Doc. A/CONF.177/20 & Add.1 (1995), para. 96.

2 Programme of Action, International Conference on Population and Development, *supra* note 1, para. 7.2.

3 Ibid., para. 7.4.

4 Beijing Declaration and Platform for Action, Fourth World Conference on Women, *supra* note 1, para. 96.

5 UN General Assembly, Keeping the Promise: A Forward-looking Review to Promote an Agreed Action Agenda to Achieve the Millennium Development Goals by 2015, Report of the Secretary-General, U.N. Doc A/64/665 (2010).

6 Ibid.

7 In this case, relevant international law includes the International Covenant on Civil and Political Rights, G.A. Res. 2200A (XXI), 21 U.N. GAOR Supp. (No. 16) at 52, U.N. Doc. A/6316 (1966), 999 U.N.T.S. 171, entered into force 23 March 1976; International Covenant on Economic, Social and Cultural Rights, G.A. Res. 2200A (XXI), 21 U.N. GAOR Supp. (No. 16) at 49, U.N. Doc. A/6316 (1966), 993 U.N.T.S. 3, entered into force 3 January 1976; Convention on the Elimination of All Forms of Discrimination against Women, G.A. Res. 34/180, 34 U.N. GAOR Supp. (No. 46) at 193, U.N. Doc. A/34/46 (1979), entered into force 3 September 1981; International Convention on the Elimination of All Forms of Racial Discrimination, G.A. Res. 2106 (XX), Annex, 20 U.N. GAOR Supp. (No. 14) at 47, U.N. Doc. A/6014 (1966), 660 U.N.T.S. 195, entered into force 4 January 1969; Convention on the Rights of the Child, G.A. Res. 44/25, Annex, 44 U.N. GAOR Supp. (No. 49) at 167, U.N. Doc. A/44/49 (1989), entered into force 2 September 1990; American Convention on Human Rights, O.A.S. Treaty Series

No. 36, 1144 U.N.T.S. 123, entered into force 18 July 1978, reprinted in Basic Documents Pertaining to Human Rights in the Inter-American System, OEA/Ser.L.V/II.82 doc.6 rev.1 at 25 (1992); Additional Protocol to the American Convention on Human Rights in the Area of Economic, Social and Cultural Rights, "Protocol of San Salvador," O.A.S. Treaty Series No. 69 (1988), entered into force 16 November 1999, reprinted in Basic Documents Pertaining to Human Rights in the Inter-American System, OEA/Ser.L.V/II.82 doc.6 rev.1 at 67 (1992); International Labour Organization, Convention 169 concerning Indigenous and Tribal Peoples in Independent Countries, entered into force 5 September 1991.

8   Committee on the Elimination of Discrimination against Women, General Recommendation 24, U.N. Doc. CEDAW/C/1999/I/WG.II/WP.2/Rev.1 (1999).

9   Committee on Economic, Social and Cultural Rights, General Comment 14, U.N. Doc. E/C.12/2000/4 (2000), para. 12.

10 International Covenant on Economic, Social and Cultural Rights, *supra* note 7, art. 2(1).

11 Convention on the Elimination of All Forms of Discrimination against Women, *supra* note 7, art. 12(1)–(2).

12 General Recommendation 24, *supra* note 8; General Comment 14, *supra* note 9.

13 Ibid., para. 21.

14 General Recommendation 24, *supra* note 8, para. 26.

15 General Comment 14, *supra* note 9, paras. 14, 44; General Recommendation 24, *supra* note 8, para. 27.

16 Paul Hunt, Report of the Special Rapporteur on the right of everyone to the enjoyment of the highest attainable standard of physical and mental health, General Assembly, U.N. Doc. A/61/338 (2006) [hereinafter Hunt Report]; Paul Hunt, Economic, Social and Cultural Rights: The right of everyone to the enjoyment of the highest attainable standard of physical and mental health, Report of the Special Rapporteur, Commission on Human Rights, U.N. Doc. E/CN.4/2004/49 (2004).

17 Human Rights Council, Resolution 11/8, Preventable Maternal Mortality and Morbidity and Human Rights, U.N. Doc. A/HRC/11/L.16 (2009); Human Rights Council, Resolution 15/17, Preventable Maternal Mortality and Morbidity and Human Rights: Follow-Up to Council Resolution 11/8, U.N. Doc. A/HRC/RES/15/17 (2010).

18 General Comment 14, *supra* note 9, para. 43.

19 Ibid., para. 43.

20 Ibid., para. 44.

21 Ibid., para. 43(f).

22 International Covenant on Economic, Social and Cultural Rights, *supra* note 7, art. 2; General Comment 14, *supra* note 9.

23 Programme of Action, International Conference on Population and Development, *supra* note 1, para. 7.2; General Comment 14, *supra* note 9, paras. 20–21; General Recommendation 24, *supra* note 8.

24 General Comment 14, *supra* note 9, para. 43.

25 India, High Court of Delhi, *Laxmi Mandal v. Deen Dayal Haringer Hospital & Ors Writ Petition,* Sentence, 2010; *Premlata w/o Ram Sagar & Ors. V. Govt. of NCT Delhi,* W.P. Civ. 7687/2010.

26 General Comment 14, *supra* note 9, paras. 12, 43(e), 44(a).

27 Hunt Report, *supra* note 16, para. 17(c).

28 General Recommendation 24, *supra* note 8.

29 General Comment 14, *supra* note 9, para. 12; Paul Hunt, Report of the Special Rapporteur on the right of everyone to the enjoyment of the highest attainable standard of physical and mental health, Commission on Human Rights, U.N. Doc. E/CN.4/2003/58 (2003), para. 75.

30 Universal Declaration of Human Rights, G.A. Res. 217A (III), U.N. Doc A/810 at 71 (1948).

31 Committee on Economic, Social and Cultural Rights, General Comment 20, U.N. Doc. E/C.12/GC/20 (2009).

32 General Comment 14, *supra* note 9, para. 19.

33 Ibid., para. 43.

34 Ibid., para. 18.

35 Committee on the Elimination of Discrimination against Women, Concluding Comments: Peru, U.N. Doc. CEDAW/C/PER/CO/6 (2007).

36 Government of Peru, Código Penal, Decreto Legislativo No. 635, 1991, arts. 114, 115.

37 Human Rights Committee, *Karen Noelia Llantoy Huamán v. Peru,* Communication No. 1153/2003, U.N. Doc. CCPR/C/85/D/1153/2003 (2005).

38 Ibid.

39 General Recommendation 24, *supra* note 8, para. 14.

40 Declaration of Alma-Ata, International Conference on Primary Health Care, Alma-Ata, USSR, 6–12 September 1978.

41 General Comment 14, *supra* note 9, para. 17.

42 Paul Hunt, Report of the Special Rapporteur on the right of everyone to the enjoyment of the highest attainable standard of physical and mental health, General Assembly, U.N. Doc. A/59/422 (2004), para. 58.

43 General Comment 14, *supra* note 9, para. 11.

44 For example, policies and programmes that have shown little evidence of success based on published literature, such as training of traditional birth attendants in the absence of a functioning referral network or programmes aimed at assigning risk status to pregnancies to predict complications, should not be considered reasonable or appropriate means to realise women's right to health nor achieve MDG 5. See, e.g., Campbell et al. (2006).

CHAPTER 7

HIV and AIDS

SOFIA GRUSKIN AND SHAHIRA AHMED

CASE STUDY: MINH, AN INJECTING DRUG USER IN VIETNAM

Minh is a 35-year-old Vietnamese male injecting drug user. He has been married to his female partner, Hang, for 10 years, and they have two small children. They would like a third child. He admits to frequenting sex workers and injecting drugs with his friends, and is not sure if he has been consistent in using condoms or clean needles in every situation. When asked about his knowledge of HIV transmission, he correctly described how HIV is transmitted—but he does not wish to seek an HIV test.

INTRODUCTION

Minh's situation is quite common in Vietnam, and his case exemplifies a typical situation in a country with a concentrated epidemic. What factors lead to Minh's refusal to test? What will it take for Minh to choose to undergo an HIV test and, if needed, change his behaviour and access the prevention, treatment, and care services that he might require? This chapter argues that the issues raised by Minh's case are best analysed and addressed through the application of a rights-based approach.

HIV remains one of the most important global health issues today. By the end of 2009, there were 33.3 million people living with HIV worldwide, more than half of them women (UNAIDS 2010a, p. 23). In addition to its epidemiological and medical implications, the social, economic, and political implications of the disease have been intensely debated and studied. The role of human rights in this work has been critical in, among many things, defining global and national policies, changing attitudes, and advocating for new resources to address the epidemic. Civil society has played a crucial role in this history. More recently, human rights approaches have been used to design, develop, and implement HIV policies and programmes. While there have been many successes, there remain challenges and gaps in the HIV response—both within countries and globally—that require attention and new frameworks and tools. This chapter will review and discuss the key health and human rights aspects of HIV, progress that has been made, and some of the remaining challenges to be addressed.

The first global strategy on AIDS was launched by the World Health Organization (WHO) in 1986 (UNAIDS 2001, p. 3). It emphasised the importance of a supportive environment and the need to implement structures and services to serve the needs of vulnerable populations. The strategy was grounded in recognition of the need to uphold human rights and recognition of the human rights violations that people living with HIV were suffering worldwide. These violations included violence within families and communities, denial of inheritance and property rights, and violations regarding access to food, housing, marriage, education, medical care, international travel, health insurance, and employment. Global strategies since that time have continued to reference the need to promote and protect human rights. Importantly, the Declaration of Commitment on HIV/AIDS (DoC), adopted by the UN General Assembly Special Session on HIV/AIDS (UNGASS) in 2001, provides concrete targets and obligations, including a global reporting mechanism that includes questions about human rights in the HIV response.[1] Countries report biannually on a set of core indicators that are used to monitor compliance by governments. This has much potential also to promote accountability at the national level, initiate dialogue with diverse actors, mobilise civil society, and facilitate regional interaction. Other international documents have played important roles in the HIV response at national and global levels, and reflect various levels of commitment to human rights. The Millennium Development Goals (MDGs), for example, provide targets related to HIV and have linked these targets to development and poverty reduction; the specific linkages to human rights, however, are not clear.

A recent review of the extent to which national HIV plans integrate human rights found that most countries explicitly refer to human rights in their national-level plans regardless of whether the country is party to relevant international human rights treaties (Tarantola and Gruskin 2008). Conversely, some countries, such as China, do not use the language of human rights explicitly, even though they have ratified international human rights treaties—but they do integrate human rights concepts, such as equity and quality of care, into their plans. However, even when countries include human rights language and concepts in their national HIV plans, generally there is limited concrete attention to human rights in their programmatic activities or monitoring frameworks.

The three sections below analyse Minh's case from three broad perspectives, with explicit attention paid to the Vietnamese context: medical and public health; ethical and legal; and application of the right to health in practice. These are followed by a section that considers key cross-cutting issues in the HIV response. The chapter concludes with some broad areas for future consideration. Each section begins by discussing the multitude of issues with human rights ramifications that require a rights-based response. Broadly, the following questions will be considered:

- What are the primary health and human rights concerns for injecting drug users? What issues might they face when accessing services regarding their drug use and beyond?
- What information and services are needed in order for a person to decide to seek an HIV test? Where is attention needed to ensure that people will stay connected to the health-care system after testing?
- What are potential strategies for reducing stigma and discrimination so that Minh, and others like him, will wish to use condoms, clean injection equipment and other prevention commodities in order to reduce the risk of infection? Will Minh feel comfortable accessing the HIV-related services available to him?
- How can we determine whether prevention, treatment, and care efforts in Vietnam are rights based? How can human rights play a more prominent role in addressing specific challenges to Vietnam's HIV response?
- Are prevention, treatment, and care services reaching everyone who needs them?
- What opportunities and challenges exist that allow for more effective rights-based approaches to countries' HIV responses?

MEDICAL/PUBLIC HEALTH ASPECTS

Vietnam's epidemic is categorised as "concentrated"—that is, the epidemic is mainly confined to injecting drug users, men who have sex with men, and sex workers and their clients. According to the latest estimates by UNAIDS (Joint UN Programme on HIV/AIDS), HIV prevalence among the general population remains low (0.53%) but is significant among key population groups, including female sex workers (3.2%), men who have sex with men (16.7%), and injecting drug users (18.4%) (2010b, p. 5).

This suggests that policies and programmes targeted towards these populations would be desirable. Yet Minh and his family do not appear to have been effectively reached. This may seem surprising: since Vietnam's first HIV case was reported in the mid-1990s, the country has expended considerable efforts to prevent and control the disease, in line with a global move to respond to the epidemic in a more comprehensive way. Yet even as the world's response to HIV has evolved over the years, with better data and research on how to prevent and treat HIV and on how it affects different populations, challenges remain in reaching vulnerable populations. There is growing consensus that a comprehensive response to HIV requires a multifaceted approach to prevention, treatment, and care that integrates rights-based approaches. This section explores prevention, treatment, and care approaches more closely and analyses how the design and implementation of policies and programmes influence whether Minh, his family, and others like them receive the HIV services they need. But first, we return to the case and discuss HIV counselling and testing.

HIV COUNSELLING AND TESTING

We return here to a key concern for Minh: he does not wish to seek an HIV test. Fundamental to the success of prevention, treatment, and care efforts is HIV counselling and testing, whose importance is undisputed. Knowing one's status gives individuals important information relevant to their ability to remain healthy, access health services, and protect others from being infected. In 2009 in Vietnam, a mere 2.3% of women and men aged 15–49 had received an HIV test within the prior year and knew their status (UNAIDS 2010b, p. 3). What will it take for more people to seek HIV counselling and testing?

Increasing the uptake of counselling and testing requires increasing the number of services available. This, in turn, will encourage people like Minh and Hang to come forward and seek testing. According to the latest reports, the number of voluntary counselling and testing sites across the country increased from 157 in 2005 to 256 in 2009, with a parallel rise in testing among key populations particularly vulnerable to infection (for example, the percentage of male injecting drug users who received an HIV test rose from 11.4% to 17.9% in 2009) (UNAIDS 2010b, p. 25). Barriers to increased testing are believed to be largely due to stigma and discrimination, as well as the perception that treatment is unavailable.

Increasing the uptake of counselling and testing thus requires activities to address stigma and discrimination at the facility and community levels. One important consideration is the impact of laws and policies on counselling and testing. There remains persistent misuse and contradictions in how language around testing is deployed by the institutions responsible for setting relevant policy at the international and national levels. Thus, how laws and policies are written, interpreted, and implemented may discourage and impede vulnerable populations, such as Minh and his family, from using testing sites. Various approaches to HIV testing are being scaled up—for example, provider-initiated testing and counselling—which are based on the well-founded urgency to expand efforts to increase the number of people being tested. However, evidence of the effectiveness and of the public health and human rights implications of such strategies is not yet clear (Bartlett et al. 2008; Mounier-Jack et al. 2008). While researchers and practitioners alike acknowledge that stigma and discrimination in relation to testing practices persist everywhere—including in resource-rich settings—this acknowledgment has not been translated sufficiently into policy and programmatic strategies that pay special attention to human rights.

If Minh seeks an HIV test, his experience while testing will be influenced by several factors. These include the following: (1) whether he is given his results on site, by whom, and how; (2) whether he will feel encouraged and supported to return to the site to collect his results; (3) whether he will seek prevention, treatment, and care services after receiving his results; and (4) whether he will continue to seek such services over time. Thus, from a health systems perspective, HIV counselling and testing should be linked to not only specific prevention, treatment, and care services but to health and health-care services more generally, including sexual and reproductive health services. Both pre- and post-test counselling is key to ensuring that people are fully informed about the implications of testing positive, including their options for treatment and care, and can serve as an important entry point for providing HIV prevention information and services to those who test negative. Thirty years into the epidemic, there is a dangerous trend away from counselling; more emphasis is being placed on testing alone— with insufficient thought being spent, for example, on how a test result is provided and what information a person needs upon hearing a result—as donors focus increasingly on the number of people being tested and not on the specifics of individual experience and how this influences an individual's engagement with the health system over time (Beckwith et al. 2005). This practice contradicts the global guidance on HIV counselling and testing, which continues to emphasise the need for counselling, informed consent, and confidentiality. The UNAIDS/WHO Policy Statement on HIV Testing states that

> the conditions of the "3 Cs", advocated since the HIV test became available in 1985, continue to be underpinning principles for the conduct of HIV testing of individuals. Such that testing of individuals must be: confidential; be accompanied by counseling; only be conducted with informed consent, meaning that it is both informed and voluntary. (UNAIDS and WHO 2004, p. 1)

In Vietnam, national- and local-level guidance on HIV counselling and testing varies in its attention to these concepts. In addition, HIV counselling and testing services are not provided in the same way across the country. For Minh and Hang, the systems in place must ensure that the client not only agrees to undergo a test but is also fully aware of the range of available options for prevention, treatment, and care.

PREVENTION

According to Vietnamese government reporting under the DoC in 2010, the country launched its National Strategy on HIV/AIDS Prevention and Control for 2010–20, which is to be implemented through nine guidance documents

196

(programmes of action) and the establishment of provincial AIDS centres (so far, fifty-eight of the sixty-four provinces have such centres). This is a positive development, particularly since the global community's attention to prevention has waned with the advent of antiretroviral drugs. At the international level, recent efforts have brought attention to the importance of strategies that give equal attention to prevention, treatment, and care, and the international community is beginning to show a renewed commitment to this approach. This shift is due to several factors. Growing evidence shows the value of "combination prevention"—efforts that not only focus on individuals, information, testing services, and behaviour change but also address the socio-economic, legal, and political context. In Vietnam and elsewhere, the human rights framework has been employed by civil society groups, researchers, governments, and public health experts concerned with prevention. There appears to be a global consensus that "HIV prevention requires locally contextualized approaches that address both individuals and social norms and structures, and are grounded in human rights" (Piot et al. 2008, p. 846). The challenge remains, however, to ensure that the range of prevention interventions are accessible to all who need them, including Minh and his family. In Vietnam, 90% of the HIV strategy is funded through international sources, including the United States President's Emergency Plan for AIDS Relief; the Global Fund to Fight AIDS, Tuberculosis and Malaria; the UK Department for International Development; the Asian Development Bank; and the World Bank (UNAIDS 2010b, p. 15). Despite this large funding base, the lack of universal access to necessary services means that if Minh lives in a community that does not receive HIV funding from either the government or these external donors, he will not have easy access to prevention services.

Minh's knowledge of HIV is adequate, yet knowledge alone has not convinced him to seek an HIV test or to consistently use condoms or clean needles. This is despite the fact that information, education, and communication (IEC) strategies are known to play an important role in HIV prevention. Included under this rubric are awareness campaigns and educational interventions aimed at achieving a range of goals, such as helping individuals increase their knowledge about HIV transmission and changing behaviours that put people at risk of infection. In Vietnam, mass media campaigns have been used to raise awareness about how infection is transmitted, but there is still a great deal of misinformation within communities, with potentially devastating implications for the prevalence of HIV among society at large. While evidence strongly supports the effectiveness of IEC strategies in increasing knowledge, the evidence is mixed regarding which IEC strategies are most likely to lead to actual changes in behaviour. This may in part be due to the quality of evaluations conducted (for example, inadequacy of research methods to evaluate behaviour change), but it may also be linked to the quality of the content of IEC strategies (this, in turn, is often related to the extent to which an understanding of local context has been adequately integrated into interventions). Globally, over 80% of all HIV transmission is sexual (UNAIDS 2010c, p. 16); therefore, ideological, cultural, religious, and social factors—and not just the evidence alone—may affect how the information is presented and understood. For example, for a number of years the IEC intervention known commonly as the "ABC approach" (for "Abstain, Be faithful, and use Condoms"), due in large part to ideologically driven U.S. government pressure and funding, resulted in an inordinate amount of money being spent on abstinence even when the evidence was clear that this alone would not be an effective strategy. Similarly, in Vietnam, concerns exist that donor funding is driving implementation, resulting in insufficient attention to all three prongs of the ABC approach.

Condom use is an accepted intervention for HIV prevention among key populations and more generally (UNAIDS 2008). Correct and consistent condom use is known to reduce the risk of HIV transmission, and currently the male condom is considered the most efficient technology available to reduce sexual transmission of HIV and other sexually transmitted infections for people engaged in penetrative sex. Global guidance therefore calls for universal access to condoms at no or very low cost and for condoms to be promoted in ways that address the social and cultural barriers to their use (importantly, female condoms have continued to remain less accessible due to cost and lack of availability, despite evidence of their efficacy) (UNAIDS 2009). In Vietnam, however, reported condom use among key populations is inconsistent, pointing to a range of barriers beyond the legal and policy realms. For example, reported condom use with clients among female sex workers ranged between 59.3% and 91.8% (UNAIDS 2010b, p. 21). Perceptions of risk, knowledge of how HIV is transmitted, and attitudes towards condom use are some of the factors that have been shown to be related to consistency in condom use. Knowledge of where to access condoms also influences the rate of use. It remains the case in Vietnam, as in other countries, that because of persistent gender inequality, women who possess correct information and access to condoms are nonetheless unlikely to be able to negotiate condom use with their male partners, even if both are aware of the risk. In fact, until they began to discuss the possibility of having a third child, Hang had wanted to suggest to Minh that they use condoms but had been afraid to do so.

In addition to comprehensive prevention policies and programmes, attention to the health and rights of injecting drug users is an important aspect of a rights-based approach to HIV prevention. In other words, it is not enough to provide HIV prevention strategies for Minh that ignore his drug use. Evidence and global guidance promotes addressing HIV and drug use simultaneously through outreach activities, access to voluntary counselling and testing, and syringe- and needle-exchange programmes as harm reduction strategies. These interventions have been shown to reduce both needle-risk behaviour and HIV transmission and, importantly, have not been shown to increase injecting drug use (Ball et al. 2005; Institute of Medicine of the National Academies 2006). Despite overwhelming public health evidence, due to stigma and discrimination at the individual and community levels, it remains difficult to ensure implementation of harm reduction programmes, even when governments are interested in doing so. In addition, lack of resources and a complex legal and policy environment may make it difficult to scale up programmes. The situation in Vietnam highlights some of these issues. While there is an explicit law protecting the ability of all populations to receive HIV services, and supporting harm reduction, the government reports that laws exist which impede implementation of harm reduction programmes since they criminalise the buying and selling of instruments used in the production and use of drugs (UNAIDS 2008). The latest Vietnamese UNGASS country report states, for example, that "despite amendments to the Law on Drugs inconsistencies remain between public security measures to control drug use and sex and public health measures to reach the populations engaged in those activities" (UNAIDS 2010b, p. 38).

Vietnam adopted a national programme of action for preventing mother-to-child transmission (PMTCT) of HIV in 2006. However, guidelines for its implementation are still in development, indicating that efforts in this area are still needed. This is despite the recognition that PMTCT is a critical prevention strategy that can also facilitate women's ability to access care and support for themselves. If Minh is HIV positive, his wife, Hang, may be also. Consequently, access to PMTCT services could provide her with a range of needed services. Despite the name, PMTCT programmes involve a comprehensive package of interventions that are not limited to the prevention of vertical transmission; these interventions include preventing primary infection among women, supporting the prevention of unintended pregnancies among women living with HIV, and providing treatment, care, and support to HIV-infected women and their families over time. These interventions require the integration of HIV services with treatment services and sexual and reproductive health services. However, in Vietnam, many PMTCT programmes still focus primarily on the prevention of transmission from mother to child, with little attention to the longer-tem need for treatment of the women themselves. This raises concerns regarding the testing of women without their full consent, inadequate post-test counselling, and programmes that fail to ensure the sustained relationship of both the woman and her infant to the health-care system. More specifically, the availability of PMTCT programmes does not imply that all pregnant women will choose to undergo HIV testing. Thus, Hang may wish to have another child with Minh and yet be afraid to engage with the services ostensibly available to her. Recent studies in other parts of the world have shown a relatively high uptake of HIV testing when offered as part of antenatal care services where PMTCT services were available; however, despite the availability of PMTCT services, 3%–30% of their users nonetheless declined to be tested (Gruskin, Ahmed, and Ferguson 2007, p. 26). Reasons given by women for refusing the HIV test include fear of the test itself, fear of the consequences of a positive test result (e.g., abandonment or abuse), knowledge that antiretroviral therapy is not available, and the need to consult their partners before testing. For many women, these factors can outweigh women's concerns related to perinatal transmission of HIV and their desire to know their own status.

An additional prevention strategy gaining global support is male circumcision. As a prevention strategy, male circumcision is considered relevant only for generalised epidemics, and therefore is not yet an issue for Minh and his family, or for other places where the epidemic is still concentrated. While not an immediate issue, the human rights implications that male circumcision will have for women (and for boys and girls coming into their sexuality) is still being determined and may be of relevance in the near future. In particular, as the perceived risk of HIV infection decreases for circumcised men, it not clear how, given gender and power dynamics, this will affect condom use. These issues must be considered in any HIV prevention strategy that includes male circumcision.

CARE AND TREATMENT

Vietnam adopted its National Plan on Care and Treatment in 2006, in which targets were set to provide antiretroviral therapies to 70% of adults in need by 2010; but to date, the reality falls far short of this goal. As Minh is likely to be unaware that he and Hang are entitled to treatment if needed, and unaware of where they could access such treatment, he will probably have a limited interest in knowing his HIV status.

Evidence from around the world has shown that people are more interested in learning their HIV status if they know that they will be able to access safe and effective treatment once they are sick. It is estimated that approximately 36% of people in need of treatment, about 5.2 million worldwide, were receiving antiretrovirals by the end of 2009 (UNAIDS 2010a, p. 95). This is approximately a thirteen-fold increase in six years. Coverage in Southeast Asia is consistent with global trends; HIV epidemics are concentrated in harder-to-reach areas and among certain populations particularly vulnerable to infection. These variations point to issues of limited access to treatment for vulnerable groups, and policies and programmes that are insufficiently targeted to the needs of local epidemics (UNAIDS 2010a).

A first step is to ensure that all people have access to the health system; but at the same time, it is also important to ensure that particularly vulnerable populations, including people like Minh, who use drugs, feel comfortable attending the health centres and can access health services free of discrimination.

The increasing availability of antiretroviral therapies is vastly changing the response to HIV in Vietnam and elsewhere. With the development of new drug therapies, such as life-saving drug cocktails and highly active antiretroviral therapy, HIV has the potential to become a chronic, treatable illness. Many countries, such as Brazil, have made dramatic progress in recent years in providing needed drugs to people living with HIV (Piot 2006). Treatment is often discussed in terms of factors that include coverage (the number of people receiving treatment), the capacity of health systems to provide treatment (including trained and sufficient numbers of health workers), integration of services within health systems (e.g., integration with tuberculosis, sexual and reproductive health, and nutrition), and the provision of care and support to orphans and vulnerable children. However, challenges remain regarding the ability of health systems to provide and sustain treatment in the long term.

The Vietnamese government is seeking to address numerous health system challenges, including that of human resource capacity. For example, while provincial AIDS centres have been established in many provinces, most are understaffed and have minimal technical capacity. In addition, antiretrovirals and other drugs are available in only a small number of provinces, largely in urban settings where donors focus their efforts (UNAIDS 2008). As resources from donors are shifted to other priorities or reduced, it is critical to ensure that those people on treatment regimens maintain access to these drugs through the health system. A successful treatment programme, therefore, must not only increase the number of individuals accessing antiretrovirals for the first time but also ensure that these individuals have the goods and services necessary to remain on treatment over time. This requires facilities with the capacity to diagnose cases, dispense drugs appropriately, and provide follow-up to patients in ways that support their adherence to their treatment regimens. Given the stigma that still exists around drug use in Vietnam, governmental efforts on this front are needed before Minh is likely to feel comfortable engaging with the health system in his province.

This situation also highlights the vulnerability of Hang, Minh's wife, not only to infection but also to receiving necessary treatment and care. One critical avenue for connecting HIV-positive individuals to comprehensive services is through the integration of health services. Vietnam has expended considerable effort in linking both tuberculosis and sexual and reproductive health services with HIV services. For example, an action programme on reproductive health and HIV prevention education for secondary school students was launched in 2007. The integration of services is essential for ensuring that individuals receive comprehensive care and has been proven effective in terms of costs and public health outcomes, as well as appropriate from a human rights perspective (Berer 2003). The integration of HIV and sexual and reproductive health services in particular is critical for ensuring that HIV-positive women, whether or not they are on treatment, receive the services and support necessary to decide if and when to become pregnant. Hang has two young children whose statuses are also unknown, and she is anxious for a third child. In Vietnam and beyond, a range of factors are known to influence HIV-positive women's desire to bear children, including age; health status; the cultural significance of motherhood; the number of living children; previous experience of a child's death from HIV-related causes; the availability of HIV treatment and PMTCT programmes; the attitudes and influence of partners, family, and health-care workers; and stigma and discrimination on the basis of HIV status, especially for women from marginalised populations.

ETHICAL AND LEGAL PERSPECTIVES

ETHICAL DILEMMAS AND CONCERNS

Ethical issues arise with respect to many aspects of HIV prevention, treatment, and care. Of particular note are concerns around privacy, confidentiality, and informed consent. A host of issues are also raised around, for example, HIV counselling and testing and access to services more broadly. Access to and use of condoms is another area that is often discussed. Although condoms represent one of the most successful interventions for HIV prevention, there are still challenges to their uptake and distribution. Stigma associated with condom use can occur in both steady and casual partnerships, leading not only to unprotected sex but to fears of disclosure when one of the partners is HIV positive. With rates of infection increasing disproportionately among young adults, the literature is increasingly discussing individual-level, programmatic, and societal barriers to access and use of condoms, as this group is known to be inconsistent in its use of condoms (Kaplan et al. 2001; Sheeran, Abraham, and Orbell 1999). A range of factors affects access to and use of condoms for this population, including issues around sexuality, peer norms and pressure, and gender dynamics. In addition to individual and societal attitudes and behaviour, the legal and policy environment within countries, as discussed further below, can also hinder effective condom use— for example, by impeding access to or use of condoms by young people, as well as by injecting drug users and sex workers. Human rights advocates have consistently pointed to the challenges of condom access and use for vulnerable populations; certainly, this would be an issue for Minh and Hang if they decided to use condoms in their marriage.

Research and clinical trials also raise a host of relevant ethical issues. For example, research over the past decade has focused on the development of new technologies to prevent HIV infection between discordant partners. If Minh and Hang eventually choose to have HIV tests and find that they are discordant (for example, he is positive and she is negative), this would raise concerns not only about disclosure but about their ability to access and use technologies that may prevent transmission, such as microbicides (WHO 2010). Microbicides, if effectively developed, would be a prevention method that women could use, even without the explicit engagement of the sexual partner. This again raises concerns about disclosure and a host of other legal and ethical issues.

LEGAL CONTEXT

The legal and policy environment shapes the availability of health services and programmes, as well as the degree to which they are responsive to individual needs. The international community is increasingly recognising the negative impacts of laws and policies that create obstacles to an effective HIV response (including laws that criminalise same-sex relations between consenting adults and various aspects of sex work and drug use, as well as those that restrict the entry, stay, and residence of people living with HIV) and is paying closer attention to improving the legal and policy context within which HIV interventions are implemented. In addition to the need for supportive policies to ensure access to and uptake of prevention, treatment, care, and support services, explicit laws and policies are needed to protect people living with HIV, and other vulnerable populations, from discrimination. While the number of countries reporting such laws is increasing, the extent to which these laws and policies are effectively implemented is not known. Furthermore, attention must be paid to obstructive and punitive laws and policies that serve as obstacles to the HIV response; indeed, according to UNAIDS, in 2010, 67% of countries reported the existence of such harmful laws and policies (UNAIDS 2010a, p. 126).

Vietnam has seen major developments in the law and policy arena in recent years. In 2006, it passed a law on HIV/AIDS that explicitly acknowledges the right of people living with HIV to be protected against stigma and discrimination.[2] Furthermore, Vietnam has signed on to a number of regional and international commitments, including the MDGs, the DoC on HIV/AIDS, Universal Access by 2010, the Asia Pacific Ministerial Declaration on HIV/AIDS Leadership and Development, and the ASEAN Declaration on the Protection and Promotion of the Rights of Migrant Workers.[3] It has also ratified several human rights treaties containing provisions relevant to HIV prevention, treatment, care and support, including the International Covenant on Economic, Social and Cultural Rights; the Convention on the Elimination of All Forms of Discrimination against Women; and the Convention on the Rights of the Child.[4]

A review of Vietnam's legal and policy context reveals the existence of laws that can, despite the best of intentions, impede implementation of what a country considers to be its rights-based HIV strategy. For example, sex work and injecting drug use remain criminal activities in Vietnam, as in many other countries. Therefore, even as harm reduction interventions are being promoted to address HIV among injecting drug users, many users, like Minh, are afraid to access the services available to them, including voluntary counselling and testing. While civil society organisations, including groups of people living with HIV, are forming in the country and advocating for change, such a restrictive legal and policy context nonetheless hinders these efforts by creating an unfavourable environment for human rights awareness and a flourishing civil society.

There is increasing attention by the international community to structural barriers that increase an individual's risk and vulnerability to HIV infection. Structural barriers can be understood to encompass contextual factors that exacerbate vulnerability to HIV infection or impede access to HIV-related services in the legal, social, political, and economic realms. Stigma and discrimination, entrenched gender inequalities, gender-based violence, laws that pose barriers to access, and lack of economic resources are all recognised to be major structural drivers that hamper HIV prevention efforts. Each of these poses problems for Minh and Hang; for example, Hang may want to get tested but may be afraid to do so because of her presumed subservient role in society and fear of violence. She may also be economically dependent on Minh.

Another concern for Minh in terms of knowing his status is a fear of the implications for his family if he tests positive. In Vietnam, schools have barred children living with HIV from attending school, despite the fact that there are no laws supporting their ability to do so (Brickley et al. 2008). Such actions demonstrate that stigma and discrimination continue to be major issues hampering the success of HIV efforts. Stigma and discrimination remain pervasive in developing and industrialised countries alike, and operate at multiple levels of society. UNAIDS defines HIV-related stigma as a "process of devaluation" of people living with or associated with HIV, and explains that "discrimination follows stigma and is the unfair and unjust treatment of an individual based on his or her real or perceived HIV status" (UNAIDS 2003, p. 1). Together they can lead to violence, ostracism, abandonment, and denial of services or legal protection. These consequences, or simply the fear of them, may mean that people will be less likely to adopt preventative behaviours and use the services available to them, including HIV counselling and testing. Distinguishing between stigma and discrimination is important for guiding programmatic activities and ensuring opportunities for redress if needed.

How can Vietnam ensure that its laws and policies are translated into rights-based strategies? Accountability is critical: governmental actors and other policy makers have a responsibility to provide rights-based policies, an infrastructure for sustainable prevention, care and treatment programmes, and a climate in which all populations will want to know their HIV status and will trust health-care providers to provide them with both the necessary information and concomitant support. Vietnam has taken important first steps in this direction, but more effort is needed.

APPLICATION OF THE RIGHT TO HEALTH IN PRACTICE

For Minh and Hang to seek HIV testing and remain linked to prevention, treatment, and care services will require efforts at the policy, programmatic, and individual levels, and by multiple actors and stakeholders. The right to health, and human rights more generally, offers a framework for action and for programming. Human rights also provide a compelling argument for governmental responsibility—not only to provide HIV-related services but also to alter the conditions that create, exacerbate, and perpetuate the poverty, deprivation, marginalisation, and discrimination associated with HIV (Gruskin and Braveman 2005). A diverse array of actors is increasingly finding innovative ways to relate human rights principles to HIV-related efforts, thereby demonstrating how a human rights perspective can yield new insights and more effective ways of addressing HIV within both countries and the policy and programmatic guidance offered at the global level.

This section looks at some of the human rights concepts and approaches currently being used in HIV-related efforts. There is no one framework or approach for integrating human rights into HIV work. That is, organisations that implement a rights-based approach use a broad range of definitions and a variety of different methods. The human rights principles generally recognised as most relevant to a rights-based approach to HIV include participation, non-discrimination, accountability, and the service-provision elements of the right to health (the accessibility, availability, acceptability, and quality of services (AAAQ); see chapters 1 and 4). A rights-based approach translates into very different interventions for actors whose work focuses on advocacy and ensuring the legal accountability of governments around their HIV commitments than it does for entities that adopt a rights-based approach in the design, implementation, or monitoring of HIV policies and programmes. Some actors have determined that a grounding in a legal framework, particularly around the right to health, is key to rights-based programming efforts; others are concerned only with the participation of affected communities; others bring attention to discrimination; others focus on transparency and accountability; and still others bring conscious attention to all these criteria and more.

While there is no consensus on what a human rights approach to HIV entails, the multiple ways that human rights are being used to address HIV can be categorised into three broad areas: advocacy, the use of legal norms and standards, and policy and programmatic frameworks (Gruskin, Mills, and Tarantola 2007). Each of these is discussed further below, both generally and in relation to the Vietnam case study specifically.

ADVOCACY FRAMEWORKS

Advocacy is a key component of many organisations' work on HIV and human rights. Efforts in the advocacy category can be described as using human rights language to draw attention to an issue, mobilise public opinion, and advocate for change. Advocacy efforts may call for the implementation of rights even if they are not yet in fact established by law—and in so doing, serve to move governmental and intergovernmental bodies closer to legitimising these issues as legally enforceable human rights claims. This means also linking up to other activists working on issues indirectly related to HIV (such as groups focused on violence against women, poverty, and global trade issues), reaching out to policy makers and other influential groups, translating international human rights norms to the work and concerns of local communities, and supporting the organising capabilities of people living with HIV. Advocacy can happen anywhere from the community to the international level. For example, activists can demand that governments explain how they are meeting their rights-related targets under the DoC or how their programmes and policies reflect the concepts embodied in the International Guidelines on HIV/AIDS and Human Rights (UNAIDS 2006). One famous example is the work of the Treatment Action Campaign in South Africa to pressure the government to make antiretrovirals available to all (Friedman and Mottiar 2005; see chapters 1 and 9). In addition, advocacy efforts have relied on action at the community level, drawing on grassroots social movements and including strong public-education components. In Vietnam, community-based efforts have raised awareness among groups of people living with HIV and other vulnerable populations about the connections between HIV and human rights in their lives through workshops, publications, and educational programmes (Hammett et al. 2008).

Returning to the case, in order to adequately address the public health, ethical, and legal aspects affecting Minh and Hang, efforts are needed that seek to change the root causes that lead to stigma, discrimination, and lack of services. Also required are interventions to ensure that data are collected and made publicly available. The Institute for Social Development Studies, a non-governmental organisation based in Hanoi, Vietnam, uses rights concepts in its advocacy efforts to reduce HIV-related stigma and discrimination in the country. Using empirical evidence from its own research, the organisation collaborates with governmental and international agencies to build the capacity of policy makers, the community, and the media around issues of stigma and discrimination facing people living with HIV (Institute for Social Development Studies 2011). The organisation's efforts contributed to the passage of Vietnam's HIV/AIDS law in 2006, which includes a commitment to the protection of the rights of people living with HIV.[5] This advocacy by the Institute for Social Development Studies demonstrates one of the important tools that can be used in the application of the right to health.

LEGAL FRAMEWORKS

Let us now assume that Minh finally decides to seek an HIV test. He goes to the nearest clinic, but his fears are realised when the health-care provider mistreats him and refuses to administer the test, claiming that Minh is a drug user and that the provider does not want to waste scarce resources on him. This occurs despite the fact that Vietnam is party to relevant international human rights treaties and has passed a law on HIV providing for the promotion and protection of the rights of people living with HIV against stigma and discrimination. In addition, Vietnam submits progress reports under the DoC that contain essential information on the country's AIDS response, including how Vietnam's laws and policies affect the human rights of key populations.

How can the law be used to assist Minh in seeking redress? Are there any legal provisions that would protect him in Vietnam?

In some countries, litigation has been used successfully for some time to promote and protect the rights of people living with HIV. Vietnam is just starting to witness the establishment of legal clinics that defend the rights of people within the context of AIDS. Discrimination in relation to access to treatment is one area where court cases have been used successfully. While such litigation is in still its infancy in Vietnam, it can draw on the examples of recent court cases in several Latin American countries, as well as in South Africa, that have won increased access to antiretroviral therapy for people living with HIV by invoking the rights to life and health, among other rights (Carrasco 2000; Nattrass 2006). In such cases, constitutional provisions and international human rights treaties were used to challenge the inaction or opposition of governments to the procurement and availability of drugs alleged to be beyond the economic means of the state or, in the case of South Africa, lacking scientific evidence of their safety and efficacy (Gruskin, Ferguson, and Bogecho 2007).

In addition to litigation, another effective strategy involves working with national-level human rights bodies, such as national human rights commissions, to encourage them to address HIV more substantially in their work. International human rights bodies and mechanisms (including human rights treaty bodies and other UN mechanisms) can also be used to promote governmental accountability for HIV-related actions, including ensuring that related legislation respects human rights.

Legal approaches use human rights law at the national and international and national levels to produce norms and standards, change laws, and ensure accountability for HIV-related efforts. These efforts also include ensuring consonance between national law and international human rights norms and standards. Pursuing accountability through national law and international treaty obligations often takes the form of analysing what a government is or is not doing in relation to HIV and how this might constitute a violation of rights, seeking remedies in national and international courts and tribunals, and focusing on transparency, accountability, and functioning norms and systems to promote and protect HIV-related rights. Legal approaches are just beginning to take shape in Vietnam, suggesting that Minh and others like him will soon be able to access and use legal frameworks to claim their rights.

POLICY AND PROGRAMMATIC FRAMEWORKS

The Vietnamese government has worked to ensure that its national AIDS plan is accompanied by guidance documents and programmes of action to aid in implementation (UNAIDS 2008). Importantly, the government has worked to improve the possibility for civil society participation in this process, recognising that such engagement, including that of people living with HIV, is key to an effective response. Efforts are nonetheless needed to ensure that civil society groups from remote areas and working on behalf of vulnerable populations are also well represented and supported. Despite these positive efforts, it remains the case that other policies exist that violate human rights; for example people from key populations, such as Minh, may be placed in "rehabilitation centres" against their will. Much national and global advocacy in this area gives hope that this practice will disappear in the coming years.

The application of human rights principles can help improve the design, implementation, monitoring, and evaluation of HIV policies and programmes, including what issues are prioritised and how, at different stages of programming. In general, work in this category refers to the inclusion of human rights components within programmatic initiatives—specifically, ensuring attention to the participation of affected communities; ensuring that discrimination is not occurring in the implementation of the programme; considering the broad range of laws and policies that could support or impede the programme (for example, laws that criminalise same-sex sexual activity may impede access to relevant services out of fear of being reported to the police) (Gruskin and Ferguson 2009); and ensuring transparency in how priorities are set and decisions made, as well as accountability for the results. Often, these efforts are carried out with the support of large international organisations, including intergovernmental and non-governmental entities.[6]

Attention to the right to health raises issues related not just to accessibility but also to the availability, acceptability, and quality of treatment services. Unless individuals can reach the services they need, afford them, and feel comfortable using them, uptake and long-term engagement will remain limited. Systematically focusing on what it takes to make services truly available, accessible, acceptable, and of quality—and, in doing so, paying specific attention to the human rights principles of interdependence, participation, non-discrimination, and accountability—may provide the key to achieving universal access to treatment. In addition, application of the right to health requires attention to processes and not just outcomes. For example, in relation to availability, a specific issue to be considered in this regard is the process by which policy makers determine which population groups will be the first to access new drugs when they become available. The need to pay more attention to such issues in relation to access to treatment is apparent in Vietnam, where the percentage of adults and children with advanced HIV infection receiving antiretrovirals was approximately 28.4% in 2007 and remains low to this day (UNAIDS 2008, p. 2). Concerns remain about the sustainability of access even where it does exist, given changing donor priorities, the mobility of populations, and persistent stigma and discrimination.

This section outlined ways in which the human rights framework is being used in HIV-related work.[7] The categorisations above provide a broad way of describing how human rights principles are conceptualised and applied to HIV. Each framework suggests a different but equally valid conceptualisation of human rights norms and standards that requires different tools and approaches for implementation and assessment.

THE HIV RESPONSE: CROSS-CUTTING ISSUES

Thus far we have shown that a rights-based response at many levels is necessary before Minh is likely to seek an HIV test and utilise available services. As stressed in this chapter, the tremendous burden of HIV and its continuously changing dynamics necessitates a response that includes prevention, treatment, and care. This section brings these pieces together and considers how human rights can be used to both highlight concerns and provide a framework to improve the response.

STIGMA AND DISCRIMINATION

Minh's case highlights the existence of factors beyond availability and accessibility that impede him and his wife from choosing to undergo an HIV test. In response to the stigma and discrimination that individuals face on multiple levels, a number of efforts have focused on advocating around specific human rights issues, such as confidentiality, informed consent, access to education and information, and reduction of the stigma and discrimination occurring at the hands of providers and communities. Discrimination in institutions, policies, and programmes also need to be addressed—for example, children who are prevented from attending school and policies that force mandatory testing of couples prior to marriage. Human rights norms and standards have been applied to address the issue of provider attitudes, for example. In addition, they have been used to advocate for both changing current non-discrimination laws and developing new ones. Instrumentally, human rights have been used in efforts to construct stigma and discrimination indicators for use in advocacy and HIV programming (Gruskin and Ferguson 2009).

VULNERABLE POPULATIONS

Minh's drug use increases his vulnerability to HIV. Even in communities where HIV has not spread widely, some individuals—such as injecting drug users—may be more vulnerable to infection than others (Gruskin and Tarantola 2008). Vulnerability in the context of HIV includes limitations on the ability of individuals and communities to minimise or modulate their risk of exposure to HIV infection and, once infected, to receive adequate care and support. Depending on the setting, vulnerable groups can include women and young people, pregnant women, injecting drug users, sex workers, men who have sex with men, prisoners, mobile populations, and uniformed personnel, among others. Attention to vulnerable populations in the HIV response is recognised as a key consideration from a human rights and public heath perspective. Realising the rights of marginalised groups also fulfils governmental obligations towards disenfranchised individuals. Arguments are also made that attention to vulnerable groups in prevention, treatment, and care efforts leads to a better response and containment of HIV (Mechanic and Tanner 2007).

INVOLVEMENT OF PEOPLE LIVING WITH HIV AND AIDS

Advocacy by Minh or other people within his community who use drugs and are living with HIV will likely lead to policies and programmes that are more responsive to their needs. Recognition of the importance of the participation of individuals living with HIV in designing and implementing the policies and programmes that concern them resulted in recognition by the international community of the now widely cited "greater involvement of people living with AIDS (GIPA) principle" (UNAIDS 1999). The GIPA principle, formally adopted by forty-two countries at the 1994 Paris AIDS Summit, was endorsed by UN member states as part of the 2001 Declaration of Commitment on HIV/AIDS.[8] The principle incorporates a human rights perspective by advocating for the meaningful participation of people living with HIV in all aspects of the HIV response. This emphasis on meaningful participation implies the need for equity and transparency, broad represen-tation and access to adequate resources, shared ownership and responsibility while simultaneously maintaining independence, and access to information and technical support to enable full participation. Much progress has been made in involving civil society in research, advocacy, and programming efforts in the HIV response at the international, regional, national, and local levels. The Global Network of People Living with HIV and the International Community of Women Living with HIV/AIDS are two examples of global networks whose primary objective is to ensure the meaningful participation of people living with HIV in the AIDS response. A review of countries' UNGASS reporting in 2010 showed significant involvement of people living with HIV (Peersman et al. 2009). Despite this progress, there are still extreme social, political, legal, and economic barriers to achieving GIPA in a meaningful way. Persistent stigma and discrimination, token representation in political processes, and lack of resources and capacity continue to challenge successful operationalisation of the principle. While Vietnam has seen a dramatic increase in the number of community networks and organisations of people living with HIV in recent years, these groups' capacity to influence governmental action remains limited.

GENDER-BASED VIOLENCE

Prevention strategies need to include explicit efforts to address gender-based violence. Considering the details of the case, one can wonder about the nature of Minh and Hang's relationship. Several studies show that violence against women is prevalent in Vietnam (Taft, Small, and Hoang 2008; Vung, Ostergren, and Krantz 2008). The reasons for this are many: gender inequality, social and economic stresses, and, as noted earlier, in some cases a woman and/or her partner's HIV status. In the past few years, there has been increasing collaboration between civil society organisations working on HIV and those working on violence against women in Hanoi; these organisations have collaborated to address these dual epidemics by integrating services, building skills and strategies, and focusing on vulnerable women who suffer from violence and HIV (Nguyen et al. 2006). However, Hang's access to such services will be limited if she lives outside the capital city. Thus, efforts to strengthen these initiatives across the country are needed.

ORPHAN AND VULNERABLE CHILDREN

What concerns should we have for Minh and Hang's two children? Children's vulnerability in the context of HIV results from a range political, economic, social, and cultural factors. This vulnerability can leave children, and their families, without the support necessary to cope with the impact of HIV. Vulnerability is heightened for children "living in refugee and internally displaced persons camps, children in detention, children living in institutions, as well as children living in extreme poverty, children living in situations of armed conflict, child soldiers, economically and sexually exploited children, and disabled, migrant, minority, indigenous, and street children."[9] Children orphaned by AIDS and children from affected families, including child-headed households, require special consideration. General Comment 3 on HIV/AIDS and the rights of the child, issued by the UN Committee on the Rights of the Child, states that "for children from families affected by HIV/AIDS, the stigmatisation and social isolation they experience may be accentuated by the neglect or violation of their rights, in particular discrimination resulting in a decrease or loss of access to education, health and social services."[10] In addition, the right to an identity, while always critical, has taken on increasing importance as children orphaned by AIDS require proof of their identity in order to exercise their rights to inheritance, to education, and to have access to other social and health services. This requires increased attention to children's legal protection both at the national level and through international mechanisms. While these issues are not considered of major concern in a country like Vietnam, where the epidemic is concentrated and the numbers are small, for affected children—potentially Minh and Hang's children, for example—they can have enormous consequences and must be addressed despite limited legal, policy, and programmatic support.

HEALTH SYSTEM CAPACITY

If Minh and Hang decide to seek an HIV test, this decision will mark the beginning of their engagement with the health system with respect to HIV-related issues. The presence of a health-care system with the capacity to scale up testing and treatment and to sustain access is a growing challenge that raises a host of human rights concerns. The incorporation of human rights elements into health systems strengthening can help address the underlying causes and inequities that lead to poor health systems performance (see chapter 4). In addition, attention to human rights can support implementation of the GIPA principle within health system strengthening and reform efforts; the full participation of affected communities in all aspects of health systems development is vital to the long-term success of the HIV response. There is also a need to focus on the myriad interactions between gender, race, and sexuality discrimination, among others, as they affect access to and use of HIV services. Even when services are scaled up, unless individuals can reach the services, can afford to access them, and feel comfortable using them, uptake and long-term engagement will remain limited. Human rights can provide norms and standards to assess the availability, accessibility, acceptability, and quality of HIV services for all sectors of a population, including those most difficult to reach. Finally, human rights direct attention to the accountability of policy makers and other decision makers for ensuring that their commitments to HIV prevention, treatment, and care remain at the forefront of any health systems strengthening efforts (see chapter 1).

CONCLUSION AND FUTURE CONSIDERATIONS

The current global framework for addressing HIV prevention, treatment, and care is based on the 2006 UN General Assembly resolution on universal access.[11] This framework is intended to address the response to HIV by "scaling up HIV prevention, treatment, care and support with the aim of coming as close to possible to the goal of universal access to treatment by 2010 for all those who need it."[12] The MDG targets related to HIV are set for review in 2015. To meet the goals of universal access and the broader development agenda of the MDGs requires continued attention to human rights through advocacy, legal, and programming efforts in all aspects of the response. Incorporating a human rights framework is not without its challenges, however. Discussed below are some of these challenges: the current lack of evidence attesting to the positive impacts of a human rights approach, scepticism around the value-added of a human rights framework, and the politics surrounding the response to the epidemic.

EVIDENCE

Sceptics from various disciplines—including epidemiological, social, and legal—cite the lack of evidence and documentation that demonstrates the value of integrating human rights in the response to HIV. Despite the pervasive use of indicators in monitoring the HIV response, indicators that specifically capture human rights concerns are not well developed, and those that exist are inconsistently used (Gruskin and Ferguson 2009). The National Composite Policy Index (NCPI), which countries report on as part of their reporting under the DoC, is one tool intended to capture specific human rights concerns. For example, the NCPI asks governments whether human rights monitoring and enforcement mechanisms exist within their countries, as well as whether countries have a mechanism to record, document, and address cases of discrimination experienced by people living with HIV. However, the NCPI does not capture implementation of existing laws, nor does it deal with the complete range of human rights issues relevant to national HIV responses. In addition, debates persist over what is meant by "evidence" and the extent to which policy decisions must therefore be "evidence-based" rather than "evidence-informed." There also remains disagreement over what is required to ensure that evidence is considered reliable and valid in both human rights and public health terms. To generate evidence requires rights-sensitive indicators that show progress and that demonstrate disparities and gaps within countries and globally; and the process of measurement matters as much as the data collected. Rights-sensitive indicators can show the extent to which governments and other entities are meeting their HIV-related human rights obligations, highlight areas where further efforts might lead to increased fulfilment of these obligations and, by extension, improve HIV outcomes. Indicators that genuinely capture both HIV and human rights concerns will ultimately help determine whether policies and programmes that are the most effective in health terms are also those that achieve the greatest level of compliance with human rights principles.

MISCONCEPTIONS OF WHAT HUMAN RIGHTS MEAN FOR THE AIDS RESPONSE

While there is general consensus on the value-added of incorporating a human rights framework into the HIV response, advocates in recent decades continue to encounter certain forms of resistance, usually arising from a lack of understanding of human rights principles combined with outright scepticism of the importance of human rights for achieving positive outcomes. The lack of general understanding of human rights (e.g., what they include, what they do not, and how they operate) is an impediment to successful incorporation of human rights into HIV work. Public health experts often misunderstand how human rights can be integrated into public health efforts, sometimes even suggesting that the two approaches are not in alignment regarding HIV prevention, treatment, and care. This tension threatens to dissipate the aims of human rights and public health experts attempting to reach common goals in the AIDS response. The human rights community must address this challenge by working to clarify concepts, simplify language, and collaborate with other sectors to raise awareness.

POLITICS

Global- and national-level politics greatly influence HIV policy and programme development and implementation. The political climate globally and within countries, the ongoing lack of awareness (or interest) in the epidemic among high-profile officials in many countries, and the extent to which HIV policy is driven by political or ideological beliefs all affect the extent to which governments commit to addressing human rights and HIV. In addition, there have been increasing calls, both globally and nationally, to redirect resources and efforts to other "more urgent" public health issues and to abandon "AIDS exceptionalism" in favour of a more medical model, which would thereby "normalise" the disease (De Cock and Johnson 1998). As global initiatives threaten to move increasingly in this direction, caution must be taken to ensure that human rights concerns are addressed and that effective approaches to addressing HIV prevention, treatment, and care are not lost.

CONCLUSION

The aim of this chapter has been threefold: to outline the approaches being used to respond to HIV and their human rights implications; to discuss how human rights have been used to address HIV and explore ways to move this approach forward; and to describe some of the key challenges for human rights in the HIV response. Very broadly, there is wide consensus on the value of human rights to the HIV response. What is meant by human rights and how their value is transferred to policy and programming, however, remain variable and inconsistent. Future efforts in Vietnam and around the world should systematically employ human rights tools and methods in order to ensure that human rights are respected in the HIV response. Using human rights principles to define the boundaries of health systems and their response to the disease can ultimately help ensure improvements in HIV prevalence, treatment outcomes, and quality of life.

REFERENCES

Ball A., G. Weiler, M. Beg, et al. 2005. "Evidence for Action: A Critical Tool for Guiding Policies and Programmes for HIV Prevention, Treatment and Care among Injecting Drug Users." *International Journal of Drug Policy* 16S:S1–S6.

Bartlett, J. G., B. M. Branson, K. Fenton, et al. 2008. "Opt-Out Testing for Human Immunodeficiency Virus in the United States: Progress and Challenges." *Journal of the American Medical Association* 300 (8): 945–951.

Beckwith, C., T. Flanigan, C. del Rio, et al. 2005. "It Is Time to Implement Routine, Not Risk-Based, HIV Testing." *Clinical Infectious Diseases* 40 (7): 1037–1040.

Berer, M. 2003. "Integration of Sexual and Reproductive Health Services: A Health Sector Priority." *Reproductive Health Matters* 11 (21): 6–15.

Braveman, P., and S. Gruskin. 2003. "Poverty, Equity, Human Rights and Health." *Bulletin of the World Health Organization* 81 (7): 539–545.

Brickley, D., D. Hanh, L. Nguyet, et al. 2008. " Community, Family, and Partner-Related Stigma Experienced by Pregnant and Postpartum Women with HIV in Ho Chi Minh City, Vietnam." *AIDS and Behavior* 13:1197–1204.

Carrasco, E. 2000. "Access to Treatment as a Right to Life and Health." *HIV/AIDS Policy and Law Review* 5 (4): 102–103.

De Cock, K., and A. Johnson. 1998. "From Exceptionalism to normalisation: a reappraisal of attitudes and practice around HIV testing." *British Medical Journal* 316:290.

Friedman, S., and S. Mottiar. 2005. "A Rewarding Engagement? The Treatment Action Campaign and the Politics of HIV/AIDS." *Politics and Society* 33 (4): 511–565

Gruskin S., S. Ahmed, and L. Ferguson. 2007. "Provider-Initiated HIV Testing and Counseling in Health Facilities: What Does This Mean for the Health and Human Rights of Pregnant Women?" *Developing World Bioethics* 8 (1): 23–32.

Gruskin, S., and L. Ferguson. 2009. "Using Indicators to Determine the Contribution of Human Rights to Public Health Efforts." *Bulletin of the World Health Organization* 87 (9): 714–719.

Gruskin S., L. Ferguson, and D. Bogecho. 2007. "Beyond the Numbers: Using Rights-Based Perspectives to Enhance Antiretroviral Treatment Scale-Up." *AIDS* 21 (suppl. 5): S13–S19.

Gruskin, S., E. Mills, and D. Tarantola. 2007. "History, Principles, and Practice of Health and Human Rights." *The Lancet* 370 (9585): 449–455.

Gruskin, S., and D. Tarantola. 2008. "Universal Access to HIV Prevention, Treatment and Care: Assessing the Inclusion of Human Rights in International and National Strategic Plans." *AIDS* 22 (suppl. 2): S123–S132.

Guenter, D., J. Esparza, and R. Macklin. 2000. "Ethical Considerations in International HIV Vaccine Trials: Summary of a Consultative Process Conducted by the Joint United Nations Programme on HIV/AIDS (UNAIDS)." *Journal of Medical Ethics* 26 (1): 37–43.

Hammett, T., Z. Wu, T. Duc, et al. 2008. "Social Evils and Harm Reduction: The Evolving Policy Environment for Human Immunodeficiency Virus Prevention among Injection Drug Users in China and Vietnam." *Addiction* 103 (1): 137–145.

Institute of Medicine of the National Academies. 2006. *Preventing HIV Infection among Injecting Drug Users in High Risk Countries: An Assessment of the Evidence. Washington, DC: The National Academies Press.*

Institute for Social Development Studies. 2011. "Institute for Social Development Studies." Accessed 4 June 2011. http://www.isds.org.vn.

Kaplan, D., R. Feinstein, M. Fisher, et al. 2001. "Condom Use by Adolescents." *Pediatrics* 107 (6): 1463–1469.

Kippax, S. 2006. "A Public Health Dilemma: A Testing Question; Based on a Presentation at AIDS Impact Conference, Cape Town, 4–7 April 2005." *AIDS Care* 18 (3): 230–235.

Mechanic, D., and J. Tanner. 2007. "Vulnerable People, Groups and Populations: Societal View." *Health Affairs* 26 (5): 1220–1230.

Mounier-Jack, S., S. Nielsen, and R. J. Coker. 2008. "HIV Testing Strategies across European Countries." *HIV Medicine* 9 (suppl. 2): 13–19.

Nattrass, N. 2006. "South Africa's Rollout of Highly Active Antiretroviral Therapy: A Critical Assessment." *Journal of Acquired Immune Deficiency Syndromes* (43) 5: 618–623.

Nguyen, V. A. T., V. A. Nguyen, S. Ahmed, et al. 2006. "HIV/AIDS and Gender-Based Violence: Linking the Response at Programmatic Level in Vietnam." Poster presentation at the XVI International AIDS Conference, Toronto, Canada, 13–18 August 2006.

Peersman, G., L. Ferguson, M. Torres, et al. 2009. "Increasing Civil Society Participation in the National HIV Response: The Role of UNGASS Reporting." *Journal of Acquired Immune Deficiency Syndromes* 52 (suppl. 2): S97–S103.

Piot, P. 2006. "AIDS: From Crisis Management to Sustained Strategic Response." *The Lancet* 368 (9534): 526–530.

Piot, P., M. Bartos, H. Larson, et al. 2008. "Coming To Terms with Complexity: A Call to Action for HIV Prevention." *The Lancet* 372 (9641): 845–859.

Sheeran, P., C. Abraham, and S. Orbell. 1999. "Psychosocial Correlates of Heterosexual Condom Use: A Meta-Analysis." *Psychological Bulletin* 125 (1): 90–132.

Taft, A., R. Small, and K. Hoang. 2008. "Intimate Partner Violence in Vietnam and among Diaspora Communities in Western Societies: A Comprehensive Review." *Journal of Family Studies* 14 (2):167–182.

Tarantola, D., R. Macklin, Z. H. Reed, et al. 2007. "Ethical Considerations Related to the Provision of Care and Treatment in Vaccine Trials." *Vaccine* 25 (26): 4863–4874.

UNAIDS (Joint UN Programme on HIV/AIDS). 1999. *From Principle to Practice: Greater Involvement of People Living with or Affected by HIV/AIDS (GIPA).* UNAIDS Best Practice Collection. Geneva: UNAIDS.

—. 2001. *The Global Strategy Framework on HIV/AIDS.* Geneva: UNAIDS.

—. 2003. *Fact Sheet: Stigma and Discrimination.* Geneva: UNAIDS. http://data.unaids.org/publications/Fact-Sheets03/fs_stigma_ discrimination_en.pdf.

—. 2005. *Intensifying HIV Prevention: UNAIDS Policy Position Paper.* Geneva: UNAIDS.

—. 2006. *International Guidelines on HIV/AIDS and Human Rights.* Geneva: UNAIDS.

—. 2007a. "The Greater Involvement of People Living with or Affected by HIV/ AIDS (GIPA)." *UNAIDS Policy Brief.* March.

—. 2007b. *Monitoring the Declaration of Commitment on HIV/AIDS: Guidelines on the Construction of Core Indicators; 2008 Reporting.* Geneva: UNAIDS.

—. 2007c. *Practical Guidelines for Intensifying HIV Prevention: Towards Universal Access.* Geneva: UNAIDS.

—. 2008. *UNGASS Progress Report: Vietnam; January 2006–December 2007.* Hanoi: Government of Vietnam. http://www.unaids.org/en/dataanalysis/mo nitoringcountryprogress/2010progressreportssubmittedbycountries/2008p rogressreportssubmittedbycountries/viet_nam_2008_country_progress_ report_en.pdf.

—. 2009. *Position Statement: Condoms and HIV Prevention.* Geneva: UNAIDS. http://www.unaids.org/en/media/unaids/contentassets/dataimport/pub/ basedocument/2009/20090318_position_paper_condoms_en.pdf.

—. 2010a. *UNAIDS Report on the Global AIDS Epidemic.* Geneva: UNAIDS.

—. 2010b. *UNGASS Progress Report: Vietnam; January 2008–December 2009.* http://aidsdatahub.org/dmdocuments/New_vietnam_2010_country_ progress_report_edited.pdf. 2010b.

—. 2010c. *2011–2015 Strategy: Getting to Zero.* Geneva: UNAIDS.

UNAIDS (Joint UN Programme on HIV/AIDS) and WHO (World Health Organization). 2004. "UNAIDS/WHO Policy Statement on HIV Testing." June. http://data.unaids.org/una-docs/hivtestingpolicy_en.pdf.

Vung, N. D., P. Ostergren, and G. Krantz. 2008. "Intimate Partner Violence against Women in Rural Vietnam: Different Socio-Demographic Factors Are Associated with Different Forms of Violence; Need for New Intervention Guidelines?" *BMC Public Health* 8 (55): 1471–2458.

Wynia, M. K. 2006. "Routine Screening: Informed Consent, Stigma and the Waning of HIV Exceptionalism." *American Journal of Bioethics* 6 (4): 5–8.

NOTES

1 Declaration of Commitment on HIV/AIDS, Resolution adopted by the General Assembly, U.N. Doc. A/RES/S-26/2 (2001).

2 Law on HIV/AIDS Prevention and Control, No. 64/2006/QH11.

3 Declaration of Commitment on HIV/AIDS, *supra* note 1; Universal Access by 2010, http://www.unaids.org/en/aboutunaids/ universalaccesstohivtreatmentpreventioncareandsupport; Ministerial Statement, Asia Pacific Ministerial Meeting, declared in Melbourne, Australia, 9–10 October

2001; ASEAN Declaration on the Protection and Promotion of the Rights of Migrant Workers, declared in Cebu, Philippines, 13 January 2007.

4 International Covenant on Economic, Social and Cultural Rights, G.A. Res. 2200A (XXI), 21 U.N. GAOR Supp. (No. 16) at 49, U.N. Doc. A/6316 (1966), 993 U.N.T.S. 3, entered into force January 3, 1976; Convention on the Elimination of All Forms of Discrimination against Women, G.A. Res. 34/180, 34 U.N. GAOR Supp. (No. 46) at 193, U.N. Doc. A/34/46 (1979), entered into force September 3, 1981; Convention on the Rights of the Child, G.A. Res. 44/25, Annex, 44 U.N. GAOR Supp. (No. 49) at 167, U.N. Doc. A/44/49 (1989), entered into force September 2, 1990.

5 Law on HIV/AIDS Prevention and Control, No. 64/2006/QH11.

6 In addition to the inclusion of human rights norms within recent global consensus documents such as the UN General Assembly Special Session on AIDS, a large and growing number of national and international entities have formulated rights-based approaches to health in the context of their own efforts. Among these are several official development assistance organisations and agencies, funds, and UN programmes (e.g., UNAIDS, UNICEF, UNDP, UNFPA, the UK Department for International Development, the Canadian International Development Agency, and Swedish International Development Cooperation Agency).

7 Although bioethical frameworks are not explicitly incorporated into the discussion in this section, the long-standing collaborations between those working in bioethics and those working in human rights in relation to HIV has contributed to the analysis and discussion.

8 Declaration of Commitment on HIV/AIDS, *supra* note 1, para. 33.

9 Committee on the Rights of the Child, General Comment 3, U.N. Doc. CRC/GC/2003/3 (2003), para. 30.

10 Ibid., para. 31.

11 Preparations for and Organization of the 2006 Follow-Up Meeting on the Outcome of the Twenty-Sixth Special Session: Implementation of the Declaration of Commitment on HIV/AIDS, Resolution adopted by the General Assembly, U.N. Doc. A/RES/60/224 (2006).

12 Ibid., para. 12.

CHAPTER 8

Mental Disability

LANCE GABLE

CASE STUDY: ANNA, A WOMAN WITH SCHIZOPHRENIA IN A HIGH-INCOME COUNTRY

Anna is a twenty-five-year-old single woman living in a major metropolitan area in a high-income country. She developed the initial symptoms of schizophrenia in her early twenties. When the condition manifested itself, her behaviour patterns changed and she suffered episodes of paranoia and hallucinations. She was assessed and treated by a psychiatrist, who prescribed medication for her condition. She responded well to the medication, and, along with regular counselling, she was able to control her symptoms without significantly affecting her day-to-day functioning.

Initially, Anna did not reveal her mental health condition to others— she was concerned that because of the stigma that often surrounds mental health problems like schizophrenia, many people would not react well to this information. Eventually, though, she informed her parents and a close friend about her diagnosis. Her friend inadvertently revealed information about Anna's schizophrenia to some mutual acquaintances, and this information subsequently was revealed to her employer and landlord. Immediately upon learning about her condition, Anna's employer fired her, despite the fact that her job performance up to that point had been excellent. Similarly, Anna's landlord proceeded to evict her from her rented apartment, where she had been living independently for several years without incident. Anna reached out to several friends who had helped her in the past, seeking emotional support and a place to live temporarily, but these friends now refused to help her.

Some portions of this chapter are based on Gable and Gostin (2009). I would like to thank Ahmad Chehab, Kunle Fadipe, and David Standish for their able research assistance.

Without employment, income, or housing, Anna was forced to move back into her parents' home in a rural area of the country. While she would have liked to continue taking medication for her condition, the sparse health infrastructure in this rural location made accessing appropriate mental health services nearly impossible. In addition, the loss of her income undermined Anna's ability to pay for care even if she could have accessed it.

With Anna's mental health condition deteriorating due to lack of treatment, her parents initiated court proceedings to have her involuntarily committed to a psychiatric institution located in another part of the country. Anna objected to the civil commitment proceedings and requested that the court provide her with access to medication. However, based on the testimony of her parents, the court deemed Anna incompetent and confined her over her objections. The conditions in the psychiatric facility were unsafe and unsanitary.

Since being committed three years ago, Anna has suffered from multiple infections and injuries inflicted by other patients. Treatment regimens have been inconsistent. Her mental health condition has further deteriorated, and she is often kept under sedation. She has gained a significant amount of weight since being institutionalised and has developed diabetes. Since her parents live far away, she rarely receives visitors and is largely isolated from the outside world. The terms of Anna's confinement have not been reviewed since her admission to the facility.

INTRODUCTION

Anna and many millions of other people around the world are affected by mental health problems. Achieving good mental health presents one of the most important and compelling challenges for global public health and for the enjoyment of the right to health and other related human rights. Mental health morbidity is a pervasive global health concern, with upwards of 450 million people around the globe affected by mental, neurological, and behavioural health conditions (WHO 2001). Neuropsychiatric disorders are "the leading cause of disability in young people" aged ten to twenty-four years in every region worldwide (Gore et al. 2011). These conditions exist along a wide continuum, from severe psychological conditions like schizophrenia[1] and bipolar disorder[2] to less harmful—but still notable—conditions like mild depression (WHO 2007b). The medical, psychological, legal, and social consequences of these conditions resonate across society, influencing population health, social policy, and, indeed, all aspects of life. Thus, mental disorder and/or disability is a concern not only for persons with mental disabilities but for the population in general.[3]

The widespread health and social effects of mental disability support the connection between mental health and human rights. Human rights scholars have long recognised the close and complex relationship between health and human rights generally (Mann et al. 1994) and mental health and human rights in particular (Gostin and Gable 2004). The link between mental health and human rights can be demonstrated in a variety of ways. First, mental health policies and practices may violate human rights, especially when state powers and systemic practices are used arbitrarily or discriminatorily to restrain persons with mental disabilities, deprive them of basic citizenship rights, or functionally impede their access to needed services and opportunities. Second, human rights violations can undermine mental health. The negative mental health implications imposed by severe human rights abuses like torture, systematic rape, and inhuman and degrading treatment are readily apparent; but even less serious human rights violations like discrimination and invasion of privacy can have enduring and damaging effects on mental health. Third, mental health and human rights are inextricably linked in a mutually reinforcing and synergistic manner. A modicum of mental health functioning is integral to engaging in political and social activities within society and to enjoying the benefits of other human rights (Gostin 2001). Recognition and support of human rights likewise provides a context within which mental well-being can flourish (Gostin and Gable 2004).

Numerous international human rights documents recognise mental health as a core component of the right to health, including the Constitution of the World Health Organization (WHO), the Universal Declaration of Human Rights, and the International Covenant on Economic, Social and Cultural Rights (ICESCR).[4] The right to mental health receives protection in the Convention on the Rights of the Child and the Convention on the Rights of Persons with Disabilities (CRPD) as well.[5] Taken together, these international instruments—along with interpretive documents, such as General Comment 14 of the UN Committee on Economic, Social and Cultural Rights (ESCR Committee) and reports issued by UN Special Rapporteurs on the Right to Health—affirm that health is a fundamental human right and that mental health comprises an integral component of overall health and well-being (Hunt 2003a, 2003b).[6] The right to health, as formulated in international human rights instruments, necessarily and clearly encompasses both physical and mental health. The relationship between rights in these international instruments suggests an additional, but equally important, conclusion: that attainment of good mental health requires the protection of the full range of human rights and that human rights themselves are interconnected. Attaining the right to health cannot occur without contemplating and upholding other related human rights (see chapter 1).

Unfortunately, the strong textual support for a right to mental health in international law and jurisprudence has not translated into consistent recognition of this right in national laws or the meaningful diminution of human rights violations affecting persons with mental and intellectual disabilities in many parts of the world.[7] Paul Hunt, former Special Rapporteur on the Right to Health, has recognised mental health as "among the most grossly neglected elements of the right to health."[8] Persons living with mental disabilities frequently confront daunting medical, legal, and social impediments to full participation in society, including discrimination, stigmatisation, disrespect, and misguided fear of persons with mental health disabilities by others. Furthermore, mental disabilities occur more frequently in poor populations and often disproportionately affect women, children, and other already disempowered groups (WHO 2003). The common convergence of mental disability with other indicators of vulnerability is particularly troubling.

Sustained political and social support for the recognition of a right to mental health remains elusive and thus undermines the attainment of human rights. In political prioritisation, the rights of persons with mental disabilities—including the rights to health, liberty, autonomy, equal treatment under the law, civic participation, education, work, and social security—are, at best, an afterthought. Politicians and policy makers often overlook the concerns of persons living with mental disabilities and in some instances actively undermine them for purposes of political expediency. This is particularly true for the approximately twenty-five million people globally who have schizophrenia (WHO 2003). Recurrent human rights violations and political inattention intensify the burden of schizophrenia and other mental disabilities throughout the population, affecting the opportunities of persons with mental disabilities to access mental health services and to live free from stigma and discrimination.[9]

MEDICAL/PUBLIC HEALTH ASPECTS

While both biological and social factors affect the onset and ongoing manifestation of all mental health disabilities, Anna's mental health condition arose independently of any specific, identifiable external stimuli. However, once her symptoms appeared, the medical and public health systems in her community and country failed to provide the support and treatment that she needed. As the following discussion demonstrates, these failures arose from both the medical and social complexities of schizophrenia and the inadequacy of health, social, and legal systems to address the needs of people in Anna's situation. This section addresses several medical and public health issues that affect mental health rights: the medical and socio-economic factors involved in accessing mental health care; the impact of both medical advances and deinstitutionalisation on medical and public health systems; and mental health care provided in community and institutional settings.

MEDICAL AND SOCIO-ECONOMIC FACTORS IN ACCESSING MENTAL HEALTH CARE

People affected by schizophrenia, like Anna, experience symptoms that can distort perceptions and thought processes and impair some types of functioning. Left untreated, these symptoms can be extremely debilitating and may result in self harm. Data suggest that despite the serious effects of the condition, approximately one-third of those with schizophrenia can recover completely with appropriate treatment. Even among individuals with chronic schizophrenia, with the assistance of medical and psychosocial treatment only about one in five encounter ongoing, serious effects to their daily activities (WHO 2001).

People with mental disabilities frequently face additional health challenges due to the simultaneous presence of more than one mental health condition or comorbidity between mental and physical health problems. Conditions like depression (more than 150 million people) and substance abuse (90 million people) comprise the most prevalent mental disabilities worldwide (WHO 2003). Often, these other mental health conditions simultaneously affect people with schizophrenia (WHO 2001). In particular, substance abuse is common among people with schizophrenia (Koyanagi 2004). Studies have demonstrated that people with serious mental disabilities generally and people with schizophrenia in particular suffer from debilitating physical health problems at a higher rate than the general population (Prince et al. 2007). Anna's significant weight gain after her institutionalisation may be attributable to insufficient physical exercise or her long-term use of anti-psychotic medications. The combination of risk factors such as high rates of smoking and obesity, infrequent opportunities for physical exercise, and recognised side effects of anti-psychotic medications render people with schizophrenia more susceptible to heart disease, cancer, diabetes, and other health problems (Koyanagi 2004). Governments must ensure that psychiatric institutions maintain adequate living standards that allow residents to live safely and in good health, rather than exacerbating their mental and physical health problems.

Social and economic determinants also significantly affect the ability of persons with mental disabilities to access mental health care. Anna's precarious economic and social position certainly contributed to her inability to maintain access to treatment when she lost her job, housing, and social support.[10] Mental health problems often coincide with other attributes of vulnerability, rendering persons with mental and intellectual disabilities especially susceptible to human rights abuses. Studies have demonstrated association between low socio-economic status, high prevalence of mental disabilities, and difficulty in accessing and maintaining treatment (Andrade et al. 2000; Lorant et al. 2003; Muntaner et al. 1998; Weich and Lewis 1998).

THE IMPACT OF TREATMENT ADVANCES AND DEINSTITUTIONALISATION

The development of more effective psychotropic medications in the 1960s revolutionised treatment options for persons with severe psychiatric conditions (like schizophrenia) and prompted changes to mental health systems that greatly affect mental health care and human rights. Prior to these discoveries, treatment options for schizophrenic patients such as Anna were limited and available only through institutional care. The introduction of these newer treatments had two immediate effects. First, the new medications more successfully controlled symptoms. Second, the availability and accessibility of these treatments spurred the deinstitutionalisation movement, enabling thousands of people with severe mental disabilities to receive treatment within their communities instead of in institutional settings. Governments had an additional incentive to strongly support deinstitutionalisation: resources previously designated for expensive psychiatric institutions could be directed towards other purposes (Frank and Glied 2006).

These changes had monumental effects on the structure and orientation of mental health systems in high-income countries, stemming primarily from substantial decreases in the numbers of patients confined to psychiatric institutions and a concomitant reduction in the capacity of these institutions. Nevertheless, the promise of more effective treatments and greater freedom embodied by the deinstitutionalisation movement never fully materialised. As Anna's case demonstrates, while many former patients were literally able to escape from the shackles of institutional confinement and live freely— and in better health—in the community, others faltered due to inadequate support for community mental health programmes and structural barriers that impeded access to necessary medications in the community setting.

The mixed success of deinstitutionalisation has medical and public health connotations. From a medical perspective, the new psychiatric medicines successfully relieved the symptoms of schizophrenia and other serious psychiatric conditions, and had fewer side effects than some earlier medications. However, when taken in high doses over long periods, these newer medications also produced significant side effects, such as increases in obesity linked to higher rates of diabetes and heart disease (Foley and Morley 2011; Hennekens 2007) and tardive dyskinesia, a debilitating neurological condition that causes uncontrollable tics and shaking (Leucht et al. 2003; Owens, Johnstone, and Frith 1982).

From a public health systems perspective, efforts to implement community mental health care and treatment have rarely received sufficient organisational, economic, or political support (Bazelon 1975; Burt 2001). Effective treatment with pharmaceuticals in the community requires a robust infrastructure to ensure that medications and other support services are available and affordable. Many countries have not created community mental health systems to support persons who have been deinstitutionalised or who are newly in need of mental health services. Even in jurisdictions with established community services, these services often have remained chronically underfunded, fragmented, and punitive (Miller 2006). Such systemic deficiencies might have contributed to the difficulties faced by Anna in accessing services in the community.

Although Anna, who lives in a high-income country, suffered serious human rights violations related to her mental disability, it is important to recognise that persons with schizophrenia in low-income and middle-income countries may face even more impediments to obtaining mental health services. Mental health services may be extremely hard to access in these countries due to the relative lack of infrastructure, trained mental health professionals, or access to medications (Bartlett 2010). Moreover, in low-income and middle-income countries, these services, when available, often are provided in more expensive centralised institutional settings instead of in the community (Saraceno et al. 2007). These countries may also continue to rely on older medications to treat schizophrenia and other mental health conditions (Patel et al. 2007).

MEDICAL AND PUBLIC HEALTH ASPECTS OF COMMUNITY-BASED MENTAL HEALTH SERVICES

Anna has a serious psychiatric condition, but fortunately it is one that can be treated in the community with medication and supportive services. Her inability to successfully access necessary mental health services in the community represents a failure of her country's medical and public health systems. It also represents a violation of the ICESCR and CRPD, which obligate governments to recognise the rights of persons with disabilities to live and work independently in the community and to have access to health services.[11] Persons with mental disabilities face a number of systemic impediments to access, including inadequate mental health infrastructure (not enough facilities, professionals, or resources); inability to pay for services (expensive care and lack of insurance coverage); insufficient access to information; perpetuation of negative social attitudes towards mental health treatment and people with mental disabilities; and legal barriers.

The failure of many countries and communities to create community-based mental health systems stems from a number of factors. The political powerlessness of persons with mental disabilities may preclude their ability to effectively advocate for sufficient services. Mental health services are often not given high priority in the development of health systems, based on the perception that such services are non-essential. Despite ample evidence demonstrating the close connection between physical and mental health outcomes, public health and health-care resources typically flow to services addressing physical health conditions (Jacob et al. 2007).

Community treatment of mental health conditions like schizophrenia can be resource intensive, and their expense affects policy decisions and access to services in several ways. First, the cost of mental health treatment can be high and therefore out of reach for many people. Insurance coverage, whether public or private, may exclude mental health care or provide only limited coverage. Anna's inability to afford her medications and treatment after losing her income narrowed her options for care outside an institutional setting. Second, mental health treatment often requires more than just medication. Components such as counselling and other support services may involve frequent interaction between people with mental disabilities and trained professionals. In addition to their cost, these professionals are often in short supply. The negligible health infrastructure in her parents' rural region constrained Anna's options for community services. Third, the chronic nature of many mental health conditions demands long-term treatment and support plans, which may impose cost obligations for patients, governments, and health systems over time. Despite these limitations, however, community-based mental health services are less costly than institutional mental health care and more consistent with individual liberty for persons with mental disabilities (Saraceno et al. 2007). These factors created a vicious cycle for Anna: without sufficient economic resources and health system infrastructure at her disposal, she was unable to obtain her needed medications; and without the medications, her mental health worsened, thereby making it more difficult for her to work and make money to fund her own care.

Given these realities, if Anna were living in a low- or middle-income country, her chances of enjoying access to community-based mental health services would be vanishingly small. In fact, even in the high-income country where Anna lives, the likelihood of her being able to access adequate mental health services in the community remains low, given the marginal political and economic priority typically given to such services.

Each of these barriers to accessing mental health treatment and supportive services can be overcome by strengthening health systems to include these services. In order for countries' health systems to be consistent with human rights norms of individual liberty and community care, these services should be available in the community rather than in institutional settings.[12] Thus, governments are obligated to develop health systems that can provide community-based mental health services to people, like Anna, who have treatable mental health conditions, and they are also obligated to fund these systems adequately (see chapter 4).

MEDICAL AND PUBLIC HEALTH ASPECTS OF INSTITUTIONAL MENTAL HEALTH SERVICES

Once confined to an institutional setting, Anna's access to appropriate treatment did not necessarily improve. Institutional settings in many countries do not meet professional standards of care for mental health treatment, nor do they uphold minimum standards of sanitation and safety. Countries often retain institutional mental health facilities in lieu of community mental health services due to inertia, entrenched interests, and other political impediments (Saraceno et al. 2007). Many psychiatric institutions, like the one that housed Anna, fail to provide necessary mental health care, use sedatives for patient management, inadequately train staff, and are in squalid condition (Mental Disability Rights International 2000, 2004, 2005). These problems are systemic problems that are the by-products of neglect, misprioritisation, and disregard for the humanity of institutionalised persons with mental disabilities. Anna's physical and mental health worsened under these deplorable conditions, which violate standards of ethics and human rights.

ETHICAL AND LEGAL PERSPECTIVES

ETHICAL DILEMMAS AND CONCERNS

A number of ethical concerns arise from this case study. Societal prejudices against persons with mental disabilities contributed considerably to the circumstances that led to Anna's firing, eviction, social ostracism, and eventual institutionalisation. The perpetuation of social stigma against persons with schizophrenia across all levels of society—whether through governmental policy decisions; the actions of Anna's employer, landlord, friends, and family; or the court ruling that led to her confinement—has ethically problematic consequences. Stigma, fear, and misperceptions fuel punitive and unjust policies and practices towards persons with mental disabilities. These factors effectively impeded Anna's access to needed health services and her full participation in society. Health systems often perpetuate these damaging social norms. These policies, practices, and behaviours may transgress core ethical principles of autonomy, beneficence, justice, and solidarity, as well as human rights legal obligations, such as the rights to liberty, autonomy, fair procedures, full participation in society, health, education, work, and social security. It is notable that many of the practices that violate ethical norms also contravene legal and human rights principles.

The ethical principle of autonomy supports individual liberty (access to treatment without confinement unless the person poses a danger to self or others, and ability to make decisions about one's life and to fully participate in all areas of life) and bodily integrity (avoiding involuntary treatment and granting informed consent prior to treatment). Since Anna did not appear to be a danger to herself or others, and since she remained competent to make life decisions when using her medication, imposing serious restrictions on her liberty through involuntary confinement over her explicit objection undermined her autonomy and violated several human rights and fundamental freedoms protected under international and regional human rights treaties. Furthermore, her autonomy was constrained indirectly as a result of systemic deficiencies that prevented her from accessing mental health treatment in the community, thus denying Anna successful treatment outside of an institutional setting and the full enjoyment of the right to physical and mental health care.

The ethical concept of beneficence demands efforts that affirmatively seek to improve the well-being of others. In this context, beneficence would oblige the government, and members of society more generally, to take steps to assist Anna to live with her schizophrenia, whether through bolstering access and support within health systems or removing impediments in these systems to achieving good mental health. Many economic, social, and cultural rights contained in international human rights treaties advance beneficent goals (Gostin 2001).

Ethical notions of justice require fair treatment of all people, including those people living with a mental disability, across all areas of life. Satisfying this principle may involve providing procedural protections against civil commitment and involuntary treatment, eliminating discriminatory practices targeting persons with mental disabilities, allocating adequate economic expenditures for necessary health and social services, and supporting the development of health, social, and legal systems conducive to improving mental health. As discussed below, the principle of justice is applied to governmental action through international human rights norms and national legal obligations prohibiting discrimination, requiring fair procedural protections, and mandating standards allowing full and equal participation in all areas of life.

Several insidious myths about persons with mental and intellectual disabilities continue to undercut these ethical considerations, in the process hampering efforts to reduce stigma and discrimination and complicating initiatives to cultivate political support for mental health services (Gable and Gostin 2008). Negative stereotypes grounded in these myths—and the misperceptions they create—are difficult to dispel and have dominated the public discourse surrounding mental disability (Pescosolido et al. 1999). Anna and others like her lack political power and do not have a well-organised and vocal constituency to combat these perceptions (Gable and Gostin 2009).

One such myth, the myth of incompetency, stems from the false assumption that persons with mental disabilities lack the competence to make decisions or grant consent. In fact, symptoms of mental disabilities vary over time and differ according to type and individual manifestation, yielding a continuum of competency. Along this continuum, some mentally disabled people lack competency, others have limited incapacity, and still others retain full competency. In our case, Anna seemed quite competent while taking her medications. Policies that presume automatic or permanent incompetency for mentally disabled individuals—or that fail to assess individually a person's competency with regard to specific services, decisions, or functions—violate human rights and the ethical principles of autonomy and justice. Anna's right to mental health was undermined when she was inappropriately denied the ability to make health-related decisions. Her subsequent confinement without periodic reassessment of her mental health provides an additional example of how the myth of incompetency can lead to onerous and potentially unwarranted restrictions on liberty and autonomy. Legal regimes should ensure periodic review of all involuntary confinement and utilise the least restrictive alternatives available (Gostin and Gable 2004).

The myth of incompetency also affected Anna's interactions with her employer, her parents, and the court. Anna's dismissal from her job was likely grounded in part in her employer's misconception that Anna could no longer competently perform her job while suffering from schizophrenia. In reality, many people with this condition and other mental health conditions function very effectively in all areas of life, provided they have access to treatment and support (Bowie et al. 2006). The employer's actions reflect stigma and animus towards Anna, which undercut her autonomy to work and make a living. With regard to her parents, it is possible that in facilitating her institutionalisation, they believed themselves to be protecting her best interests. However, they also may have had other motivations related to not wanting to bear the economic and personal burdens of assisting their daughter in dealing with the symptoms and effects of schizophrenia. Their conclusions may have been further influenced by their own misperceptions about Anna's capacity and potential to harm herself or others. Finally, the court's finding that Anna was not competent to contest her confinement also presumes, without apparent evidence beyond her parents' assertions about her condition, that Anna could not grant consent due to her condition. This determination further denied Anna her autonomous desire to avoid confinement and subjected her to legal proceedings that violated her rights to liberty, autonomy, and fair process, as guaranteed under international human rights law.

Additional myths attached to mental disability are the myth of dangerousness and the competing myths of institutionalisation and deinstitutionalisation. The myth of dangerousness inaccurately presumes that people with serious mental disabilities such as schizophrenia pose a substantial threat to themselves or others. Yet numerous studies, described in more detail below, have debunked this notion. Anna's eviction from her apartment was likely predicated on stereotypical assumptions about the effect of her schizophrenia on the safety and well-being of herself and others. Her subsequent civil commitment also may reflect these presumptions, as the court may have falsely assumed—based solely on her medical diagnosis—that she posed a threat.

The myth of institutionalisation, building on the myths of incapacity and dangerousness, concludes that institutions provide an appropriate setting for anyone with a serious mental health problem. While institutionalisation is necessary for some patients, most people with mental health problems—even serious conditions like schizophrenia—can live in the community as long as they can access appropriate treatment. Prolonged civil commitment often arises from a further facet of this myth—namely, the tendency to assume that once an individual is committed, that individual should remain institutionalised indefinitely. Since competency can improve over time, especially with treatment, institutionalisation without procedures for periodic review, as in the case of Anna, violate human rights norms and ethical principles of autonomy. Additionally, the institutional setting potentially can give rise to tensions between the ethical principles of autonomy and beneficence, since the goal of institutional care is putatively treatment for the benefit of the patient, even though it limits the patient's autonomy.

The related myth surrounding the effects of deinstitutionalisation, discussed above, is predicated on the idea that the process of deinstitutionalisation, which greatly enhanced liberty for many previously institutionalised individuals, was sufficient for states to meet their ethical and human rights obligations regarding people with mental disabilities. Ethical notions of beneficence and justice, however, suggest that additional effort is needed to ensure that community mental health services are available to those who need them, especially since many of those in need are already vulnerable because of their mental health and other factors. One outcome of deinstitutionalisation has been a surge in the number of mentally disabled people either rendered homeless without any access to health services or reinstitutionalised in jails, prisons, remand centres, and nursing homes where appropriate treatment may not be available (Grob 1992; Langle et al. 2005). In many countries around the world, prisons have become the de facto mental health system, leaving this population isolated, forgotten, and deprived of its human rights.

It is incumbent upon governments and others to combat the pervasive myths and misunderstandings that perpetuate punitive policies against persons with mental disabilities. Persons with mental disabilities can be a convenient political scapegoat. Media-driven retrogressive and reactionary policies may inflame these narratives. The failure of governmental officials and others in society to correct these pernicious stereotypes represents a violation of ethical obligations of fairness, equality, and solidarity.

While a number of other ethical considerations come into play, they are beyond the scope of this chapter. One final area worth mentioning, however, concerns the medical ethics employed by the health-care professionals treating Anna in the psychiatric institution, as well as those responsible for operating the institution. Medical ethics and human rights law obligations require health workers to adhere to professional standards of care, including monitoring the patient's mental and physical health conditions, prescribing medication that is in the patient's best interest, and treating the patient with dignity and respect. Obtaining informed consent from patients prior to administering medical treatment is also required, although exceptions can be made when the patient is deemed incompetent to grant consent. Nevertheless, findings of incompetence often occur without adequate justifications, based on mistaken perceptions that presume an inherent lack of decisional capacity for a person diagnosed with schizophrenia or that fail to recognise that competency is fluid and may vary over time. Each of these ethical requirements was violated in Anna's case: her health condition deteriorated as a direct consequence of subpar treatment, and both the inconsistent administration of medication and the overuse of sedation violated good practice standards and contravened ethical goals of autonomy and beneficence (Stroup, Swartz, and Appelbaum 2002). In addition, the fact that Anna was repeatedly exposed to infections and injury raises similar concerns about the dangerous and unsanitary institutional conditions. The operators of the institution were similarly responsible for violations of autonomy and beneficence due to the conditions of the facility, which undermined Anna's ability to receive necessary care and worsened her health. Further, each of these ethical violations gives rise to similar legal and human rights violations.

LEGAL CONTEXT

The legal landscape applicable to Anna in her interactions with her employer, landlord, the mental health-care system, and society at large will vary depending on the extent to which her country has embraced international human rights treaties and whether national legislation contains enforceable human rights protections. Throughout the globe, national mental health legislation varies considerably. Approximately 62% of the world's countries do not have mental health legislation or have legislation more than ten years old (WHO 2005). In older legislation, human rights protections are generally absent or, when such protections do exist, under-enforced (Gostin and Gable 2004). High-income countries often boast more comprehensive mental health systems supported by detailed legal systems (Gostin et al. 2010; Hale 2010), while low-income countries often have neither robust mental health systems nor legal systems (Bartlett 2010). Many countries have adopted legal provisions protecting the human rights of persons with mental disabilities. These provisions derive from regional and international human rights treaties to which the countries are party, as well as from national legislation and jurisprudence. However, national-level legal infrastructures do not adopt uniform human rights approaches to mental health. Legal systems at the national and sub-national levels often disproportionately and unfairly penalise persons with mental disabilities. These systems may not provide much protection for human rights, especially affirmative rights claims for health-related services. People like Anna, who are affected by schizophrenia, may be subjected to involuntary confinement without fair process, limited in their ability to access needed care and treatment, and confronted with perpetual social and economic barriers that limit their opportunities across many areas of life.

National mental health legislation, unfortunately, can propagate and solidify destructive myths about persons with mental disabilities and create even greater obstacles for them to attain care, dignity, and normalcy. The presupposition that persons with mental disabilities in general—and persons with schizophrenia in particular—are unreasonably dangerous towards others often guides legal decision making in the context of civil commitment. Research on this issue demonstrates that persons with mental disabilities are no more likely to commit violent acts than persons without mental disabilities (Appelbaum,

Robbins, and Monahan 2000; MacArthur Violence Risk Assessment Study 2001). Comorbidity between mental disorder and alcohol and drug dependency is the key variable in predicting dangerousness (Fazel et al. 2009). Moreover, people who do not have a mental disability commit most violent acts (Fazel and Grann 2006). Nevertheless, the rare cases when a mentally disabled person commits a violent crime often garner disproportionate media and political attention (Smith 1997). Two recent examples illustrate how a single incident of this nature can outrage the public, intensify stigma against persons with mental disabilities, and provide the impetus to enact punitive mental health laws. In reaction to a highly publicised violent crime, the British Parliament enacted the Mental Health Act 2007, which embraces the aforementioned stereotypes about dangerousness and enhances governmental powers of preventive confinement at the expense of patients' rights (Gostin 2007). Another recent example arises from the state of Virginia in the United States, which passed legislation enacting civil commitment reform after a tragic shooting spree by a mentally disordered student at Virginia Tech University. This legislation contained detailed involuntary commitment processes, which could intensify stigma against persons with mental disabilities. Unlike the British Parliament, however, savvy policy makers were able to adopt more restrained civil commitment provisions that balanced issues of autonomy and procedural due process with concerns about public safety and secured additional funding for community mental health services in the state (Bonnie et al. 2009).

It is possible that Anna's eviction from her apartment was predicated on fears of her dangerousness. Legal protections against discrimination could have supported a challenge by Anna to this eviction, presuming that relevant laws apply to persons with disabilities and cover discrimination in the housing sector. The judicial determination that led to Anna's civil commitment also may have reflected such presumptions about both her competency and her potential dangerousness. Courts should not subject a person to involuntary confinement based solely on a diagnosis of schizophrenia. Involuntary confinement is warranted only under very limited circumstances, such as when the person cannot consent and poses a serious risk of harming herself or others and when less restrictive alternative settings for treatment are not available. Moreover, once a legal order for involuntary commitment is issued, the ongoing need for commitment must be reviewed periodically. None of these legal procedural protections were applied to Anna.

Most of the legislative, jurisprudential, and advocacy activity around human rights violations related to persons with mental disabilities has addressed infringements of civil and political rights: issues involving liberty, dignity, and, to a lesser extent, equality (Bonnie 2001). Relevant jurisprudence from regional human rights courts has focused on issues related to the involuntary confinement of persons with mental disabilities, including ensuring scientific criteria and fair procedures for admission and release,[13] appropriate review processes,[14] and adequate conditions of confinement and treatment.[15] Cases such as these may create precedents for legal claims in which Anna invokes her rights to life, liberty, anti-discrimination, fair process, and freedom from cruel and unusual punishment. However, these rulings, drawn from regional human rights courts in Europe and the Americas, do not recognise affirmative access to mental health services in the community. Only more recently have initiatives sought to take the additional step of formulating a right to mental health that acts also as an entitlement to the conditions necessary for good mental health.

An increasing number of recently drafted national constitutions and legislation, such as those of Brazil and South Africa, establish a right to health. These newer legal provisions follow a clear trajectory: more recent definitions of the right to health are more likely to include detailed descriptions of the contents of the right, and many of these definitions explicitly invoke a right to mental health as a component of the right to health (Gable 2007). National legislation may also address related areas such as anti-discrimination law applicable to work, education, health, and housing sectors. In addition, some national courts have begun to uphold the right to health (see Yamin and Gloppen 2011). Courts in Argentina and South Africa, for example, have required their respective governments to provide access to specific medical treatments in order to fulfil the right to health (see chapters 1, 7, and 9).[16] If Anna's country recognises a right to health through constitutional or statutory provisions, she could invoke these provisions to challenge the system that led to her eventual institutionalisation. She may have a strong case that her right to health was violated when mental health-care services were not available to her in the community or that her firing and eviction were examples of discrimination based on her mental disability.

Finally, all of these issues will be affected by whether her country has explicitly incorporated international human rights provisions into its domestic law. As described below, international human rights law extensively recognises and develops legal and normative rights to mental health—which directly affects the legal landscape for Anna and others in similar circumstances.

APPLICATION OF THE RIGHT TO HEALTH IN PRACTICE

CORE ASPECTS OF THE RIGHT TO MENTAL HEALTH

The right to mental health, as broadly recognised in international human rights law and analogous national laws implementing human rights principles, imposes a series of obligations on states. The contours of this right, however, continue to evolve, leaving states with daunting challenges to ensure that good mental health thrives and to prevent human rights violations that undercut the dignity, equality, and health of persons with mental disabilities. It is important to recognise that states will need to pursue multiple strategies to respect, protect, and fulfil the right to mental health, particularly in circumstances similar to those faced by Anna, whose right to mental health was disregarded in numerous contexts.

The linkage between health and human rights has gained increasing recognition in international human rights law, in part due to the proliferation of human rights norms and infrastructure related to the right to health across many jurisdictional levels (Gable 2007). Indeed, this increasing acceptance of the connection between health and human rights represents an important outcome of the collective efforts of the human rights movement and the disability rights movement, two of the great international social movements of the last sixty years (Herr, Gostin, and Koh 2003). Nevertheless, legal and social acceptance of an affirmative right to mental health has developed relatively slowly, especially in comparison with other aspects of the right to health. Aspects concerning physical health have received much more attention and support than have mental and intellectual disabilities, even within the disability rights movement. Thus, the rights of individuals like Anna often remain marginalised, even when protections against disability discrimination exist in national law.

The right to mental health is firmly grounded in numerous international human rights documents. The WHO Constitution recognises that "health is a state of complete physical, mental, and social well-being and not merely the absence of disease or infirmity."[17] The Universal Declaration of Human Rights acknowledges the right to health as a component of "a standard of living adequate for the health and well-being of [a person and that person's] family, including ... medical care and necessary social services, and the right to security in the event of ... sickness."[18] The ICESCR adopts a broad concept of health as a human right, declaring "the right of everyone to the ... highest attainable standard of physical and mental health."[19] The Principles for the Protection of Persons with Mental Illness and the Improvement of Mental Health Care (MI Principles), drafted by the UN in 1991, afford a right to the "best available mental health care."[20]

In solidifying mental health as an explicit component of the right to health, article 12 of the ICESCR establishes a binding obligation on ratifying governments to respect, protect, and fulfil the right to mental health. As described in detail in the following section, this article could allow Anna to condemn her government for failing to prevent discrimination against her and for failing to ensure access to mental health services in the community. Furthermore, if Anna's country has ratified the Optional Protocol to the ICESCR, she could bring a claim to the ESCR Committee directly.[21]

Other contemporary international human rights instruments have expanded on the inclusion of mental health as a core aspect of the right to health and applied this right to specific demographic groups. The Convention on the Rights of the Child states that a "mentally or physically disabled child should enjoy a full and decent life, in conditions which ensure dignity, promote self-reliance, and facilitate the child's active participation in the community."[22] The Convention further requires "effective access to ... education, training, health care services, rehabilitation services ... in a manner conducive to the child's achieving the fullest possible social integration and individual development," a provision that would seem to support access to mental health services for children in the community. The more general language of the Convention on the Elimination of All Forms of Discrimination against Women (CEDAW), which provides for the elimination of "discrimination in the field of health care to ensure ... access to health care services,"[23] can be interpreted to implicitly encompass a right to mental health. Indeed, the human rights treaty bodies charged with overseeing implementation of various human rights conventions have interpreted these conventions as supporting the human rights of persons with mental disabilities (Degener 2003). The case study does not suggest explicitly that Anna, as a woman, received less access to mental health services than a man would have in her position; however, the tendency of many societies to offer women fewer opportunities in general could have contributed to her overall opportunity to access mental health services and may have constituted a de facto violation of this CEDAW provision. Moreover, Anna's exposure to violence and mistreatment while institutionalised may implicate other human rights protections contained in CEDAW.

The CRPD provides the most extensive articulation of the right to mental health of any international human rights treaty. The CRPD affirms the right to health, access to habilitation and rehabilitation services, and inclusion in the community for persons with physical and mental disabilities.[24] Notably, the Convention defines persons with disabilities broadly as those with "long-term physical, mental, intellectual or sensory impairments" (art. 1). Article 25 expands the right to mental health by requiring states to both uphold "the right the enjoyment of the highest attainable standard of health without discrimination on the basis of disability" and "provide those health services needed by persons with disabilities specifically because of their disabilities, including … services designed to minimize and prevent further disabilities." These health services must be provided "as close as possible to people's own communities." Thus, the CRPD not only prohibits discrimination against persons with mental disabilities regarding access to existing health services but also requires the provision of health services needed by persons with mental disabilities. To properly meet these obligations in the case of Anna, her national government would have to expand health systems to create additional capacity for mental health services in the community. Support for a right to community-based services is bolstered by other provisions in the CRPD requiring independent living and full participation in the community; moreover, the Convention requires that persons with disabilities participate in the implementation of the enumerated rights and, like other international human rights treaties, creates a monitoring body to oversee implementation. The CRPD is also notable because it was negotiated rapidly, with extensive participation from non-governmental organisations and representatives of disability rights advocacy groups (Lewis 2010). If Anna's government has ratified the Optional Protocol to the CRPD, she will be able to bring complaints of violations of the Convention on her own behalf.

The legal basis for a right to mental health therefore comes from both international treaties and domestic laws. Thus, depending on Anna's geographic location, she may either have substantial opportunities for mental health care and well-developed legal protections or lack both of these options. Three additional sources, however, have played an important role in explaining the application of a right to mental health to state actions: General Comment 14 of the ESCR Committee; the work of the Special Rapporteurs on the Right to Health; and jurisprudence recognising rights to health at the regional and national levels.

General Comment 14 provides an authoritative examination of the scope and meaning of the right to health under article 12 of the ICESCR. It adopts a broad normative interpretation of the right to health that encompasses public health, health care, and the underlying determinants necessary for healthy living, including those required to maintain good mental health. The right to health also contains both "freedoms and entitlements,"[25] and states must guarantee that services, goods, facilities, and determinants meet standards of availability, accessibility, acceptability, and quality (AAAQ).

Paul Hunt, the first person to serve as Special Rapporteur on the Right to Health, published a report in 2005 examining the right to health in the context of mental and intellectual disabilities, which provides a detailed, thoughtful assessment of the significance of mental health as a component of the right to health.[26] While the Special Rapporteur's findings are not legally binding on states, they carry great weight in assessing whether countries have appropriately complied with their human rights obligations with respect to mental health.

Considered together, General Comment 14 and the Special Rapporteur's report on mental disability provide clarity on the application of the right to mental health under article 12 of the ICESCR. These documents recognise a right to mental health that goes beyond entitlements to mental health services and the availability of underlying determinants of mental health. The right also encompasses freedoms encapsulated in other human rights, such as prohibitions against discrimination, involuntary detention without due process, and non-consensual medical treatment—several freedoms that were denied to Anna. The involuntary commitment order imposed on

Anna by the court precluded her from exercising control over her health and body, deprived her of liberty, and subjected her to additional non-consensual exposure to medical treatment. The apparent overuse of sedation by workers clearly violated her rights to informed consent, freedom from interference in health decision making, and freedom from discrimination based on disability status (Hunt 2005). The entitlements cited in General Comment 14 contain an affirmative "right to a system of health protection which provides equality of opportunity for people to enjoy the highest attainable level of health" (para. 8). Certainly, the mental health system failed Anna in numerous ways, providing inadequate care and resulting in an outcome much more restrictive and less therapeutic than could have been achieved through community care. Indeed, Special Rapporteur Hunt framed these entitlements broadly, imploring states to "take steps to ensure a full package of community-based mental health care and support services conducive to health, dignity, and inclusion."[27]

An additional avenue open to Anna to judicially challenge her confinement and compel access to community-based care may exist through regional human rights systems. Regional human rights instruments have incorporated variations of the right to health into their respective texts. Both the European Social Charter and the Protocol of San Salvador include expansive conceptions of a right to health that encompass rehabilitation and social resettlement of people with mental or physical disabilities[28] and "satisfaction of the health needs of the highest risk groups."[29] The African Charter on Human and Peoples' Rights protects "the right to enjoy the best attainable state of physical and mental health," requiring states to "take the necessary measures to protect the health of their people and to ensure that they receive medical attention when they are sick."[30] Thus, regional human rights treaties may provide additional pathways for asserting rights in countries that recognise the jurisdiction of their respective regional systems.

Several notable cases in these regional systems have expanded jurisprudential recognition of the rights to health and to the conditions necessary to maintain health. The Inter-American Human Rights System has been particularly progressive in this regard. In *Victor Rosario Congo v. Ecuador*, the Commission found a violation of the right to humane treatment when a mentally disabled person was denied health services in a state-run facility.[31] A key aspect of this decision was the Commission's willingness not only to apply human rights standards from the American Convention on Human Rights[32] but also to refer to and incorporate norms from other sources, including the MI Principles and decisions of the European Court of Human Rights (Gable et al. 2005). In a later case, *Damiao Ximenes v. Brazil*, the Inter-American Court of Human Rights went further and found violations of the right to health based on standards found in the American Convention, the Protocol of San Salvador, and a number of international declarations and interpretive guidance sources.[33] If Anna's country is bound by the jurisprudence of the Inter-American Human Rights System, these judicial decisions provide a strong precedent to challenge the deplorable conditions and intermittent care endured by Anna in the psychiatric institution. More broadly, the types of legal theories advanced in these cases—grounded in assertions of the rights to life, health, and freedom from inhuman and degrading treatment—could provide a template for national-level challenges to her conditions of confinement.

IMPLEMENTING THE RIGHT TO MENTAL HEALTH: THE ROLE OF HEALTH SYSTEMS

Implementation of the right to mental health presents a difficult challenge for two reasons. First, the complex social, political, and psychological factors described above that affect mental health policies, the structure of mental health systems, and the treatment of persons with mental disabilities are hard to change. These factors negatively influenced Anna's options for accessing care, finding employment and housing, and making autonomous decisions about her life. Second, the "entitlement" components of the right are subject to a country's economic realities and consequently to "progressive realisation,"[34] which may additionally undermine their justiciability. Yet even under the progressive realisation standard, countries must take meaningful steps to implement the right to health. Nevertheless, the expansive and ambitious articulations of the right to mental health developed by General Comment 14, the Special Rapporteur's mental health report, the CRPD, and emerging right-to-health jurisprudence provide a road map and a set of parameters to respect, protect, and fulfil the right to health in the context of mental disability. Persons with mental disabilities, like Anna, and their advocates, could utilise these standards to insist that governments deliver on their obligations related to the right to mental health, including by providing community-based preventive mental health services, treatment facilities, and rehabilitation services; reforming health systems to better address mental health needs; reforming legal infrastructures to protect the right to mental health; and eliminating discrimination and stigma attached to mental disability.

Health systems play an integral role in governmental efforts to implement the right to mental health. While the standard of "progressive realisation" affords states time to construct health systems according to available national resources, General Comment 14 nevertheless enacts substantial parameters on the use of public health systems to apply the right to health by requiring all states—even those that are quite poor—to take immediate, targeted measures to strengthen systems to support the right to health (Freedman 2009). Human rights scholars have begun to assess whether state efforts to develop national plans, benchmarks, and indicators have made measurable progress towards realising the right to health (Backman et al. 2008). The Special Rapporteur on the Right to Health has recognised that "a strong health system is an essential element of a healthy and equitable society."[35] Additionally, the Special Rapporteur has assessed the connection between WHO's six building blocks for a health system (health services; health workforce; health information systems; medical products, vaccines, and technology; health financing; and leadership, governance, and stewardship) (WHO 2007a) and the right to health.[36] Health systems should be linked to a national health strategy, which governments are required to adopt as a core obligation under the right to health.[37] The national health plan should provide for a range of mental health services and allocate specific amounts in the budget for mental health programmes (Backman et al. 2008; see chapter 4).

Implementing the right to mental health obligates states to comply with at least three different, but interrelated, aspects of the right to health, which are explored below.

A Right to Mental Health as an Affirmative Right

Recognition of affirmative entitlements to health is a notable feature of contemporary understandings of the right to mental health. While scholars have long sought the inclusion of affirmative requirements for states regarding the provision of health services, consensus on the scope and potential for operationalising these entitlements has been elusive. Considerable disagreement persists around the issue of whether the concept of entitlement is too amorphous compared with concepts of liberty and dignity (Gostin 2001). Under the rubric created by General Comment 14 and the CRPD, Anna clearly would have an entitlement to a broad system of health protection comprised of medical and social support services. The state should fulfil Anna's right to health through the development of a community-based system of mental health care and support designed to avoid unnecessary institutionalisation; such a system may include "medication, psychotherapy, ambulatory services, hospital care for acute admissions, residential facilities, rehabilitation for persons with psychiatric disabilities, … supported housing and employment, income support, … and respite care for families looking after a person with a mental disability 24 hours a day."[38] The state must also ensure that the mental health-care system has adequate capacity and a sufficiently large workforce with appropriate professional expertise.

Underlying Determinants of Mental Health

Many of the health system features mentioned above extend beyond traditional categories of health-care facilities, supplies, and personnel. Rather, the right to mental health as outlined in General Comment 14 requires governments to assure that both mental health services and the underlying determinants of good mental health—which include safe homes and workplaces, adequate access to nutritious food and uncontaminated drinking water, healthy environmental conditions, and sufficient sanitation—are available, accessible, acceptable, and of appropriate quality. The recognition that underlying determinants play a vital role in fulfilling health rights is a major conceptual breakthrough. The application of a right to health based on and connected to underlying determinants of health increases the likelihood that national and local governments will augment the mental health services available to the public, undertake public education initiatives about mental and intellectual disabilities to reduce stigma, and implement other preventive and population-based mental health services. Additionally, the protection of underlying determinants of health potentially broadens the reach of health systems, links health systems with other social support systems, and fosters equality by providing a range of foundational social supports for those in the population, like Anna, who may need social support in additional to direct health services.

Upholding Other Human Rights to Support the Right to Mental Health

General Comment 14 and the Special Rapporteur's mental health report also highlight the linkages between the right to health and other human rights. Normatively, this correlation of rights grants the right to health equal standing with other rights. Practically, it expands the options for mental health promotion through other human rights claims. Many of the actions and inactions that violate the right to mental health may also be seen as violations of other human rights. For instance, Anna's firing and eviction arguably violated the strong anti-discrimination provisions found in international human rights conventions. The CRPD, for example, obligates governments to prohibit discrimination in employment and housing on the basis of disability (arts. 19, 27). Further, it requires states to take steps to protect the ability of persons with disabilities to live independently, including reasonable accommodations and equal access to housing and financial assistance (arts. 19, 28). Thus, if Anna's country is party to the CRPD or has similar national-level anti-discrimination protections, the government's failure to protect Anna from firing and eviction would have constituted rights violations.

The connection with the right to mental health here is the clear impact of these discriminatory acts on Anna's ability to access mental health services. Indeed, another way to conceptualise the interconnected relationship between the right to mental health and other human rights is to view the protection of other human rights as themselves underlying determinants of mental health. Strong and consistent protections for liberty, equality, and dignity are beneficial not only for their own sake: these conditions are likely to reduce stress, anxiety, discrimination, and depression. The availability of robust social services and community engagement even beyond the health sector can also foster good mental health in addition to other goals, such as community integration, social participation, equality, autonomy, and dignity.[39] These synergistic results suggest that upholding all human rights can positively affect mental health in numerous ways (Mann et al. 1994).

Barriers to Implementation

Despite the compelling need for mental health systems to address the significant health problems generated by mental health disabilities, and despite the clear legal and ethical obligations around the protection of mental health, numerous barriers to implementation persist. Economic constraints loom large in efforts to strengthen mental health systems and access to mental health services, and competing priorities for limited resources may prevent mental health systems from obtaining adequate resources or sufficient attention from policy makers. Political opposition to expenditures on mental health, driven by social and cultural stigma against persons with mental disabilities, has also been quite difficult to overcome in many countries. The relative lack of political power of mental health advocates helps perpetuate this reality in many countries, as more powerful interests sustain the status quo and undermine initiatives to bolster the mental health system. Integrating mental health services into the health-care system and ensuring the availability of a trained workforce also poses an economic and practical challenge (Saraceno et al. 2007).

In addition, the legal requirements for realising the right to mental health may not be sufficiently robust to advance policy and practice within a country's mental health system. As discussed above, international human rights law—through the rubric of "progressive realization"—grants governments considerable leeway in making progress on satisfying these obligations, often resulting in rights protections for mental health advancing at a slower rate than advocates might hope. Moreover, human rights obligations are difficult to enforce in many countries, particularly if national law does not provide justiciable causes of action in national courts for rights violations.

HEALTH SYSTEMS AND THE RIGHT TO MENTAL HEALTH: A SUMMARY

The impacts of health systems on mental health and human rights cannot be understated. Mental health outcomes are strongly influenced by the structure and application of health systems and legal systems. Health systems may enhance mental health by providing access to necessary mental health services and other supportive infrastructure that can bolster mental health, or these systems may undermine mental health by failing to provide these services and support. Relatedly, persons with mental disabilities may face difficulty in accessing available services within the health system due to a lack of support within their communities or due to legal and social impediments exacerbated by human rights violations, stigmatisation, and the pernicious effects of social opprobrium.

Anna's psychiatric condition, while serious, is one that can be treated in the community with proper medication and supportive services. Her inability to successfully access necessary mental health services in the community represents a failure of the medical, public health, and legal systems in her country. Together, common systemic impediments to access—such as inadequate mental health infrastructure (not enough facilities, professionals, or resources); inability to pay for services (expensive care and lack of insurance coverage); insufficient access to information; perpetuation of negative social attitudes towards mental health treatment and people with mental disabilities; and legal impediments—violated Anna's right to mental health.

At the national level, lawmakers can take steps to alleviate each of these threats to human rights. Governments must ensure that mental health services, particularly community-based services, receive adequate funding from public or private sources. The availability of these resources in her community could have allowed Anna to receive treatment while living independently and continuing to work and participate in all areas of life. In addition, social services that support mental health and the underlying determinants of health should be supported to the maximum extent of a country's available resources. Promising initiatives include providing decent economic conditions, education and health information, opportunities for meaningful employment, social and welfare services, primary and secondary mental health care, community mental health services, and hospital-based treatment and services. Governments can also support mental health by improving underlying societal conditions—for example, by implementing policies that favour humane working conditions, time and space for recreation and relaxation, and assistance with stress-causing circumstances such as child rearing and debt. The creation of a comprehensive and coordinated national plan for developing and supporting the health system can facilitate this process.

These efforts should be coupled with law reform initiatives that establish enforceable legal protections for persons with mental and intellectual disabilities. Legal systems can either perpetuate or eliminate barriers to mental health care and full social participation for persons with mental disabilities. Likewise, mental disabilities often challenge the legal system to address complicated issues of rights, inclusion, and justice, and to adapt accordingly. Legal protections grounded in human rights principles should be enacted at the national level. In particular, legal protections against discrimination can provide a vital bulwark against the sort of blatant discrimination demonstrated towards Anna by her landlord and employer. Legal protections enforcing human rights norms of due process for civil confinement, informed consent for medical treatment, adequate conditions of care in institutional settings, and periodic review of detention orders should also be enacted to avoid unnecessary institutionalisations, like the one faced by Anna.

CONCLUSION AND FUTURE CONSIDERATIONS

The persistent violations of human rights that continue to affect persons with mental disabilities will be reduced only through diligent efforts to recognise and remedy these violations at all levels. Countries should ratify international and regional human rights treaties that include the right to health and pass legislation implementing an affirmative right to mental health. Courts should enforce this right consistently and expansively. Countries should also take practical measures to disarm societal barriers that hinder full social participation of persons with mental disabilities; eliminate stigma and discrimination; encourage understanding, cooperation, and participation; uphold dignity and equality; and provide mental health services in settings that are less restrictive and more humane. The international community should continue to work towards expanding recognition of mental health disabilities as an important public health concern, such as through the inclusion of mental health indicators in future iterations of the Millennium Development Goals.

Furthermore, health workers and non-governmental organisations should adopt a central role in these initiatives. Health workers can use their expertise and direct involvement with the health system to advocate for greater inclusion of mental health services in health programmes.

Non-governmental organisations can serve as both advocates for the human rights of persons with mental disabilities and monitors to detect violations and hold governments accountable.

The widespread adoption of policies, plans, laws, and practices consistent with the right to mental health and other related human rights can help address the enduring inequity and injustice faced by this population. Moreover, these efforts can provide the impetus at long last to eliminate the insidious myths and stigma that surround mental disabilities.

REFERENCES

American Psychiatric Association. 2000. Diagnostic and Statistical Manual of Mental Disorders, Fourth Edition, Text Revision (DSM-IV-TR). Washington, DC: American Psychiatric Association.

Andrade L., J. J. Caraveo-Anduaga, P. Berglund, et al. 2000. "Cross-national Comparisons of the Prevalences and Correlates of Mental Disorders." *Bulletin of the World Health Organization* 78 (4): 413–426.

Appelbaum, P. S., P. C. Robbins, and J. Monahan. 2000. "Violence and Delusions: Data from the MacArthur Violence Risk Assessment Study." *American Journal of Psychiatry* 157:566–572.

Backman, G., P. Hunt, R. Khosla, et al. 2008. "Health Systems and the Right to Health: An Assessment of 194 Countries." *The Lancet* 372 (9655): 2047–2085.

Bartlett, P. 2010. "Mental Health and Rights Outside the 'First World.'" In *Rethinking Rights-Based Mental Health Laws*, ed. B. McSherry and P. Weller, 397–418. Oxford: Hart Publishing.

Bazelon, D. L. 1975. "Institutionalization, Deinstitutionalization and the Adversary Process." *Columbia Law Review* 75 (5): 897–912.

Bonnie, R. J. 2001. "Three Strands of Mental Health Law: Developmental Mileposts." In *The Evolution of Mental Health Law*, ed. L. E. Frost and R. J. Bonnie, 31–54. Washington, DC: American Psychological Association.

Bonnie, R. J., J. S. Reinhard, P. Hamilton, et al. 2009. "Mental Health System Transformation After the Virginia Tech Tragedy." *Health Affairs* 28 (3): 793–804.

Bowie, C. R., A. Reichenberg, T. L. Patterson, et al. 2006. "Determinants of Real-World Functional Performance in Schizophrenia Subjects: Correlations With Cognition, Functional Capacity, and Symptoms." *American Journal of Psychiatry* 163 (3): 418–425.

Burt, R. A. 2001. "Promises to Keep, Miles to Go: Mental Health Law Since 1972." In *The Evolution of Mental Health Law*, ed. L. E. Frost and R. J. Bonnie, 11–30. Washington, DC: American Psychological Association.

Degener, T. 2003. "Disability as a Subject of International Human Rights Law and Comparative Discrimination Law." In *Persons with Intellectual Disabilities: Different But Equal*, ed. S. S. Herr, L. O. Gostin, and H. H. Koh, 151–184. Oxford: Oxford Univ. Press.

Fazel, S., and M. Grann. 2006. "The Population Impact of Severe Mental Illness on Violent Crime." *American Journal of Psychiatry* 163:1397–1403.

Fazel, S., N. Langstrom, A. Hjern, et al. 2009. "Schizophrenia, Substance Abuse, and Violent Crime." *Journal of the American Medical Association* 301: 2016–2023.

Foley, D. L., and K. I. Morley. 2011. "Systematic Review of Early Cardiometabolic Outcomes of the First Treated Episode of Psychosis." *Archives of General Psychiatry* 68 (6): 609–616.

Frank, R. G., and S. A. Glied. 2006. *Better But Not Well: Mental Health Policy in the United States Since 1950*. Baltimore: The Johns Hopkins Univ. Press.

Freedman, L. P. 2009. "Drilling Down: Strengthening Local Health Systems to Address Global Health Crises." In *Realizing the Right to Health*, ed. A. Clapham and M. Robinson, 249–261. Zurich: Rüffer and Rub.

Gable, L. 2007. "The Proliferation of Human Rights in Global Health Governance." *Journal of Law, Medicine and Ethics* 35 (5): 534–544.

Gable, L., and L. O. Gostin. 2008. "Global Mental Health: Changing Norms, Constant Rights." *Georgetown Journal of International Affairs* IX (1): 83–92.

—. 2009. "Mental Health as a Human Right." In *Realizing the Right to Health*, ed. A. Clapham and M. Robinson, 249–261. Zurich: Rüffer and Rub.

Gable, L., J. Vásquez, L. O. Gostin, et al. 2005. "Mental Health and Due Process in the Americas: Protecting the Human Rights of Persons Involuntarily Admitted to and Detained in Psychiatric Institutions." *Pan American Journal of Public Health* 18 (4/5): 366–373.

Gore, F. M., P. J. N. Bloem, G. C. Patton, et al. 2011. "Global Burden of Disease in Young People Aged 10–24 Years: A Systematic Analysis." *The Lancet* 377 (9783): 2093–2102.

Gostin, L. O. 2007. "From a Civil Libertarian to a Sanitarian." *Journal of Law and Society* 34:594–616.

—. 2001. "Beyond Moral Claims: A Human Rights Approach in Mental Health." *Cambridge Quarterly of Healthcare Ethics* 10 (3): 264–274.

Gostin, L. O., and L. Gable. 2004. "The Human Rights of Persons with Mental Disabilities: A Global Perspective on the Application of Human Rights Principles to Mental Health." *Maryland Law Review* 63 (1): 20–121.

Gostin, L. O., J. McHale, P. Fennell, et al. 2010. *Principles of Mental Health Law and Policy.* Oxford: Oxford Univ. Press.

Grob, G. N. 1992. "Mental Health Policy in America: Myths and Realities." *Health Affairs* 1 (3): 7–22.

Hale, B. 2010. *Mental Health Law.* 5th ed. London: Sweet and Maxwell.

Hennekens, C. H. 2007. "Increasing Global Burden of Cardiovascular Disease in General Populations and Patients with Schizophrenia." *Journal of Clinical Psychiatry* 68 (suppl. 4): 4–7.

Herr, S. S., L. O. Gostin, and H. H. Koh, eds. 2003. *Persons with Intellectual Disabilities: Different But Equal.* Oxford: Oxford Univ. Press.

Hunt, P. 2003a. "The UN Special Rapporteur on the Right to Health: Key Objectives, Themes, and Interventions." *Health and Human Rights* 7:1–26.

Hunt, P. 2003b. *Report of the Special Rapporteur on the right of everyone to the enjoyment of the highest attainable standard of physical and mental health,* 13 February 2003, UN Doc. E/CN.4/2003/58.

Jacob, K. S., P. Sharan, I. Mirza, et al. 2007. "Mental Health Systems in Countries: Where Are We Now?" *The Lancet* 370 (9592): 1061–1077.

Koyanagi, C. 2004. *Get It Together: How to Integrate Physical and Mental Health Care for People with Serious Mental Disorders.* Washington, DC: Bazelon Center.

Langle, G., B. Egerter, F. Albrecht, et al. 2005. "Prevalence of Mental Illness among Homeless Men in the Community: Approach to a Full Census in a Southern German University Town." *Social Psychiatry and Psychiatric Epidemiology* 40:382–390.

Leucht, S., K. Wahlbeck, J. Hammann, et al. 2003. "New Generation Antipsychotics Versus Low-Potency Conventional Antipsychotics: A Systematic Review and Meta-Analysis." *The Lancet* 361 (9369): 1581–1589.

Lorant, V., V. Deliege, W. Eaton, et al. 2003. "Socioeconomic Inequalities in Depression: A Meta-Analysis." *American Journal of Epidemiology* 157 (2): 98–112.

MacArthur Violence Risk Assessment Study. 2001. "Executive Summary." Accessed 9 November 2011. http://www.macarthur.virginia.edu/risk.html.

Mann, J. M., L. Gostin, S. Gruskin, et al. 1994. "Health and Human Rights." *Health and Human Rights* 1:7–23.

Mental Disability Rights International. 2000. *Human Rights and Mental Health: Mexico.* Washington, DC: Mental Disability Rights International.

—. 2004. *Human Rights and Mental Health in Peru*. Washington, DC: Mental Disability Rights International.

—. 2005. *Behind Closed Doors: Human Rights Abuses in the Psychiatric Facilities, Orphanages and Rehabilitation Centers of Turkey*. Washington, DC: Mental Disability Rights International.

Miller, G. 2006. "The Unseen: Mental Illness's Global Toll." *Science* 311 (5760): 458–461.

Muntaner, C., W. W. Eaton, C. Diala, et al. 1998. "Social Class, Assets, Organizational Control and the Prevalence of Common Groups of Psychiatric Disorders." *Social Science and Medicine* 47 (12): 2043–2053.

Owens, D. G. C., E. C. Johnstone, and E. D. Frith. 1982. "Spontaneous Involuntary Disorders of Movement: Their Prevalence, Severity, and Distribution in Chronic Schizophrenics with and without Treatment with Neuroleptics." *Archives of General Psychiatry* 39:452–461.

Patel, V., R. Araya, S. Chatterjee, et al. 2007. "Treatment and Prevention of Mental Disorders in Low-Income and Middle-Income Countries." *The Lancet* 370 (9591): 991–1005.

Pescosolido, B. A., J. Monahan, B. G. Link, et al. 1999. "The Public's View of the Competence, Dangerousness, and Need for Legal Coercion of Persons with Mental Health Problems." *American Journal of Public Health* 89:1339–1345.

Prince, M., V. Patel, S. Saxena, et al. 2007. "No Health without Mental Health." *The Lancet* 370 (9590): 859–877.

Saraceno, B., M. van Ommeren, R. Batniji, et al. 2007. "Barriers to Improvement of Mental Health Services in Low-Income and Middle-Income Countries." *The Lancet* 370 (9593): 1164–1174.

Smith, M., 1997. "Role of the Popular Media in Mental Illness." *The Lancet* 349 (9067): 1779.

Stroup, S., M. Swartz, and P. Appelbaum. 2002. "Concealed Medicines for People with Schizophrenia: A U. S. Perspective." *Schizophrenia Bulletin* 28:537–542.

Weich, S., and G. Lewis. 1998. "Poverty, Unemployment, and Common Mental Disorders: Population Based Cohort Study." *British Medical Journal* 317: 115–119.

WHO (World Health Organization). 2001. *The World Health Report: Mental Health; New Understanding, New Hope*. Geneva: WHO.

—. 2003. *Investing in Mental Health*. Geneva: WHO.

—. 2005. *Mental Health Atlas 2005*. Geneva: WHO.

—. 2007a. *Everybody's Business: Strengthening Health Systems to Improve Health Outcomes; WHO's Framework for Action*. Geneva: WHO.

—. 2007b. "International Statistical Classification of Diseases and Related Health Problems, 10th Revision (ICD-10)." Accessed 9 November 2011. http://apps. who.int/classifications/apps/icd/icd10online/.

Yamin, A. E., and S. Gloppen, eds. 2011. *Litigating Health Rights: Can Courts Bring More Justice to Health?* Boston: Human Rights Program, Harvard Law School.

NOTES

1 Schizophrenia is a disorder with several sub-types—catatonic, disorganised, paranoid, residual, and undifferentiated—typically associated with delusions, hallucinations, disorganised behaviour and/or speech, and, as the disorder progresses, flattening and inappropriate affect. Treatment is possible through a combination of medication and therapy, but a cure does not exist; therefore, treatment must be consistent and long term (American Psychiatric Association 2000, sec. 295.20).

2 Bipolar disorder (colloquially known as manic-depression) is a mental health disorder characterised by periods of mania or hypo-mania usually followed by periods of depression. The effects of these periods should be pronounced enough to have an impact on one's life. Treatment is possible through medication and therapy to establish coping mechanisms and facilitate a support system, but there is no cure (American Psychiatric Association 2000, sec. 296.8).

3 "Persons with disabilities include those who have long-term physical, mental, intellectual or sensory impairments which in interaction with various barriers may hinder their full and effective participation in society on an equal basis with others" (Convention on the Rights of Persons with Disabilities, G.A. Res. 61/106, Annex I, U.N. GAOR, 61st Sess., Supp. No. 49, at 65, U.N. Doc. A/61/49 (2006), entered into force 3 May 2008, art. 1).

4 Constitution of the World Health Organization, signed 22 June 1946; Universal Declaration of Human Rights, G.A. Res. 217A (III), U.N. Doc A/810 at 71 (1948), art. 25; International Covenant on Economic, Social and Cultural Rights, G.A. Res. 2200A (XXI), 21 U.N. GAOR Supp. (No. 16) at 49, U.N. Doc. A/6316 (1966), 993 U.N.T.S. 3, entered into force 3 January 1976, art. 12.

5 Convention on the Rights of the Child, G.A. Res. 44/25, Annex, 44 U.N. GAOR Supp. (No. 49) at 167, U.N. Doc. A/44/49 (1989), entered into force 2 September 1990; Convention on the Rights of Persons with Disabilities, *supra* note 3.

6 Committee on Economic, Social and Cultural Rights, General Comment 14, U.N. Doc. E/C.12/2000/4 (2000); Paul Hunt, Report of the Special Rapporteur on the right of everyone to the enjoyment of the highest attainable standard of physical and mental health, Commission on Human Rights, U.N. Doc. E/CN.4/2005/51 (2005) [hereinafter Hunt Report].

7 This chapter uses the term "mental disability" to refer to people with both mental disabilities and intellectual disabilities. While these two terms are often used to describe people with different psychological and neurological conditions, for brevity and consistency, both categories are included under the term "mental disability."

8 Hunt Report, *supra* note 6, para. 6.

9 It should be reiterated that persons with all varieties of mental disabilities suffer from stigma and discrimination. While persons with schizophrenia can face some of the most significant social consequences, persons with unipolar depression—which occurs much more frequently in the population—also face social ostracism and human rights violations that undermine their health and other life activities.

10 The lack of employment protections and an adequate social support infrastructure, as described in this case study, may be less problematic in countries that provide sickness and disability benefits, as well as legal protections against discrimination in the workplace on the basis of mental disability.

11 International Covenant on Economic, Social and Cultural Rights, *supra* note 4, art. 12; Convention on the Rights of Persons with Disabilities, *supra* note 3, arts. 19, 25, 27.

12 Hunt Report, *supra* note 6, paras. 83–86.

13 *Winterwerp v. The Netherlands,* European Court of Human Rights, judgment of 24 October 1979, paras. 53–68.

14 *X v. United Kingdom*, European Court of Human Rights, judgment of 5 November 1981, paras. 48–62.

15 *Victor Rosario Congo v. Ecuador*, Case 11.427, Inter-American Commission on Human Rights, judgment of 13 April 1999.

16 *Mariela Viceconte v. Argentina Ministry of Health and Social Welfare*, Case No. 31.777/96, Court of Appeals, 1998; *Minister of Health and Others v. Treatment Action Campaign and Others*, Constitutional Court of South Africa, 2002 (5) SA 721 (CC) (see chapter 9 for details on the *Treatment Action Campaign* case).

17 Constitution of the World Health Organization, *supra* note 4.

18 Universal Declaration of Human Rights, *supra* note 4, art. 25.

19 International Covenant on Economic, Social and Cultural Rights, *supra* note 4, art. 12.

20 Principles for the Protection of Persons with Mental Illness and the Improvement of Mental Health Care, Resolution adopted by the General Assembly, U.N. Doc. A/RES/46/119 (1991).

21 The Optional Protocol allows for individual communications alleging violations of ICESCR rights to be considered by the ESCR Committee. This permits individuals, or those working on their behalf, to raise right violations directly with the Committee, to which the Committee can respond with a variety of investigation and intervention steps (see Optional Protocol to the International Covenant on Economic, Social and Cultural Rights, G.A. Res. A/RES/63/117 (2008)).

22 Convention on the Rights of the Child, *supra* note 5, art. 24.

23 Convention on the Elimination of All Forms of Discrimination against Women, G.A. Res. 34/180, 34 U.N. GAOR Supp. (No. 46) at 193, U.N. Doc. A/34/46 (1979), entered into force 3 September 1981, art. 12.

24 Convention on the Rights of Persons with Disabilities, *supra* note 3, arts. 19, 25, 26.

25 General Comment 14, *supra* note 6, para. 8.

26 Hunt Report, *supra* note 6.

27 Hunt Report, *supra* note 6, para. 43.

28 European Social Charter, 529 U.N.T.S. 89, entered into force 26 February 1965, arts. 11, 15.

29 Additional Protocol to the American Convention on Human Rights in the Area of Economic, Social and Cultural Rights, "Protocol of San Salvador," O.A.S. Treaty Series No. 69 (1988), entered into force 16 November 1999, reprinted in Basic Documents Pertaining to Human Rights in the Inter-American System, OEA/Ser.L.V/II.82 doc.6 rev.1 at 67 (1992), arts. 10(2)(a)–(f).

30 African (Banjul) Charter on Human and Peoples' Rights, adopted June 27, 1981, OAU Doc. CAB/LEG/67/3 rev. 5, 21 I.L.M. 58 (1982), entered into force 21 October 1986, art. 16.

31 *Victor Rosario Congo v. Ecuador, supra* note 15.

32 American Convention on Human Rights, O.A.S. Treaty Series No. 36, 1144 U.N.T.S. 123, entered into force 18 July 1978, reprinted in Basic Documents Pertaining to Human Rights in the Inter-American System, OEA/Ser.L.V/II.82 doc.6 rev.1 at 25 (1992).

33 *Damiao Ximenes v. Brazil*, Inter-American Court of Human Rights, judgment of 4 July 2006.

34 General Comment 14, *supra* note 6, paras. 30–31.

35 Paul Hunt, Report of the Special Rapporteur on the right of everyone to the enjoyment of the highest attainable standard of physical and mental health, Human Rights Council, U.N. Doc. A/HRC/7/11 (2008), para. 12.

36 Ibid., paras. 67–73.

37 General Comment 14, *supra* note 6, para. 43(f).

38 Hunt Report, *supra* note 6, para. 43.

39 Ibid., paras. 51–61, 83–90.

CHAPTER 9

Essential Medicines

HANS V. HOGERZEIL

CASE STUDY: ADELQUI, AN ARGENTINIAN CHILD WITH A LIFE-THREATENING DISEASE[1]

Adelqui Santiago Beviacqua, a four-year-old boy in Argentina, had suffered since birth from a severe congenital blood disease. In 2000, his parents filed a case (an *amparo*) before the Constitutional Court when the free medicine treatment that their son had been receiving for the past two years from a governmental agency was stopped on the grounds that the previous provisions were made on humanitarian grounds and that the agency was able to decide to stop it at its discretion. The parents based their claim primarily on international treaties that Argentina has ratified, including those protecting the rights of the child and the right to health.

INTRODUCTION

Since the 1970s, the World Health Organization (WHO) has promoted equitable access to basic health services through the concepts of essential medicines and primary health care. The first Model List of Essential Medicines, published in 1977, preceded the famous 1978 Alma-Ata Declaration[2] and is widely regarded as one of WHO's most influential public health achievements from the last quarter of the twentieth century. The universally accepted definition of essential medicines is as follows:

> Essential medicines are those that satisfy the priority health care needs of the population. They are selected with due regard to public health relevance, evidence on efficacy and safety, and comparative cost-effectiveness. Essential medicines are intended to be available within the context of functioning health systems at all times in adequate amounts, in the appropriate dosage

forms, with assured quality and adequate information, and at a price the individual and the community can afford. (WHO 2006, p. 54).

Since 1977, the concept of essential medicines has become truly global. By the turn of the century, over one hundred fifty countries had a national list of essential medicines and over one hundred countries a national medicines policy. Although initially aimed at developing countries, the concept of essential medicines is increasingly seen as relevant for middle- and high-income countries as well (Hogerzeil 2004). In more recent years, access to, quality of, and rational use of essential medical products has been seen as one of the six pillars of health systems (WHO 2007).

Despite this progress, lack of access to essential medicines is still widespread. A recent study found that in thirty-six low- and middle-income countries, public health facilities had essential medicines in stock only one-third of the time, while private facilities had them less than two-thirds of the time (Cameron et al. 2009). This first exact measurement of access, combined with the results of recent household surveys, comes uncomfortably close to the longstanding WHO estimate that one-third of the world's population lacks access to essential medicines—a figure that rises to one-half in some of the poorest areas of Africa and Asia (WHO 2004, p. 14).

There has been a shift in recent years towards a rights-based approach to ensuring access to essential medicines, especially in Latin America. Following the development of an international normative legal framework that includes explicit recognition of the right to health, many governments are now moving towards practical implementation of their right-to-health commitments. In particular, civil society movements in countries such as Brazil, India, Malaysia, South Africa, and Thailand, in their struggles for access to treatment for people living with HIV, have helped raise global awareness of the inequitable access to essential medicines in general. In Thailand, for example, a patients' movement, together with other civil society organisations, promoted its own version of the National Security Health Act. The new government, at that time, had agreed to create a universal access scheme. Three years later, HIV treatment was included in the scheme. In South Africa, the landmark 2001 case filed by the Treatment Action Campaign, which was supported by several grassroots groups and received extensive press coverage, proved that governmental medicine policies could successfully be challenged in court on human rights grounds (see box 9.1; see also chapters 1 and 7).[3]

SOUTH AFRICA: GOVERNMENTAL HEALTH POLICIES SUCCESSFUL CHALLENGED IN COURT

In 2001, the Treatment Action Campaign (TAC), a social movement in South Africa whose mission is "to ensure that every person living with HIV has access to quality comprehensive prevention and treatment services to live a healthy life" (Treatment Action Campaign 2011), challenged one of the South African government's most controversial actions: the restriction of the prophylactic use of nevirapine to prevent mother-to-child transmission of HIV. TAC's main argument was that the government, by restricting nevirapine's use to eighteen public hospitals conducting a pilot study, violated the rights to health, life, equality, and human dignity; TAC further argued that the Ministry of Health's failure to take actions to promote the availability of the medicine was also a breach of its obligations under constitutional and international law. In its defence, the Ministry of Health argued that the effects of nevirapine were not yet clearly established and that the eighteen pilot studies were a reasonable temporary solution.

The court stated that the restriction of nevirapine's availability "is not reasonable and is an unjustifiable barrier to the progressive realization of the right to health care" as enshrined into the Constitution, and ordered the government and provincial health officials to make nevirapine available in all public health facilities. It also demanded that the government develop a comprehensive programme to prevent mother-to-child HIV transmission and that the programme include the provision of nevirapine.

The government decided to seek leave to appeal. In response, TAC filed an application for an execution order, arguing that an "irreparable harm" was imminent and that "every day in which the implementation of paragraphs one and two of the order is delayed, results in unnecessary infection and death of 10 children." These applications were heard together before the Pretoria High Court, which, ten days later, decided in favour of TAC.

The government decided again to seek leave to appeal, this time directly before the Constitutional Court. On 5 July 2002, the Constitutional Court handed down its final judgment on this case, stating that "the policy of confining nevirapine to research and training sites fails to address the needs of mothers and their newborn children who do not have access to these sites."[4] It held that the restriction of nevirapine's availability was unconstitutional and ordered the government "without delay" to assure the availability of this medicine.

Discussion question:

Should a court of justice be able to order a government to execute a certain health programme? Or should this fall under the parliament's responsibilities?

This change to implementation has three main implications. Firstly, the discussion about strict legal principles must now transform itself into a political process that requires a careful balancing of interests and priorities. Secondly, as Amartya Sen has described, "the richness of practice … is also critically relevant for understanding the concept and reach of human rights" (2004, p. 356).

In this regard, WHO's essential medicines programme and its decades-long focus on sustainable, universal access to essential medicines has always been in line with the human rights principles of non-discrimination and care for the poor and disadvantaged. This also applies to WHO's more recent focus on good governance. For example, the careful selection of essential medicines, good quality assurance, procurement and supply management, and rational use all serve to optimise the value of limited governmental funds, and thereby empower and support governments in making basic services available to all. Other aspects of good governance work towards the same goal, such as standardised procedures for monitoring inequities in the pharmaceutical situation, and management tools to assess and reduce vulnerability to corruption.

This chapter will explore access to essential medicines in the context of the right to health. In doing so, it will address the following questions:

- Does Adelqui have the right to receive free treatment for his life-threatening disease?
- Should an expensive medicine be provided to this one child even if it means that other children may not receive cheap but life-saving essential medicines for their diseases?
- Who should decide whether and which medical products are made available by the government to individual patients—for example, doctors, health facilities, reimbursement schemes, or courts of justice?
- How can the interests of the individual be balanced against the interests of the population as a whole?
- Does the right to health include all life-saving medicines, even the most expensive ones?

MEDICAL/PUBLIC HEALTH ASPECTS

From a medical point of view, we can assume that Adelqui, who suffers from a serious congenital blood disease, will become seriously ill and probably die if his treatment is interrupted. In this sense, therefore, the treatment is life saving to him. Let us also assume that Adelqui's family cannot pay for the treatment themselves, that they are not part of an insurance scheme that covers the treatment, and that they are dependent on governmental subsidies or public supply for the treatment. From the patient's point of view, the treatment is absolutely essential. However, from a public health point of view, one must consider that governmental resources are not infinite and that paying for Adelqui's treatment might require sacrificing funding for other treatments or preventive measures. This is where public health may not necessarily be in line with individual patient needs. For example, Argentina's government may now have to choose between paying either for Adelqui's continued treatment or for the monthly vaccination of one hundred poor children in a slum area, which may be much more cost-effective in terms of "cost per life-year saved." From a public health perspective, governmental monies should be prioritised towards vaccinating all children at a low cost and high benefit before treating individual children at a high cost.

ETHICAL AND LEGAL PERSPECTIVES

ETHICAL DILEMMAS AND CONCERNS

In all countries of the world, including rich industrialised countries, the health needs and expectations of individuals will always exceed financial resources. This is, of course, especially the case in low- and middle-income countries. In such a situation, the common good must be balanced against individual needs; this ethical dilemma can be summarised as "Whom do we choose to ignore?"

The ethical dilemma is one of human solidarity—but with whom? (see chapter 5) Is it with the individual patient who is physically sitting in front of the health worker and expects to be treated (a direct beneficiary), or with the group of anonymous poor children who could benefit from cheap treatment for their disease but whose "claim" is less personal and less visible? Some would argue that health workers have, first and foremost, a direct responsibility to cater to the needs of those who ask them directly. But the Hippocratic Oath fails to guide doctors in the wider context of their responsibility to the health needs of the whole community, the economic concept of opportunity costs, or the public health objective of "the best benefit for the largest number of people." In this regard, the concept of *statistical morality* may be helpful; this is the idea that something can be morally good even if we do not know exactly which individual person will benefit (Waddington 1960). Responding to invisible collective claims can be just as good as fulfilling visible individual demands.

But what about the right to health? Does Adelqui as an individual not have a right to life and a right to life-saving treatment? Is the right to health restricted by high costs or by limited resources? Has an individual in a rich country more right to health, or a right to more health?

LEGAL CONTEXT

Most countries in the world have acceded to or ratified at least one international or regional treaty confirming the right to health. Ratifying such treaties creates binding legal obligations for state parties, including an obligation to promote access to essential medicines. But do such legal commitments mean anything in practice? For example, could any individual health-care entitlement be enforced through the courts?

In some countries, litigation that draws on this legal framework has indeed helped advance equitable access to essential medicines. In 2006, WHO presented the results of a systematic search to identify completed court cases in low- and middle-income countries in which individuals or groups had claimed access to essential medicines with reference to either the right to health generally or to specific human rights treaties ratified by their government (Hogerzeil et al. 2006). Seventy-one court cases from twelve countries were identified, mostly from Latin America. In fifty-nine cases, half of which related to life-saving HIV treatment, the courts ruled that access to essential medicines was indispensible for fulfilment of the right to health. These successful cases tended to rely on constitutional provisions on the right to health, with additional references to human rights treaties. Other success factors included a link between the right to health and the right to life, and support by public interest non-governmental organisations (NGOs). A general analysis of the successful cases showed that some individual cases generated entitlements across a population group, that the right to health was not restricted by limitations in social security coverage, and that governmental policies were successfully challenged in court. The study concluded that skilful litigation can help ensure that governments fulfil their constitutional and international treaty obligations. This is especially valuable in countries where social security systems are still being developed.

In Adelqui's case, the Constitutional Court required the social security agency of the Ministry of Health to continue providing medicine to the child, basing its decision largely on international human rights provisions, including article 3 of the Convention on the Rights of the Child (best interest of the child as a primary consideration); article 25 of the Universal Declaration of Human Rights; articles 10 and 12 of the International Covenant on Economic, Social and Cultural Rights (ICESCR); and articles 4(1) and 19 of the American Convention on Human Rights.[5] The Court also insisted on the federal government's responsibility for the fulfilment of the right to health and strongly refuted the Ministry of Health's discretionary approach.

There are at least three different routes through which the right to health can be recognised in national legal frameworks. The strongest governmental commitment is created by including the right to health in the national constitution. The second approach is constitutional recognition that international treaties ratified by the state (e.g., the ICESCR) override or acquire the status of national law. Globally, this option is available to thirty-one countries and was also used in Adelqui's case. The third option, inclusion of the right to health in other national legislation, is easier to create but also easier to change or cancel.

Constitutional recognition of the right to access to essential medicines is an important sign of national values and commitment, but is neither a guarantee nor an essential step—as shown by many countries with failing health systems despite good constitutional language, as well as many countries with good access without such constitutional recognition. Yet the many court cases in the Americas have shown that constitutional recognition of the right to access to essential medicines and services creates an important supportive environment, especially in middle-income countries where health insurance systems are being created and where patients are growing more aware of their rights and more vocal in demanding them. More recent constitutional texts seem to include some of the strongest commitments to the right to health yet, possibly reflecting the positive influence of the global development of this right over the last fifty years. For example, the Philippine Constitution declares that "the State shall ... endeavour to make essential goods, health and other social services available to all people at affordable cost."[6] South Africa's Constitution states that

> everyone has the right to have access to health-care services, including reproductive health care, sufficient food and water and social security, including, if they are unable to support themselves and their dependants, appropriate social assistance. The State must take reasonable legislative and other measures, within its available resources, to achieve the progressive realization of each of these rights. No one may be refused emergency treatment.[7]

While judicial redress mechanisms are an essential function in any society, they should preferably be used as a last resort. Rather, policy makers should ensure that human rights standards guide a country's health policies and programmes from the outset.

The final question is therefore, whom do we ask to make decisions on allocating limited health resources? The individual doctor is not in a good position to do this, as (s)he is close to the individual patient and is rarely in charge of the overall district, provincial, or national health budget. A court of justice on the other hand, important as its role is, is also not the best candidate, as aptly described by Justice Albie Sachs in a case in South Africa in which the Constitutional Court denied renal dialysis to a patient because of national resource constraints:

> The courts are not the proper place to resolve the agonizing personal and medical problems that underlie these choices. Important though review functions are, there are areas where institutional incapacity and appropriate constitutional modesty require us to be especially cautious … Unfortunately the resources are limited and I can find no reason to interfere with the allocation undertaken by those better equipped than I to deal with the agonizing choices that had to be made in this case.[8]

In order to ensure equal rights for all citizens, such difficult decisions are therefore better taken centrally for the country as whole, and they should be based on proper evidence of efficacy, safety, and comparable cost-effectiveness, with a dedicated professional review committee constituted for that purpose. This brings us back to the concept of a national process to identify a list of essential medicines, which does just that. The next section explores how a rights-based approach to essential medicines can be further developed.

APPLICATION OF THE RIGHT TO HEALTH IN PRACTICE

RECENT DEVELOPMENTS

As stated above, most countries in the world have acceded to and/or ratified at least one of the global or regional covenants or treaties confirming the right to health. For example, 160 countries are party to the ICESCR (UN 2011). Implementation of the ICESCR, which is binding, is monitored by the UN Committee on Economic, Social and Cultural Rights (ESCR Committee), which regularly issues authoritative but non-binding comments clarifying the nature and content of individual rights and state obligations. In its General

Comment 14, the Committee states that "medical service," as described in article 12(2)(d) of the ICESCR, includes, as a core obligation, the provision of essential drugs "as defined by the WHO Action Programme on Essential Drugs" (see chapters 1 and 2).[9]

Especially with regard to universal access to essential medicines, it is important to note that human rights law does not require that the right to health be realised overnight—and indeed resource constraints may prevent state parties from doing so. The principle of "progressive realization" enshrined in article 2 of the ICESCR acknowledges the limits of available resources and requires state parties to commit "to the maximum of [their] available resources... to achieving progressively the full realization of the rights recognized" in the Covenant. While this principle may allow some delays to be justified on grounds of resource constraints, the Covenant also imposes two *immediate* obligations on state parties. Firstly, they must guarantee that the right to health will be exercised without discrimination of any kind (art. 2(2)). Secondly, they must take deliberate, concrete, and targeted steps (art. 2(1)) towards the full realisation of article 12. There is a strong presumption that retrogressive measures are not permissible, which means that once states have taken steps towards the fulfilment of the right to health, these cannot be withdrawn.

To demonstrate that they have taken steps to progressively realise the right to health, state parties have a core obligation to adopt and implement national public health strategies and plans of action, which should be based on epidemiological evidence and should address the health concerns of the whole population. These plans should also make reference to an essential medicines list.[10] By 2009, 135 countries had incorporated aspects of the right to health into their national constitutions; of these, eighty-seven constitutions refer to the right to goods and services, and four specifically mention access to medical products and technologies (Perehudoff, Laing, and Hogerzeil 2010, p. 800).

Adelqui's case is noteworthy in this regard. Because the Argentinian Constitution does not explicitly mention the right to health, a constitutional right to health could not be invoked in Adelqui's defence. Instead, the Court listed all of the international treaties to which Argentina is a signatory and used this as its main argument to rule that life-saving treatment of the child could not be interrupted. Within the aforementioned series of court cases compiled by WHO, this decision is the only clear ruling in which international human rights treaties have created a state obligation regarding an individual entitlement in the absence of a constitutional right to health.

An important international development took place in April 2002, when the then UN Commission on Human Rights established the mandate of a Special Rapporteur on the Right to Health. The first Special Rapporteur, Paul Hunt, who served from 2002 to 2008, worked closely with many stakeholders (see chapter 1). In close collaboration with WHO, he prepared several reports on access to essential medicines and the role of the pharmaceutical industry (see box 9.2). These reports have promoted international recognition of the issue and have provided useful guidance on the practical implications of human rights obligations and simple indicators to measure progress. They have also prompted relevant treaty monitoring bodies to request state parties to provide information on progress in ensuring access to essential medicines in their regular reports.

BOX 9.2

SPECIAL RAPPORTEUR ON THE RIGHT TO HEALTH: REPORTS ADDRESSING THE ISSUE OF ACCESS TO ESSENTIAL MEDICINES

Intellectual property and access to medicines. U.N. Doc. E/CN.4/2004/49/ Add.1 (2004)

The human right to medicines. U.N. Doc. A/61/338 (2006), pp. 10–18

The responsibilities of pharmaceutical companies. U.N. Doc. A/61/338 (2006), pp. 19–21

Guidelines for pharmaceutical companies. U.N. Doc. A/63/263 (2008)

Health systems and the right to the highest attainable standard of health. U.N. Doc. A/HRC/7/11 (2008)

Mission to GlaxoSmithKline. U.N. Doc. A/HRC/11/12/Add.2 (2009)

In practice, the core objectives of WHO's Action Programme on Essential Drugs have always been in line with human rights principles. However, the link between universal access and the right to health was for the first time explicitly recognised as a new priority in the WHO Medicines Strategy of 2004–07 (WHO 2004). WHO now actively promotes access to essential medicines as part of the right to health through studies, advocacy, and policy guidance.

In 2006, WHO formulated five questions aimed at reviewing the extent to which a given national essential medicines policy or programme is in line with human rights principles (Hogerzeil 2006; see box 9.3).

This approach was used for the first time in 2007 to assess the human rights aspects of the Philippines' national medicines policy. An important observation made as a result of this exercise was that a focus on the right to health within a national medicines policy automatically moves the focus of policy discussion towards promoting equity, universal access, and solidarity with the poor and disadvantaged. A rights-based approach provides a strong foundation for promoting universal access to health care.

BOX 9.3

FIVE QUESTIONS FOR ASSESSING WHETHER A COUNTRY'S ESSENTIAL MEDICINES PROGRAMME IS CONSISTENT WITH THE RIGHT TO HEALTH

1. **Which medicines are covered by the right to health?** Does the national constitution, or any other national law, recognise the right of everyone to the enjoyment of the highest attainable standard of health? Are there laws that specify the government's responsibility in ensuring equitable access to essential medicines? Is there a national list of essential medicines updated within the last two years?

2. **Have all beneficiaries of the medicines programme been consulted?** Is there a national medicines policy updated within the last ten years? Were patients' organisations and rural communities consulted when the national medicines policy and programme were developed?

3. **Are there mechanisms for transparency and accountability?** Does the national medicines policy describe the obligations of the various stakeholders? Are there baseline and target data on access to essential medicines against which progress can be measured?

4. **Do all vulnerable groups have equal access to essential medicines? How do you know?** Are disaggregated access statistics available for girls, boys, women, and men, and for urban and rural populations? Are essential medicines available in prisons? Are training materials and drug information leaflets available in all common ethnic languages?

5. **Are there safeguards and redress mechanisms in case human rights are violated?** Are legal mechanisms available and have they been used to file complaints about lack of access to essential medicines?

Source: Hogerzeil (2006)

Since 2007, the WHO indicator for measuring access to essential medicines has included governmental recognition of access to essential medicines as part of the right to health in the constitution or national legislation. This same country progress indicator is also included in WHO's Medium-Term Strategic Plan for 2008–13, approved by the World Health Assembly in 2007 (WHO 2008). Governmental recognition of access to essential medicines as part of the right to health therefore has become one of the core indicators for access to essential medicines.

Access to essential medicines has also become an indicator of a government's commitment to the right to health. The UN High Commissioner for Human Rights has created sets of indicators for twelve human rights, including the rights to housing and shelter, to education, to freedom of expression, and to health. The indicators for the fulfilment of the right to health refer to five areas: (1) sexual and reproductive health; (2) child mortality and health care; (3) natural and occupational environment; (4) prevention, treatment, and control of diseases; and (5) access to health facilities and essential medicines. In addition, in 2008, the *Lancet* published the first independent assessment of the fulfilment of the right to health in all countries of the world, using a set of seventy-two indicators (Backman et al. 2008). Of these, eight indicators were used to measure access to essential medicines, largely taken from those developed by WHO and the High Commissioner for Human Rights.

In 2010, the 50th Directing Council of the Pan American Health Organization adopted a resolution in which all countries of the Americas committed to working with governmental human rights agencies to evaluate and monitor the implementation of international treaties and standards, particularly as they relate to the right to health for vulnerable groups, including people with mental disorders or disabilities, older people, women and adolescents, people living with HIV, and indigenous peoples.[11]

In particular, the countries committed to strengthening the technical capabilities of governmental health and human rights agencies to monitor health services' compliance with international human rights treaties and standards; promoting systematic technical cooperation in the design of health legislation, plans, and policies; strengthening health workers' knowledge and skills in the use of international human rights instruments; adopting legislative, administrative, and educational measures to improve the dissemination of international norms and standards protecting the right to health; and strengthening civil society organisations and combating stigma and discrimination.

CONCLUSION AND FUTURE CONSIDERATIONS

Despite the advances described above, inequity and discrimination in access to essential medicines remain a key public health challenge of our times. Inequity in access to medicines is part of inequity in health care. Many governments continue to rely on medicine supply through the private sector and on health-care financing through out-of-pocket payments. In doing so, these governments choose to ignore the fact that such practices largely exclude the poor and vulnerable from obtaining even the most basic essential medicines. Those sections of the population who need essential medicines the most include the poor, women and girls, the elderly, the internally displaced, people with disabilities, religious and ethnic minorities, and prisoners. The documentation of such inequities in access through disaggregated statistics or targeted surveys is rarely performed, again reflecting a lack of political attention to these groups.

Recognition and implementation of the right to health would help address such inequities. However, while many countries have ratified the ICESCR, there still remain more than thirty countries that have not done so—and of those who have, many do not implement the treaty in practice. One-third of the world's countries do not recognise the right to health in their national constitutions, and a similar number lack an updated national medicines policy. Over fifty countries do not have an updated list of essential medicines as the basis for public supply or reimbursement. Only four countries (Mexico, Panama, the Philippines, and Syria) have made a explicit constitutional commitment to ensuring access to essential medicines to their populations, although it should be noted that the number of countries that have made other legally binding commitments is not known (Perehudoff, Laing, and Hogerzeil 2010). While pharmaceutical systems seem to work effectively in most countries of Latin America, they are either ineffective or absent altogether in most African, Asian, and Middle Eastern countries.

The norms, standards and principles of the international human rights system must be integrated into the plans, policies and processes of pharmaceutical development. These basic principles include participation, accountability, non-discrimination, and attention to vulnerable groups. The human rights implications of any new medicines policy, legislation, or programme must also be assessed in advance.

Governments and health policy makers should be aware of the increasing trend whereby populations are demanding justice as a right, not as a charity. While the use of judicial redress is an important means for ensuring human rights accountability, a more effective approach is for governments to ensure, from the outset, that their health programmes are in line with human rights principles. The concept of essential medicines—with its focus on equity, solidarity, and social justice—is already very much in line with such principles. As governments develop their essential medicines policies and programmes, they should take heed of the growing human rights movement and its emphasis on transparency, accountability, and freedom from discrimination.

REFERENCES

Backman, G., P. Hunt, R. Khosla, et al. 2008. "Health Systems and the Right to Health an Assessment of 194 Countries." *The Lancet* 372 (9655): 2047–2085.

Cameron, A., M. Ewen, D. Ross-Degnan, et al. 2009. "Medicine Prices, Availability, and Affordability in 36 Developing and Middle-Income Countries: A Secondary Analysis." *The Lancet* 373 (9659): 240–249.

Hogerzeil, H. V. 2004. "The Concept of Essential Medicines: Lessons for Rich Countries." *British Medical Journal* 329 (7475): 1169–1172.

—. 2006. "Essential Medicines and Human Rights: What Can They Learn from Each Other?" *Bulletin of the World Health Organization* 84 (5): 371–375.

Hogerzeil, H. V., M. Samson, J. V. Casanovas, et al. 2006. "Is Access to Essential Medicines as Part of the Fulfilment of the Right to Health Enforceable through the Courts?" *The Lancet* 368 (9532): 305–311.

Perehudoff, S. K., R. O. Laing, and H. V. Hogerzeil. 2010. "Access to Essential Medicines in National Constitutions (Editorial)." *Bulletin of the World Health Organization* 88 (11): 800.

Sen, A. 2004. "Elements of a Theory of Human Rights." *Philosophy and Public Affairs* 32 (4): 315–356.

Treatment Action Campaign. 2011. "About the Treatment Action Campaign." Accessed 9 November 2011. http://www.tac.org.za/community/about.

UN. 2011. "United Nations Treaty Collection: Chapter IV; Human Rights." Accessed 9 November 2011. http://treaties.un.org/pages/Treaties.aspx?id=4.

Waddington, C. H. 1960. *The Ethical Animal*. London: Allan and Unwin.

WHO (World Health Organization). 2004. *WHO Medicines Strategy: Countries at the Core; 2004–2007*. Geneva: WHO.

—. 2006. *The Selection and Use of Essential Medicines; Report of the WHO Expert Committee, 2005 (including the 14th Model List of Essential Medicines)*. WHO Technical Report Series, No. 933. Geneva: WHO. http://whqlibdoc.who.int/trs/WHO_TRS_933_eng.pdf.

—. 2007. *Everybody's Business: Strengthening Health Systems to Improve Health Outcomes; WHO's Framework for Action*. Geneva: WHO.

—. 2008. *Medium-Term Strategic Plan 2008–2013*. Geneva: WHO.

NOTES

1 *Campodonico de Beviacqua, Ana Carina v. Ministerio de Salud y Acción Social*, Constitutional Court, File C.823.XXXV, 24 October 2000.

2 Declaration of Alma-Ata, International Conference on Primary Health Care, Alma-Ata, USSR, 6–12 September 1978.

3 *Treatment Action Campaign, Dr. Haron Sallojee and Children's Rights Centre v. RSA Ministry of Health*, High Court of South Africa, Transvaal Provincial Division, 12 December 2001.

4 *Minister of Health and Others v. Treatment Action Campaign and Others*, Constitutional Court of South Africa, 2002 (5) SA 721 (CC), para. 67.

5 Convention on the Rights of the Child, G.A. Res. 44/25, Annex, 44 U.N. GAOR
   Supp. (No. 49) at 167, U.N. Doc. A/44/49 (1989), entered into force 2 September 1990;
   Universal Declaration of Human Rights, G.A. Res. 217A (III), U.N. Doc A/810 at
   71 (1948); International Covenant on Economic, Social and Cultural Rights, G.A.
   Res. 2200A (XXI), 21 U.N. GAOR Supp. (No. 16) at 49, U.N. Doc. A/6316 (1966), 993
   U.N.T.S. 3, entered into force 3 January 1976; American Convention on Human Rights,
   O.A.S. Treaty Series No. 36, 1144 U.N.T.S. 123, entered into force 18 July 1978, reprinted
   in Basic Documents Pertaining to Human Rights in the Inter-American System,
   OEA/Ser.L.V/II.82 doc.6 rev.1 at 25 (1992).
6 Constitution of the Philippines, 1987, art. II sec. 11.
7 Constitution of South Africa, 1996 art. 27(3).
8 *Soobramoney v. Minister of Health*, KwaZulu-Natal 1998 (1) SA 765 (CC), 1997 (12)
   BCLR 1696 (CC).
9 Committee on Economic, Social and Cultural Rights, General Comment 14, U.N.
   Doc. E/C.12/2000/4 (2000), para. 43.
10 Ibid., para. 43(f).
11 Pan American Health Organization, Resolution CD50.R8, Health and Human Rights
   (2010).

CHAPTER 10

Undocumented Migrants

SUSAN WRIGHT AND HENRY ASCHER

CASE STUDY: KAGAAN, AN UNDOCUMENTED MIGRANT IN THE UK[1]

Kagaan left Turkey after a family member and friend died at the hands of the government. Kagaan had been imprisoned as a result of his political opposition, and he feared for his own safety. Upon arrival in the UK in 2002, he claimed asylum, but his claim was ultimately refused in 2003. Kagaan remained in the UK as undocumented and fell ill in 2004. In 2005, at the age of forty-seven, he was diagnosed with bowel cancer. Kagaan was told that surgery was necessary and that he would have to pay the full cost in advance for it. As an undocumented migrant living in poverty, this was impossible for him.

Kagaan tried many avenues to obtain treatment, and even received a supportive letter from his Member of Parliament, but was ultimately refused. Day by day, his condition worsened, as he experienced abdominal pain, distension, and frequent bleeding. Kagaan was so distressed and depressed about his condition that he was referred for psychiatric treatment. The doctors noted that Kagaan's psychiatric condition was a consequence of not receiving treatment for his deteriorating physical condition. Yet authorities declined to provide the surgery that would have improved both his physical and psychiatric conditions. Instead, he was institutionalised at a cost that far exceeded the price of surgical intervention.

After being discharged from psychiatric treatment, Kagaan's condition continued to deteriorate. He was forced to visit the emergency room a number of times before he finally received the surgery, which was more complicated and more costly as a result of the delay.

INTRODUCTION

Much of the focus on the right to health is placed on developing countries. However, there are numerous examples of developed countries falling short of their right-to-health obligations under the International Covenant on Economic, Social and Cultural Rights (ICESCR).[2] Across Europe, such failures have been documented (Chauvin 2007), particularly with regard to migrants, a group that has largely been excluded from society, welfare, and human rights. Migrants constitute modern Europe's *homo sacer* (Agamben 1998), perhaps together with the Roma people.

This chapter will focus on undocumented migrants' access to health services in the UK and Sweden. First, the chapter will provide background information on migration, including the definition of migration and an overview of the phenomenon. It will then highlight the barriers that migrants face in accessing health services, as well as some of the progress that has been made in increasing this access. Kagaan's case will then be analysed from the perspectives of medicine and public health, ethics and law, and the right to health.

DEFINITION OF MIGRANTS AND REFUGEES

Migrants vs. Refugees

The reasons for leaving one's native country are often mixed, extremely complex, and unique for every individual. Separating genuine refugees from various other groups through fair asylum procedures, in accordance with the 1951 Refugee Convention,[3] can thus be difficult (UNHCR 2008), as the traditional categories of migrants are often not clear-cut. The Convention was framed mainly to cope with European refugees as a consequence of World War II. However, as global migration patterns began to change, the international community adopted the 1967 Protocol, which removed the geographical and temporal restrictions from the Convention.[4] The Convention is the primary international legal document that defines who is a refugee, what refugees' rights are, and what states' corresponding legal obligations are. Article 1 defines a refugee as a person who (1) is outside his or her country of nationality or habitual residence; (2) has a well-founded fear of persecution because of his or her race, religion, nationality, membership of a particular social group or political opinion; and (3) is unwilling to avail himself or herself of the protection of that country, or to return there, for fear of persecution.

Together, the Convention and the 1967 Protocol have influenced the development of important regional instruments, such as the 1969 OAU Refugee Convention in Africa and the 1984 Cartagena Declaration in Latin America (UNHCR 2008).[5]

With today's changing patterns of global migration, new political developments, and increasing numbers of people on the move, the Convention's relevance has sometimes been called into question. One criticism is that the Convention's definition of a refugee—which fits to a middle-aged, politically active man—may have been relevant in the 1950s but is not adequate for representing more modern forms of persecution, such as those directed towards female activists or children. Nevertheless, the Convention was the first truly international agreement covering the most fundamental aspects of a refugee's life. It spelled out a set of basic human rights that are equivalent to freedoms enjoyed by foreign nationals living legally in a given country and, in many cases, by citizens of that state. It recognised the international scope of refugee crises and the need for international cooperation, including burden sharing among states, in order to tackle the problem (UNHCR 2008) (for more on international assistance between states, see chapter 2).

What Is a Migrant?

Within the international community, there is no universally accepted definition of migrants. The Oxford Dictionary defines a migrant as a "person who moves from one place to another in order to find work or better living conditions." The UN defines a migrant as "an individual who has resided in a foreign country for more than one year irrespective of the causes, voluntary or involuntary, and the means, regular or irregular, used to migrate" (Perruchoud and Redpath-Cross 2011).

Migrants themselves are divided into several sub-groups, including the following:

- Asylum seekers (whose claims for asylum are pending)
- Recognised refugees (whose claims have been successful)

- Individuals with residence permit due to protection needs
- Individuals with residence permit due to humanitarian reasons
- Refused asylum seekers (who have exhausted their claims without success)
- Undocumented migrants (who have overstayed their visas, who have entered the country without permission, or who are rejected asylum seekers living in hiding to avoid deportation). Various terms are used to describe this group, each with different advantages and disadvantages (see box 10.1).

BOX 10.1

DIFFERENT TERMS USED TO CLASSIFY A PERSON RESIDING IN A COUNTRY WITHOUT PERMISSION

"Illegal"

Rarely used and not recommended. No person in and of himself or herself can be illegal. The term risks leading to an undesirable association between migration and criminality.

"Irregular"

At times used internationally. The drawback to this term is its technical nature, which overlooks the individual behind the term.

"Undocumented"

Often used internationally (in French, *sans papier*). This term implies that a person lacks the paper providing the right to stay in a country. However, many who are labelled "undocumented" do have some type of documentation, albeit not of a type accepted by migration authorities.

"Hidden," "underground," or "clandestine"

Often used in reference to a sub-group of undocumented migrants who have applied for asylum but have been rejected and now live in a country without permission. The drawback to these terms is that they may be improper since many such migrants lead more or less open lives.

Source: Ascher (2011, p. 6)

This chapter will use the term "undocumented migrants," as it is the most accurate and the least controversial.

THE SIZE OF MIGRATION

The total number of people living outside the country where they were born has increased in the last ten years, from about 150 million in 2000 to 214 million in 2011 (IOM 2011, p. 1). This means that 3.1% of the world's people are migrants. Although the absolute number of migrants has increased over the last decade, the percentage of migrants as the share of the total population has increased by only 0.2% during the same time period. However, the patterns of migration are shifting. The European Union (EU) has seen an overall net gain in its population from international migration in the last decade. Today, migrants and ethnic minorities constitute approximately 64.1 million people in the EU, equivalent to 9% of its total population. The health situation of this group thus significantly affects public health in Europe (UN 2009). In 2005 alone, inward migration accounted for more than 1.8 million people and almost 85% of Europe's total population growth (IOM 2011). Other countries with high percentages of migrants include Qatar (87%), United Arab Emirates (70%), Jordan (46%), Singapore (41%), and Saudi Arabia (28%) (IOM 2011, p. 1).[6] It is worth noting that 49% of migrants worldwide are women (IOM 2011, p. 1).

The exact number of undocumented migrants is, for obvious reasons, extremely difficult to estimate. The United States estimates its population of undocumented migrants to be 11 million ("Delstat vill inte invänta reform för papperslösa" 2011), while in Europe estimates vary between 2.8 and 8 million (Commission of the European Communities 2009; Vogel and Kovacheva 2008).

Across Europe, there is evidence that migrants of all categories face substantial barriers when attempting to access health care. Even where access is guaranteed in theory, practical obstacles are common. Due to limited space, this chapter focuses on undocumented migrants and the barriers that they face.

UNDOCUMENTED MIGRANTS AND ACCESS TO HEALTH SERVICES: BARRIERS AND CONSEQUENCES

Numerous barriers hinder undocumented migrants' access to health services. Of these, two fundamental obstacles are (1) structural barriers and (2) lack of recognition and knowledge of the group, the circumstances in which they live, and their rights.

Structural Barriers

Within European countries, structural barriers vary greatly for undocumented migrants (PICUM 2007). Spain and Italy provide a card that enables access to free health care for undocumented migrants who sign a special register. France, Belgium, and the Netherlands provide health care to undocumented migrants in their public health services, although the procedures for accessing those services are more complex. The UK and Portugal, on the other hand, have restrictive and unclear legal frameworks, which lead to a high degree of uncertainty for undocumented migrants. Hungary and Germany offer free health care in very limited cases, and Austria and Sweden offer only "immediate" health care and demand full payment from the undocumented patient (PICUM 2007).

While governments have a variety of reasons for establishing such structural barriers, one important factor is money. Governments across Europe claim that it would be too expensive to offer free access to health care, as undocumented migrants would overuse the health system (PICUM 2007). Other countries, such as the UK, have argued that their health services would be besieged by a stream of overseas visitors coming as "health tourists" to receive free medical treatment. These arguments in favour of barriers are often discussed in the context of "pull factors," suggesting that access to health care works as a magnet to attract migrants. Restricting health care for undocumented migrants would thus operate as a "push factor" whereby limited access to health care becomes a reason to leave the country. The empirical basis for such conceptions is, however, very weak (for an overview, see SOU 2011, pp. 279–291).

The consequences of barriers. Sweden's strict laws have had negative effects on people seeking health care. Surveys in the country have demonstrated that 70%–80% of undocumented migrant patients have experienced difficulties in seeking care. The main reasons cited were fear of being captured; fear of being denied health care; and difficulties at reception, such as excessive questions about the patient's address, identification, ability to pay, and health situation (Médecins du Monde 2009; Médecins Sans Frontières 2005; Ohlson 2006). Other reasons highlighted were administrative barriers and high fees (see table 10.1).

TABLE 10.1 Patient costs for health care in Sweden: Citizens vs. undocumented migrants.

Treatment	Swedish Nationals	Undocumented Migrants
Consultation with a doctor in the emergency room	260 SEK (27 euros)	2,000 SEK (209 euros)
Consulation with a doctor at a primary health-care clinic	140 SEK (15 euros)	1,400 SEK (146 euros)
Consultation with a midwife at a maternity centre	0 SEK	500 SEK (52 euros)
Labour and delivery	0 SEK	21,000 SEK (2,197 euros)
Insulin treatment for diabetes (type 1)	1,800 SEK per year* (188 euros)	13,200 SEK per year (1,381 euros)

* This sum is equal to the maximum cost for all medications in one year for Swedish residents with a personal identity number, according to the medication subvention system.

Data from PICUM (2007, p. 91).

It has been reported that some undocumented migrants try to sidestep this problem in Sweden by borrowing the personal identity number[7] of a friend or relative who has a residence permit or Swedish citizenship. In other countries, undocumented migrants have been reported to use insurance cards belonging to family members or friends in order to access health services. These actions can have severe medical consequences for both the patient and the lender, as vital information may be included in the wrong medical record (Ascher 2010; PICUM 2007).

Because undocumented migrants in Sweden are obliged to pay the full price when accessing health services, they are often indebted (see figure 10.2). A 2005 survey showed that one-third of the patients visiting the clinic run by Médecins Sans Frontières for undocumented migrants in Stockholm had debts between 2,000 SEK and 75,000 SEK (approximately 209 euros and 7,836 euros, respectively) (Médecins Sans Frontières 2005). If these migrants' legal status is later altered and they are given permission to stay, they begin their new life as legally indebted.

Knowledge Barriers among Health Workers

A large number of health workers also lack information on and a basic understanding of the different categories of migrants (migrants, undocumented migrants, asylum seekers, etc.) and undocumented migrants' entitlements to health care, often due to unclear policies, laws, and regulations in the country. This leads to misconceptions and to unlawful limitations of patients' rights. At the same time, migrants sometimes move rapidly between these groups: they may be undocumented one week, asylum seekers the next, and later undocumented again. A study by the Platform for International Cooperation on Undocumented Migrants (PICUM) noted that hospital administrations sometimes wrongly believe that their duty to check entitlements is also a duty to report to immigration authorities. The study also reported that hospitals in some European countries perceive undocumented migrants as synonymous with the loss of income, and therefore are reluctant to treat them (PICUM 2007).

Patients' Barriers

The lack of knowledge and information is also reflected among undocumented patients themselves. Patients are often not fully aware of their rights, leading to fear of and abstention from searching for health care, even when it is needed. As Paul Hunt, former UN Special Rapporteur on the Right to Health, has noted, "undocumented people fear being reported to authorities by medical staff and thus they often refrain from seeking medical assistance even in the most serious cases."[8] In Austria, which has strict laws like Sweden, health professionals have pointed out that "undocumented migrants only come to hospital when they are in an extreme situation. Some of them come only to die" (PICUM 2007, p. 18).

IMPROVING THE RIGHT TO HEALTH FOR UNDOCUMENTED MIGRANTS: TWO EUROPEAN APPROACHES

Many undocumented migrants do not access health care at all, or else access it at a very late and perilous stage. In Europe, improving access to health care for undocumented migrants is an urgent priority. One reason is that this group is commonly a victim of discrimination and exclusion. A second reason is that undocumented migrants constitute precisely the kind of vulnerable group that human rights are especially meant to protect. This section presents initiatives that the UK and Sweden have undertaken to improve the situation.

UK

In 2004, the UK government limited undocumented migrants' access to secondary care, including specialist care and hospital care. At the same time, the government proposed changing the law to also limit undocumented migrants' access to primary health care. This proposal sought to prevent doctors from being able to exercise their discretion in determining whether to accept new patients regardless of their immigration status. This, in turn, would have resulted in even greater exclusion for undocumented migrants seeking health services. Insecurity and uncertainty about entitlements have meant that many migrants fall outside the mainstream health services, turning to clinics run by non-governmental organisations (NGOs). One such organisation is Doctors of the World UK, which runs a clinic in London that provides assistance to thousands of patients who need to see a general practitioner and need help registering with a general practitioner within the UK's National Health Service. Clinic staff also collect and analyse data to provide a clear picture of the health situation of migrants in London. These data were used by a network of NGOs, health professionals, and other stakeholders seeking to use a rights-based approach to defeat the government's proposal.

The UK government acknowledged that there was no evidence of the projected cost of migrants accessing primary care, or even of the predicted numbers of migrants (Johnson 2005). Moreover, a study by Doctors of the World indicated that the government's fear of "health tourism" was not evidence based. Five years of data showed that patients in the London clinic had, on average, been living in the UK for three years before they visited the clinic to see a doctor or seek help accessing health care (Doctors of the World UK 2010). Furthermore, the vast majority of migrants living with HIV were not aware of their disease before arriving to the UK. Two-thirds were not even aware that they were entitled to free testing in the UK.

The results of this study mirrored those of a study performed in the London Borough of Newham, which has a very diverse population and sizeable migrant population. The Newham study found that the impact of "overseas visitors" on primary health care was "minimal in terms of absolute numbers" (Hargreaves et al. 2006, p. 65). The results of both of these studies are further consistent with a 2007 Audit Commission study in the UK, which states that "most migrant workers are relatively young and healthy" and have little need for public services (Audit Commission 2007, p. 33).

Other studies have been carried out indicating that the health problems experienced by undocumented migrants closely reflect the conditions seen among the general population. The most common health problems among undocumented migrants mirror the ten most common reasons that British citizens consult a general practitioner, according to the last national survey of ill health in primary care (McCormick, Fleming, and Charlton 1995). The only deviation is related to psychological problems, which are more commonly reported by migrants. This is not surprising, given the conditions that led them to migrate to the UK, the poor living conditions in which they live in the UK, and the stress caused by uncertain immigration status.

Furthermore, in relation to medical needs, undocumented migrants' medical requirements are in fact quite routine and modest. According to Doctors of the World UK (2007), fewer than 50% of the undocumented migrant service users who had a medical consultation at their clinic even needed prescriptions. The vast majority required access to basic primary care or antenatal services rather than expensive, specialised treatment.

The government's proposal prompted NGOs to submit evidence to the UK's Joint Committee on Human Rights and the Health Select Committee. It also sparked debate among the medical community, with nearly 750 doctors registered to practise in the UK signing a petition opposing the policy on the grounds that it caused conflict between ethics and the law. The petition was published in the *Lancet* (see box 10.2).

PETITION BY UK DOCTORS

This [changes of the law] would impose serious health risks on [undocumented migrants] and on the general public. It would also interfere with our ability to carry out our duties as doctors. It is not in keeping with the ethics of our profession to refuse to see any person who may be ill, particularly pregnant women with complications, sick children or men crippled by torture. No one would want such a doctor for their GP. We call on the government to retreat from this foolish proposal, which would prevent doctors from investigating, prescribing for, or referring such patients on the NHS. We pledge that, in the event this regulation comes into effect, we will: (a) continue to see and examine asylum seekers and to advise them about their health needs, whatever their immigration status; (b) document their diagnoses and required clinical care; (c) with suitable anonymisation and consent, copy this documentation to the responsible ministers, [members of parliament] and the press; (d) inform the public of the human costs, to harness popular disgust at what is being ordered by the government in their name; (e) campaign to speedily reverse these ill-advised policies.

Sources: Arnold (2007); Arnold et al. (2007)

At the international level, NGOs submitted shadow reports to the UN Committee on Economic, Social and Cultural Rights (ESCR Committee). In its final recommendations to the British government, the Committee referred extensively to data submitted by NGOs that raised concerns over the difficulties in access to health care for refused asylum seekers. The Committee urged the UK to review the provisions regulating essential services for rejected asylum seekers and undocumented migrants, including the availability of HIV treatment (for more on HIV, see chapter 7).[9]

In addition, at the national level, the Home Affairs Committee issued final recommendations to the government in which it made reference to the evidence provided by Doctors of the World, stating that "the evidence we received during consideration of the Draft (Partial) Immigration and

Citizenship Bill cautioned against any future restrictions on access to primary health services for those subject to immigration control" (Home Affairs Committee 2009, p. 10).

As a result of advocacy efforts involving data collection and references to human rights law, a clear picture was painted for national, European, and UN-level bodies. This influenced the policy landscape in the UK and convinced the government drop its proposal to limit undocumented migrants' access to primary care.

Sweden

Sweden has a tax-financed health system that provides universal access to those who have a personal identity number. Such numbers are granted to all citizens and to people with permanent residence. Health care in Sweden is the responsibility of county councils. In accordance with the 2008 Health and Medical Care for Asylum Seekers and Others Act, adult asylum seekers are entitled only to "immediate care" and "care that could not be deferred,"[10] a term not clearly defined, in addition to antenatal care, abortions, and contraceptive counselling. Undocumented adults are not covered in the law, which means that they have a right to "immediate care" only. However, the county councils can claim reimbursement from the undocumented patients for the full cost.

In 2000, the Swedish Parliament passed new legislation granting asylum-seeking children and undocumented children who were formerly asylum seekers the same rights to health care (including dental care) as Swedish children. This change came about as a result of advocacy around children's rights by NGOs and Swedish paediatricians, as well as critiques of Sweden by the UN Committee on the Rights of the Child. Undocumented children in Sweden, however, still face significant barriers to realising their right to health. Firstly, although these children have access to health services, they must pay the full cost of medicines, equipment such as blood and urine glucose tests for children with diabetes, and special foods—a requirement that is impossible for many undocumented families to fulfil. Secondly, knowledge of this legislation is limited within the health system, especially outside of paediatric clinics, leading to the erroneous denial of health care for many undocumented children. Thirdly, this law does not cover undocumented children who have not previously been asylum seekers—these children have the same restricted access to health care as undocumented adults.

In response to undocumented migrants' limited access to health care, health professionals—in some instances together with NGOs—have opened clinics in Stockholm, Gothenburg, Malmö, and smaller cities in which health professionals attend undocumented patients on a voluntary basis.

In 2006, Paul Hunt, then Special Rapporteur on the Right to Health, visited Sweden. In his report, he strongly criticised Sweden for its violation of international human rights by restricting asylum seekers and undocumented migrants' right of access to health care on an equal basis with Swedish residents, thus constituting discrimination against them.[11] The Special Rapporteur's report, together with advocacy conducted by the voluntary clinics, sparked a wide debate. As one result, a number of medical associations and NGOs joined forces to create the Right to Health Care-Initiative, which sought to pressure the Swedish government to adopt a new law granting health care on an equal basis for all, including undocumented migrants, on the sole basis of medical needs.[12] The initiative included over forty member organisations, among them civil society organisations, religious organisations, humanitarian organisations, trade unions, and nearly all of Sweden's professional health associations.

Two years later, and following a split between the coalition partners in Sweden's government, a governmental inquiry was launched with the aim of proposing a new and more generous law. The final proposal, made public in the summer of 2011, suggested changing the law so that undocumented migrants would be entitled to health care on equal conditions with other patients (SOU 2011, English summary, pp. 31–46). Such a change would mean that patients' medical needs—and not their legal status—would influence medical decisions about investigations and treatments. At the time of writing, the inquiry, which should have been referred to Swedish organisations and authorities for consideration and a public debate before a decision by the Parliament, has been halted by the migration minister.

Another effect of the debate is that several hospitals and most county councils have adopted individual policies that are more generous towards undocumented migrants, expanding the indications for treatment and offering more flexibility regarding payment (Ascher 2010, 2011).

Also as a result of the debate, the Swedish Medical Association (*Läkarför-bundet*) proposed expanding the World Medical Association's (WMA) Statement on Medical Care for Refugees by adding a new, last paragraph.[13] The WMA General Assembly adopted this suggestion in 2010 (WMA 2010; see box 10.3).

BOX 10.3

WMA STATEMENT ON MEDICAL CARE FOR REFUGEES

International and civil conflicts as well as poverty and hunger result in large numbers of refugees, including asylum seekers, refused asylum seekers and undocumented migrants, as well as internally displaced persons (IDPs) in all regions. These persons are among the most vulnerable in society.

International codes of human rights and medical ethics, including the WMA Declaration of Lisbon on the Rights of the Patient, declare that all people are entitled without discrimination to appropriate medical care. However, national legislation varies and is often not in accordance with this important principle.

Statement

Physicians have a duty to provide appropriate medical care regardless of the civil or political status of the patient, and governments should not deny patients the right to receive such care, nor should they interfere with physicians' obligation to administer treatment on the basis of clinical need alone.

Physicians cannot be compelled to participate in any punitive or judicial action involving refugees, including asylum seekers, refused asylum seekers and undocumented migrants, or IDPs or to administer any non-medically justified diagnostic measure or treatment, such as sedatives to facilitate easy deportation from the country or relocation.

Physicians must be allowed adequate time and sufficient resources to assess the physical and psychological condition of refugees who are seeking asylum.

National Medical Associations and physicians should actively support and promote the right of all people to receive medical care on the basis of clinical need alone and speak out against legislation and practices that are in opposition to this fundamental right.

Source: WMA (2010)

The examples from the UK and Sweden demonstrate how different account-ability mechanisms were used to push for change. These mechanisms, along with multisectoral collaboration (e.g., among health professionals, human rights professionals, civil rights organisations, religious organisations, unions, and media) and the application of arguments based on human rights law and empirical data succeeded in convincing the British government to drop its proposal for a more restrictive law and pressuring the Swedish government and other authorities towards a policy of improving the right to health for a vulnerable and marginalised group.

The next section will analyse Kagaan's case from medical and public health, ethical and legal, and right-to-health perspectives.

MEDICAL/PUBLIC HEALTH ASPECTS

ACCESS TO HEALTH SERVICES

Kagaan's exclusion from health care is part of a general policy of exclusion towards undocumented migrants in the UK. Through this practice, the government puts itself in conflict with its own policies, including the founding principles of the National Health Service (2011):

- meet the needs of everyone
- be free at the point of delivery
- be based on clinical need, not ability to pay

Under international human rights law, the UK is obligated to ensure Kagaan's access to health care on the primary, secondary, and tertiary levels. Since 2004, the government has consistently sought to increase barriers to access rather than to progressively realise this commitment.

The British Medical Association (2007) itself issued a directive requiring that managers within health services identify and provide training for staff wherever there is evidence that patients are receiving irregular or inappropriate administrative treatment.

CONSEQUENCES OF DENYING ACCESS

Restricted access to health care for undocumented migrants leads to their increased suffering and even death (Ascher et al. 2008). Denying or delaying examination or treatment of Kagaan, who suffers from cancer, means that he is not treated according to basic scientific principles. Generally speaking, a time delay leads to an increased risk of the cancer spreading, which in turn increases morbidity and mortality risks.

Denying access to health services for undocumented migrants can also have indirect consequences—for example, word may spread to other undocumented persons, who may come to believe that they, too, cannot access services. This may lead to an increase in the already demonstrated under-utilisation of health care by undocumented migrants (Doctors of the World UK 2010). The under-treatment of vulnerable groups thus affects public health indirectly by increasing the burden of ill health within society.

Limited access also has direct effects on public health. The fight to control epidemics, such as bird influenza and "swine flu," faces decisive obstacles when certain population groups are disregarded. The same goes for global efforts to control the spreading of resistant bacterial strains, such as tuberculosis.

CONSEQUENCES OF DELAYING TREATMENT: INCREASE IN INEQUALITY

Delaying or rejecting treatment for individuals like Kagaan sends signals to society, which affects public health in several ways. One message is that some people, like undocumented migrants, do not have the same value that "we" have. This means an implicit sanctioning of discrimination and a belief that limiting the welfare and human rights of vulnerable people is okay; and when such principles are accepted for one group, the danger of expanding them to other groups becomes more real. Homeless persons, long-term unemployed people, and single mothers are examples of groups that may be at risk—groups that, in fact, are precisely the type of vulnerable groups that human rights are designed to protect (Hunt 2008).

Furthermore, excluding undocumented people like Kagaan from health care contributes to increased inequality in society. That such exclusion will lead to increasing health gaps in society and impaired health for the groups affected probably comes as no surprise; but several studies have also convincingly demonstrated a strong correlation between the level of inequality in a society and worse outcomes for a long list of health indicators and social indicators for the whole society (Marmot 2004; Pickett and Wilkinson 2009). Even the most well-off in a society do worse in societies with large inequality gaps (Pickett and Wilkinson 2009.)

FINANCIAL IMPACT

An examination of independent research makes it clear that providing preventive and early care through primary care is a means of avoiding costly hospital treatment at a later date (Doctors of the World UK 2007).

In 1978, the Alma-Ata Declaration moved the agenda forward by highlighting "the need for urgent action by all governments, all health and development workers, and the world community to protect and promote the health of all the people of the world."[14] The World Health Organization recommends concrete steps to address patterns of exclusion within the health-care sector, noting that "the starting point is to create or strengthen networks of accessible quality primary-care services that rely on pooled pre-payment or public resources for their funding" (WHO 2008, p. 32).

ETHICAL AND LEGAL PERSPECTIVES

ETHICAL DILEMMAS AND CONCERNS

Ethical obligations lie at the heart of the medical profession, evidenced by the fact that most, if not all, medical professions have formulated ethical guidelines. The core is to sometimes cure, often alleviate, and always console. According to the UK's General Medical Council, which regulates medical professionals practising in the country, "All patients are entitled to care and treatment to meet their clinical needs" (2006, para. 11). The 1948 WMA Declaration of Geneva[15] is expressed as a physician's oath:

> I will not permit considerations of age, disease or disability, creed, ethnic origin, gender, nationality, political affiliation, race, sexual orientation or social standing to intervene between me and my patient ... I will maintain

the utmost respect for human life from its beginning even under threat and will not use my medical knowledge contrary to the laws of humanity. (WMA 2010, p. D-1948-01-2006)

Physicians must provide treatment in a non-discriminatory manner that disregards a patient's non-medical status and ability to pay.

Even if ethical principles are very clear on the fact that all patients should be treated equally on the sole ground of their medical needs, laws and regulations may counteract these principles. In Sweden, decentralisation of the economy made it more difficult for health professionals to treat patients without a personal identity number, since no one had the responsibility for reimbursement and the corresponding debts were thus made the responsibility of each health facility. At the same time, increased computerisation in Sweden made it increasingly difficult for doctors to treat patients "outside" the official system (Ascher 2010). This was the case with Kagaan as well. How should a health professional deal with this?

The WMA Declaration of Lisbon on the Rights of the Patient[16] states that "every person is entitled without discrimination to appropriate medical care" and urges physicians to uphold these rights, even when laws stand in the way:

> Physicians and other persons or bodies involved in the provision of health care have a joint responsibility to recognise and uphold these rights. Whenever legislation, government action or any other administration or institution denies patients these rights, physicians should pursue appropriate means to assure or to restore them. (WMA 2010, p. D-1981-01-2005)

The actions taken by health professionals in the UK, in which they took a stand against the government's proposal to further restrict access to health care for undocumented migrants (see box 10.2), may be seen as such a means of restoring the rights of their patients.

According to PICUM, it is uncommon to find doctors and nurses openly denying health care to a patient (PICUM 2007). However, administrative staff, such as those working at the registration desks, are usually the first point of call. These staff members are usually not involved in professional medical-ethical discussions and may view themselves more as administrators than as health personnel. Administrators may thus have a lower threshold for denying a patient access to health care if the patient does not fulfil certain bureaucratic criteria (PICUM 2007). One example can be found in Germany, where regulations require health-care centres to report undocumented migrants seeking health care to the authorities. However, this requirement is formulated as a duty for administrative—not medical—staff, probably to avoid a discussion about ethics with the medical profession.

LEGAL CONTEXT

The UK has the National Health Service, which provides health care to those who are eligible or entitled. Determining eligibility or entitlement is sometimes complicated and depends on the type of care (e.g., primary care or secondary care) and the status of the patient (e.g., UK citizen, EU citizen, or undocumented migrant). It is left to health-care professionals to make these determinations. When doing so, they must be mindful of their contractual obligations with the government, which require them to provide care on a non-discriminatory basis. If care is provided on a discriminatory basis, this amounts to a breach of contract.

Through the Human Rights Act of 1998 and the Equality Act of 2010, the UK's national legal framework obligates the government to ensure freedom from discrimination. The country has also ratified a number of international treaties that recognise the right to health: the International Covenant on Economic, Social and Cultural Rights; the International Covenant on Civil and Political Rights; the Convention against Torture; the International Convention on the Elimination of All forms of Racial Discrimination; the Convention on the Elimination of All Forms of Discrimination against Women; and the Convention on the Rights of the Child.[17] By ratifying these treaties, the state is obliged to give effect to the right to health at the national and international levels.

The right to health is a progressive right and acknowledges that there are limitations to realising the right to health immediately due to resource availability. It is thus important to note that while the right to health is qualified in this way, it does impose some obligations of immediate effect, such as non-discrimination.[18] As articulated by the ESCR Committee,

> By virtue of article 2.2 and article 3, the Covenant proscribes any discrimination in access to health care and underlying determinants of health, as well as to means and entitlements for their procurement, on the grounds of race, colour, sex, language, religion, political or other opinion, national or social origin, property, birth, physical or mental disability, health status (including HIV/AIDS), sexual orientation and civil, political, social or other status, which has the intention or effect of nullifying or impairing the equal enjoyment or exercise of the right to health.[19]

The Committee also states that although the right to health is a progressive right, states have a continuing obligation, with some exceptions, "to move as expeditiously and effectively as possible towards the full realization of article 12" (see chapters 1, 2, and 4).[20] If Kagaan's case is any indication, it is clear that the UK is out of step with its legal obligations.

APPLICATION OF THE RIGHT TO HEALTH IN PRACTICE

Like many states, the UK has ratified treaties and conventions that obligate the government to give effect to the right to health to the maximum extent of its available resources. The government is likewise bound to make a concerted effort to operationalise the right over a period of time.

Furthermore, the UK is part of the EU—and it is notable that the right to health is one of the EU's core values, together with the principle of equity in health. The EU has highlighted the importance of equity, social cohesion, and growth, which has put migrant and ethnic minority health on the agenda (Padilla and Miguel 2007).

Several developments in the UK have cast doubt on the extent to which the government has met its obligations.

RESPECT, PROTECT, AND FULFIL

International human rights law requires that the UK respect, protect, and fulfil its right-to-health obligations.[21]

Respect

The ESCR Committee, which monitors states' compliance with and interprets the ICESCR, has noted that "states are under an obligation to respect the right to health by refraining from denying or limiting equal access for all persons, including … asylum-seekers and illegal immigrants, to preventive, curative and palliative health services."[22] Moreover, it has stated that "the ground of nationality should not bar access to Covenants rights … The Covenant rights apply to everyone including non-nationals, such as refugees, asylum-seekers, stateless persons, migrant workers and victims of international trafficking, regardless of legal status and documentation.[23]

The British government is interfering with respect for Kagaan's right to health when primary care trusts (the entities responsible for implementing the Department of Health's regulations and policies, as well as providing oversight of general practitioners) are able to advise general practitioners not to register Kagaan due to his status as an undocumented migrant, effectively cutting him off from access to primary care.

Protect

By making a decision about Kagaan's cancer treatment according to eligibility rather than standards based on medical evidence, the UK is failing to protect his health and life. This places the government out of step with its international obligations as a signatory to the ICESCR.

Fulfil

The British government fails to fulfil Kagaan's human rights when it seeks to introduce changes to the law that represent not a progressive realisation but increasing restrictions of the right to health.

HEALTH SYSTEM: AVAILABLE, ACCESSIBLE, ACCEPTABLE, AND GOOD QUALITY

In order for countries to respect and realise the right to health, they must have a functioning health system that is available and accessible to all, acceptable, and of good quality (AAAQ). This health system must include services for both physical and mental health (see chapter 4).

Accessible

While health services appeared to be available to Kagaan, they were not accessible. The right to health requires that health services be accessible to all without discrimination. This principle, together with equality, is a core obligation of the right to health—that is, it is non-derogable (see chapter 1).

Kagaan suffered discrimination. He could not access the services because he was an undocumented migrant. The right to health requires states to pay particular attention to vulnerable and marginalised sections of the population.[24] As an undocumented migrant, Kagaan is himself vulnerable. Health services should also be economically accessible—that is, affordable.[25] In Kagaan's case, free treatment, which is a cornerstone of the National Health Service, was withheld on a discriminatory basis as a result of his migration status. Any governmental policy that requires, encourages, or tolerates the refusal of treatment on a discriminatory basis violates international human rights law—and it is clear that the UK's laws, policies, and procedures regarding undocumented migrants' access to health care fall into this category. Although Kagaan received psychiatric care, it was for involuntary inpatient treatment and failed to treat the underlying cause of his psychiatric condition—namely, his worsening cancer. Accessibility also refers to the accessibility of information, which was not in dispute in Kagaan's case.[26]

By denying Kagaan access to health services, the UK's laws and practices regarding access to health services for undocumented migrants are in violation of international human rights law.[27]

Acceptable

Acceptability means that health services must respect medical ethics, ensure cultural appropriateness, and be sensitive to age and gender. By placing health-care professionals in a position where they are encouraged to refuse treatment, and thus violate their ethical duties, the UK has failed to ensure acceptability.

Good Quality

Quality requires that treatment be medically appropriate. The decision to deny cancer surgery to Kagaan was based not on scientific evidence but on his legal status. It put Kagaan's health at risk, since the longer he waited to receive treatment, the greater the likelihood that his cancer would spread. For Kagaan, the very refusal of treatment caused additional complications— namely, severe depression. Rather than treat his depression through ongoing care, medical personnel determined that Kagaan posed a threat to himself and others and committed him against his will to a secure facility. This was an avoidable and medically unacceptable consequence of his refused cancer treatment. In this way, the UK failed to fulfil the quality demands of the right to health.

PROGRESSIVE REALISATION

The ICESCR provides for the progressive realisation of the right to health, meaning that while states may not be able to immediately achieve the right to health due to resource constraints, they must demonstrate continuous movement towards improvement. The UK government's proposal to further restrict access to health care for undocumented migrants violated this principle and was a clear attempt to counteract the progressive realisation of the right to health. In a rich country like the UK, rejection of treatment on the basis of his residency status constitutes discrimination in application of the right to health. Moreover, the right to health contains certain obligations that are not subject to progressive realisation and that require immediate implementation. One of these is non-discrimination. If not all people can be treated—due to the availability of resources, for example—the decision not to treat someone should be based on sound medical guidelines and should not be an ad hoc decision. This was how the Constitutional Court of South Africa reasoned in a case where a man was denied dialysis treatment and he tried to argue that he was discriminated against.[28]

MONITORING, ACCOUNTABILITY, AND REDRESS

When a person's human rights are violated, it can sometimes be difficult to determine who is directly responsible for the wrongdoing. In Kagaan's case, there is a shared responsibility between the British Parliament (responsible for making the laws and regulations that govern access to primary care, as well as allocating funds to the same), the Department of Health (responsible for implementing Parliament's decisions and formulating complementary policies, as well as distributing funds to and providing oversight of primary care trusts), primary care trusts (responsible for implementing the Department of Health's regulations and overseeing general practitioners), and general practitioners (responsible for accepting or refusing patients and providing an adequate standard of care). Despite these different levels of responsibility, however, the state is ultimately responsible for ensuring protection of the right to health. In a similar situation in Sweden, the Special Rapporteur on the Right to Health urged the Swedish government to improve coordination between the different levels, "with a view to the better protection of the right to health and the implementation of the goals set out" (for more on accountability, see chapters 1 and 3).[29]

A Swedish case could be used as a positive illustration of accountability and shared responsibility. An undocumented male migrant, who was middle-aged and a smoker, visited the volunteer-run clinic for undocumented migrants to seek help for his longstanding hoarseness. He was referred to the ear, nose, and throat (ENT) department at the university hospital. However, he returned to the voluntary clinic several times, as he was too afraid to visit the hospital despite its generous policy of providing treatment to undocumented migrants. After several months, he finally went to the hospital, where he was diagnosed with larynx cancer. He was referred to irradiation treatment, but during his first visit, the doctor told him that the radiation was too expensive and that he ought to go back to his "home" country. The man reported the incident to the voluntary clinic; in turn, the clinic contacted the hospital's ethics board, which was responsible for education, training, and support. The ethics board reached out to the hospital's medical director, and subsequently the hospital offered the patient an apology, a new scheduled appointment, and a promise not to assign him to the same physician. Furthermore, the ethics board offered education on medical ethics, human rights, and health-care needs for refugees and undocumented migrants to the ENT staff. Much later, after undergoing his cancer treatment, the patient encountered the physician who had initially denied him treatment. The doctor apologised to the patient for his behaviour and asked for forgiveness (Ascher 2010).

CONCLUSION AND FUTURE CONSIDERATIONS

The UK and Sweden are resource-rich settings, and it is tempting to think that governments operating within more resource-poor settings cannot necessarily draw on the lessons from this chapter. But it is clear that patients in the UK and Sweden fight the same battles as people throughout the world who cannot access the health services they need. They encounter multiple barriers to care, compounded by discrimination and fear of detection and referral to governmental authorities—circumstances all too common in the developing world. Regardless of the context, certain common lessons can be drawn: the right to health is meant be enjoyed by all, without discrimination, and it has a practical application. The right to health in all countries is especially important for vulnerable individuals and groups. Asylum seekers and undocumented migrants are among the most vulnerable people in the UK and Sweden, and "they are precisely the sort of disadvantaged groups that the international human rights law is designed to protect."[30]

An important lesson from the British and Swedish experiences in improving access to health care for undocumented migrants is that human rights, especially in combination with medical ethics, can be an important tool. When health professionals, human rights lawyers, civil society representatives, and other stakeholders work together on a participatory and human rights basis, they can become a powerful force in stopping retrogressive changes and pushing for improvements in the realisation of the right to health.

REFERENCES

Agamben, G. 1998. *Homo Sacer: Sovereign Power and Bare Life*. Stanford, CA: Stanford Univ. Press.

Arnold, F. 2007. "Medical Justice for Asylum Seekers." Petition. 9 December. http://www.gopetition.com/petitions/medical-justice-for-asylum-seekers. html.

Arnold, F., I. Chalmers, A. Herxheimer, et al. 2007. "Medical Justice for Undocumented Migrants." *The Lancet* 371 (9608): 201.

Ascher, H. 2010. "Rätten till hälsa för papperslösa migranter i Sverige." In *Mänskliga Rättigheter-juridiskt perspektiv*, ed. A. Lundberg, 267–292. Malmö: Liber.

—. 2011. "Sverige diskriminerar papperslösa i vården." *Göteborgs Fria Tidning* 21–27 May, 6–10. http://bit.ly/jC59GF.

Ascher, H., A. Björkman, L. Kjellström, et al. 2008. "Diskriminering av papperslösa i vården leder till lidande och död. Nytt lagförslag hot mot patienterna, vården och samhället." *Läkartidningen* 105 (8): 538–541.

Audit Commission. 2007. *Crossing Borders: Responding to the Local Challenges of Migrant Workers*. London: Audit Commission.

British Medical Association. 2007. *BMA Directive on Training*. London: British Medical Association.

Chauvin P., I. Parizot, N. Drouot, et al. 2007. *European Observatory on Undocumented Migrants' Access to Healthcare*. Paris: Médecins du Monde.

Commission of the European Communities. 2009. Communication from the Commission to the European Parliament and the Council. "An area of freedom, Security and Justice Serving the Citizen." 10 June. COM (2009) 262 final.

"Delstat vill inte invänta reform för papperslösa". 2011. *Sveriges Radio Ekot*, 31 May.

Doctors of the World UK. 2007. *Improving Access to Healthcare for the Community's Most Vulnerable: Report and Recommendations 2007*. London: Doctors of the World UK.

—. 2010. *Impact Report 2009–2010*. London: Doctors of the World.

General Medical Council. 2006. *Good Medical Practice*. London: General Medical Council.

Hargreaves, S., J. S. Friedland, A. Holmes, et al. 2006. *The Identification and Charging of Overseas Visitors at NHS Services in Newham: A Consultation; Final Report*. London: Newham Primary Care Trust.

Home Affairs Committee. 2009. *Borders, Citizenship and Immigration Bill [HL]: Fifth Report of Session 2008–09*. London: The Stationery Office Limited.

Hunt, P. 2008. "Remarks by Paul Hunt, UN Special Rapporteur on the Right to the Highest Attainable Standard of Health." Seminar on the Right to Health for Undocumented Migrants, Stockholm, 13 February. http://www.snabber. se/files/vardforalla/paul_hunts_tal_hearingen_080213.pdf.

IOM (International Organization for Migration). 2011. "Fact and Figures: Global Estimates and Trends." Accessed 2 October 2011. http://www.iom.int/jahia/ Jahia/pid/241.

Johnson, M. 2005. Evidence of Minister for Public Health to Health Select Committee Enquiry (Questions 211–215) in Health Select Committee (2005) "New Developments in Sexual Health and HIV/AIDS Policy." House of Commons, Oral and Written Evidence, HC252-II.

Marmot, M. 2004. *The Status Syndrome: How Social Standing Affects Our Health and Longevity*. New York: Owl Books.

McCormick, A., D. Fleming, and J. Charlton. 1995. *Morbidity Statistics from General Practice: Fourth National Study 1991–2; Office For Population Censuses and Surveys*. Series MB5 No. 3. London: HMSO.

Médecins du Monde. 2009. *Access to Healthcare for Undocumented Migrants in 11 European Countries*. Report from the European Observatory, Médecins du Monde.

Médecins Sans Frontières. 2005. *Gömda in Sweden: Exclusion from Health Care for Immigrants Living Without Legal Status; Results from a survey by Médecins Sans Frontières*. Stockholm: Médecins Sans Frontières.

National Health Service. 2011. "NHS Core Principles." Last modified April 11. http://www.nhs.uk/NHSEngland/thenhs/about/Pages/nhscoreprinciples.aspx.

Ohlson, M. 2006. "Irreguljära immigranter – osynlig-gjorda och diskriminerande inom sjukvården." In *Hälsa, vård och strukturell diskriminering*, ed. A. Groglopo and B. M. Ahlberg, 137–170. Rapport av Utredningen om makt, integration och strukturell diskriminering. SOU 2006:78. Stockholm: Fritzes.

Padilla, B., and J. P. Miguel. 2007. "Health and Migration in the European Union: Building a Shared Vision for Action." In *Health and Migration in the European Union: Better Health for All in an Inclusive Society*, ed. A. Fernandes and J. P. Miguel, 15–22. Lisbon: Instituto Nacional de Saúde Doutor Ricardo Jorge.

Perruchoud, R., and J. Redpath-Cross, eds. 2011. *International Migration Law No. 25: Glossary on Migration*. 2nd ed. Geneva: International Organization for Migration.

Pickett, K., and R. Wilkinson. 2009. *The Spirit Level: Why Greater Equality Makes Societies Stronger.* New York: Bloomsbury Press.

PICUM (Platform for International Cooperation on Undocumented Migrants). 2007. *Access to Health Care for Undocumented Migrants in Europe.* Brussels: PICUM.

SOU (Statens offentliga utredningar). 2011. *Vård efter behov och på lika villkor: En mänsklig rättighet.* Stockholm: Fritzes. http://www.regeringen.se/download/1ce2f996.pdf?major=1&minor=169815&cn=attachmentPublDuplicator_0_attachment.

UN. 2009. *World Migrant Stock: The 2005 Revision Population Database.* Geneva: UN.

—. 2010. *The Millennium Development Goals Report 2010.* New York: UN.

UNHCR (UN High Commissioner for Refugees). 2008. *The 1951 Refugee Convention: Questions and Answers.* Geneva: UNHCR.

Vogel, D., and V. Kovacheva. 2008. "Classification Report: Quality Assessment of Estimates on Stocks of Irregular Migrants." Hamburg Institute of International Economics, Database on Irregular Migration, Working Paper No. 1.

WHO (World Health Organization). 2008. *The World Health Report: Primary Health Care; Now More Than Ever.* Geneva: WHO.

WMA (World Medical Association). 2010. *Handbook of WMA Policies.* Vancouver: World Medical Association.

NOTES

1 This case study is based on the work of Project:London, the drop-in clinic and advisory service run by the international humanitarian organisation Doctors of the World UK (Médecins du Monde UK).

2 International Covenant on Economic, Social and Cultural Rights, G.A. Res. 2200A (XXI), 21 U.N. GAOR Supp. (No. 16) at 49, U.N. Doc. A/6316 (1966), 993 U.N.T.S. 3, entered into force 3 January 1976.

3 Convention Relating to the Status of Refugees, 189 U.N.T.S. 150, entered into force 22 April 1954.

4 Protocol Relating to the Status of Refugees, 606 U.N.T.S. 267, entered into force 4 October 1967.

5 OAU Convention Governing the Specific Aspects of Refugee Problems in Africa, OAU Doc. CAB/LEG/24.3 (1969), entered into force 20 June 1974; Cartagena Declaration on Refugees, adopted by the Colloquium on the International Protection of Refugees in Central America, Mexico and Panama, 22 November 1984.

6 It is difficult to estimate the number of refugees. According to the UN High Commissioner for Refugees (UNHCR), the number was 15.9 million in 2000 and 15.2 million in 2009 (UN 2010, p. 15). However, due to changes in classification and estimation methodology in a number of countries, figures after 2007 are not fully comparable with those prior to 2007. In addition, Palestinian refugees are under the mandate of the UN Relief and Works Agency and not UNHCR (see http://www.unrwa.org). Internally displaced persons (i.e., refugees fleeing one part of their native country for another part but who remain within the borders of their country) are also not included in these figures, as they are outside the mandate of UNHCR.

7 In Sweden, all citizens and those with a residence permit have a unique personal identity number. The first six digits are based on the person's date of birth, the following three digits are a serial number, and the last digit is a checksum. For example, a person born on 6 January 1990 would have a personal identity number of 900106-XXXX.

8 Paul Hunt, Report of the Special Rapporteur on the right of everyone to the enjoyment of the highest attainable standard of physical and mental health, Mission to Sweden, Human Rights Council, U.N. Doc. A/HRC/4/28/Add.2 (2007), para. 71 [hereinafter Hunt Report].

9 Committee on Economic, Social and Cultural Rights, Concluding Observations: United Kingdom, U.N. Doc. E/C.12/GBR/CO/5 (2009), para. 27.

10 Lag om hälso- och sjukvård åt asylsökande m. fl. Lag om hälso- och sjukvård åt asylsökande m. fl. [The Health and Medical Care for Asylum Seekers and Others Act] SFS 2008:344SFS 2008:344, para. 6.

11 Hunt Report, *supra* note 8, paras. 67–91.

12 See the Initiative's website, http://www.vardforpapperslosa.se.

13 The WMA is an international organisation consisting of ninety-five national medical associations. The organisation was founded after World War II to ensure the independence of physicians and to work towards achieving the highest possible standards of ethical behaviour and care by physicians at all times. WMA Statement on Medical Care for Refugees, including Asylum Seekers, Refused Asylum Seekers and Undocumented Migrants, and Internally Displaced Persons, adopted by the 50th World Medical Assembly, Ottawa, Canada, October 1998.

14 Declaration of Alma-Ata, International Conference on Primary Health Care, Alma-Ata, USSR, 6–12 September 1978.

15 WMA Declaration of Geneva, adopted by the 2nd General Assembly of the World Medical Association, Geneva, Switzerland, September 1948.

16 WMA Declaration of Lisbon on the Rights of the Patient, adopted by the 34th World Medical Assembly, Lisbon, Portugal, September/October 1981.

17 International Covenant on Economic, Social and Cultural Rights, *supra* note 2; International Covenant on Civil and Political Rights, G.A. Res. 2200A (XXI), 21 U.N. GAOR Supp. (No. 16) at 52, U.N. Doc. A/6316 (1966), 999 U.N.T.S. 171, entered into force 23 March 1976; Convention against Torture and Other Cruel, Inhuman or

Degrading Treatment or Punishment, G.A. Res. 39/46, Annex, 39 U.N. GAOR Supp. (No. 51) at 197, U.N. Doc. A/39/51 (1984), entered into force 26 June 1987; International Convention on the Elimination of All Forms of Racial Discrimination, G.A. Res. 2106 (XX), Annex, 20 U.N. GAOR Supp. (No. 14) at 47, U.N. Doc. A/6014 (1966), 660 U.N.T.S. 195, entered into force 4 January 1969; the Convention on the Elimination of All Forms of Discrimination against Women, G.A. Res. 34/180, 34 U.N. GAOR Supp. (No. 46) at 193, U.N. Doc. A/34/46 (1979), entered into force 3 September 1981; Convention on the Rights of the Child, G.A. Res. 44/25, Annex, 44 U.N. GAOR Supp. (No. 49) at 167, U.N. Doc. A/44/49 (1989), entered into force 2 September 1990.

18 Committee on Economic, Social and Cultural Rights, General Comment 14, U.N. Doc. E/C.12/2000/4 (2000), para. 30.

19 Ibid., para. 18.

20 Ibid., para. 31.

21 Ibid., paras. 34–36.

22 Ibid., para. 34.

23 Committee on Economic, Social and Cultural Rights, General Comment 20, U.N. Doc. E/C.12/GC/20, (2009), para. 30.

24 General Comment 14, *supra* note 18, para. 12(b).

25 Ibid.

26 Ibid.

27 Hunt Report, *supra* note 8.

28 *Soobramoney v. Minister of Health*, KwaZulu-Natal 1998 (1) SA 765 (CC), 1997 (12) BCLR 1696 (CC).

29 Hunt Report, *supra* note 8, para. 20.

30 Hunt Report, *supra* note 8, para. 73.

CHAPTER 11

Palliative Care

GUNILLA BACKMAN AND JAN STJERNSWÄRD

CASE STUDY: LUCAS, A CANCER PATIENT IN SWEDEN

In June 2011, Lucas passed away from cancer in a university hospital in South Sweden. He was fifty-eight years old and married with two children. From his initial diagnosis until his death, about ten months passed—ten months of regular visits to the hospital and of numerous tests, treatments, and medications.

21 June 2010 – After suffering from a stiff neck, constant headaches, and unsteady balance for over a month, Lucas decided to visit the accident and emergency department at the hospital in South Sweden. He explained to doctors that he had stopped smoking and drinking twenty years ago and had been a sober alcoholic ever since. Lucas also explained that he had been in a motorbike accident in April 2010 in which he injured his back and that, as a result, was consequently sick listed due to back problems. He was admitted to the hospital, where he spent the night. Lucas underwent numerous tests, including a computed tomography (CT) head scan,[1] which showed an expanded mass of tissue in his cerebellum,[2] confirmed by magnetic resonance imaging (MRI);[3] in addition, the doctors performed surgery, opening his skull to remove a tissue sample (biopsy) for further analysis.

After studying the biopsy, the pathologist determined that the mass was a metastasis from an adenocarcinoma[4] of the lung found in the cerebellum. The hospital performed additional tests on Lucas, including a CT-thorax scan, which identified a tumour in Lucas's left lung lobe that had spread to

The authors gratefully acknowledge the expertise and contributions of Dr. Carl-Magnus Edenbrandt, consultant in palliative medicine, and Dr. Lars Ek, consultant in thorax oncology, University Hospital of Lund, Sweden.

the regional lymph nodes.[5] In response to Lucas's back pain, an MRI of his spine was also performed, which showed multiple metastases.[6] Lucas was consequently referred to the outpatient lung clinic, where further tests were performed. He was told to come back on 9 August to retrieve the test results.

9 August – Lucas returned to the hospital's outpatient lung clinic for his appointment, where he met Dr. Johansson, who was to be his doctor from then on. Dr. Johansson told him, "Lucas, we have found a tumour in your lung, and the tests show that you have primary lung cancer. However, to be certain, I want a bronchoscopy to be performed to verify the diagnosis of primary lung cancer."

The bronchoscopy confirmed that Lucas had primary lung cancer. There was no time for Lucas to ask questions. He was immediately referred to the Radiotherapy and Oncology Department for irradiation of the metastases in his cerebellum and spine. Dr. Johansson requested that an epidermal growth factor receptor (EGFR) mutation test[7] be performed on the previously biopsied tumour.

12 August – Lucas visited the outpatient clinic to receive his remaining test results. The EGFR mutation test was negative. Dr. Johansson told Lucas that the type of lung cancer he had was aggressive and recommended chemotherapy. "We can offer you chemotherapy treatment, and I would advise you to accept this."

Lucas accepted and then asked, "How long do I have?"

Dr. Johansson answered, "It is difficult to tell, as it depends on a number of things, such as your response to the treatment." No additional conversation was held regarding Lucas's situation.

Dr. Johansson thus decided to give Lucas chemotherapy (in the form of cisplatin + Alimta) every twenty-one days in the day clinic. He was to receive a total of four cycles, in addition to radiotherapy. The chemotherapy treatment was set to begin in four weeks' time.

7 September – Lucas went to the thorax oncology day clinic to receive his first chemotherapy cycle. However, Lucas informed Dr. Johansson that he and his wife, Emilia, wished to take a holiday before Lucas's chemotherapy was to begin—they wished to spend some time together. From Dr. Johansson's point of view—that is, from a medical perspective—Lucas needed to begin his chemotherapy treatment immediately. However, Dr. Johansson reluctantly agreed to postpone Lucas's appointment until 21 September.

21 September – Lucas returned to the hospital to initiate chemotherapy as planned. However, his thrombocyte values[8] were found to be too low to commence chemotherapy, so his treatment was postponed. In order to understand the cause(s) of Lucas's observed thrombocytopenia, a bone marrow aspiration (removal of bone marrow) was carried out. Dr. Johansson discussed the test results with other colleagues at the hospital, and they concluded that Lucas's low thrombocyte count might have been due to the radiotherapy that he had received to date. Dr. Johansson informed Lucas of the complications and said that he had decided to administer chemotherapy the following week.

1 October – Lucas received his first cycle of chemotherapy. About two weeks later, his health began to deteriorate. His haemoglobin, normally around 130 g/L, fell to 91 g/L. Most likely as a result of his low haemoglobin, Lucas felt tired and had to receive two blood transfusions.

22 October – Lucas received his second cycle of chemotherapy. He complained of increased breathlessness with physical activity. Dr. Johansson asked Lucas about his pain, and Lucas responded that there was good control of earlier pain.

12 November – As it was difficult to find an available peripheral vein, Lucas was asked to return to the hospital to have a portacath implanted to secure access to a central vein for future intravenous infusions. During this visit, Lucas received his third cycle of chemotherapy. He also received an x-ray, which showed partial remission of the tumour in his lung; the tumour had been reduced to half of its original diameter, corresponding to one-eighth of its original volume. Yet Lucas's perception of his condition remained the same—he told Dr. Johansson that with excellent support from his family, he functioned well at home. However, he continued to experience movement-related back pain.

26 November – Lucas returned to see Dr. Johansson, saying that he felt very tired. Dr. Johansson ordered more tests, which showed that Lucas was anaemic. As a result, he received two blood transfusions, and his dose of opioids (pain relief) was increased (from OxyContin10 mg 1×2 to 2×2).

2 December – Lucas received his fourth and final planned cycle of chemotherapy. He was positive and in good spirits, as he felt less tired after blood transfusions. Yet his pain remained unchanged. The doctor ordered a CT scan to be performed on Lucas's thorax and upper abdomen before his next visit, in order to evaluate Lucas's tumour and overall clinical status. Lucas received a new appointment for mid-January to receive the results of these tests.

However, only two weeks later, Lucas contacted the clinic because his back pain and nausea had increased. Dr. Johansson decided to increase Lucas's prescribed medication (OxyContin 10 mg, to 3×2). Dr. Johansson also ordered a new MRI and referred Lucas for additional radiation therapy to reduce the tumour and pain.

Another two weeks passed, and it was New Year's Eve. Lucas went to the hospital because he was experiencing severe pain in his lower abdomen. However, investigations showed that Lucas had no residual urine in his bladder after urinating, which might have explained his increased pain. No other tests were performed. Lucas was sent home.

Mid-January – Lucas went to his initially scheduled appointment to receive the results of his MRI and CT scan that were carried out in December. Lucas said that he was feeling better again, as his pain had decreased. Yet, the test results were not encouraging—they showed more sclerosis, or hardening, in the bone metastases. As a result, Dr. Johansson prescribed Zometa (a type of bisphosphonate), to strengthen the bone, every fourth week. Dr. Johansson asked Lucas to come back in two months.

One week later – Lucas was already back in the hospital. His pain had increased dramatically, indicating that previous treatment with a Matrifen patch (fentanyl) for pain relief had been ineffective. Lucas also continued to complain about nausea. To exclude the possibility of the tumour progressing in his skull, Dr. Johansson requested a CT scan of Lucas's head. The results were negative—that is, no progress could be seen.

During the spring, Lucas visited the outpatient clinic every four weeks to receive Zometa to strengthen his bones. Lucas had lost ten kilograms, the majority of which had been additional weight gained due to steroid treatment. He had also lost weight due to a decrease in muscle mass, despite his attempts at routine exercise with the help of his son. Lucas was now back to his normal weight.

In April, Lucas met with Dr. Johansson, who informed Lucas that his tumour was considered to be "stable." However, Dr. Johansson put Lucas on a new anti-tumour treatment (Tarceva) in the form of a daily pill. Furthermore, in order to diminish any possible neuropathic pain, Lucas was given Lyrica, a pain-relief medication that acts against neurological pain when morphine is not sufficient.

Three weeks later, Lucas called the outpatient clinic because he felt burning pain radiating down into his left buttock. No varicella zoster vesicles[9] were observed in his skin, thus excluding shingles as a potential source of the pain. The clinic doubled Lucas's prescribed dosage of Lyrica.

Lucas's deteriorating health and increased pain began to have consequences beyond the well-being of Lucas. *In May,* Emilia, his wife, had to take sick leave from her job due to psychological exhaustion. Emilia also decreased her working hours in order to take care of Lucas at home. She was informed that she could claim economic compassionate leave support[10] as Lucas's caretaker.

While Emilia's psychological health deteriorated, Lucas's health also worsened. He suffered from increased breathing problems and was consequently equipped with an oxygen concentrator at home.

In mid-May, Lucas returned to his doctor. Dr. Johansson decided to continue Lucas's steroids and pain therapy. Lucas could use the oxygen when needed. He was told to continue with Zometa infusions every fourth week, as well as with the anti-tumour treatment (Tarceva). Lucas was sent home.

One week later, Lucas was forced to go to the hospital again. He had mucous in his bronchia that was causing severe breathing problems. He was sent home with antibiotics and portable oxygen.

31 May – Lucas was back in the hospital. He went to the emergency unit due to deterioration in his breathing, once again. Lucas was hospitalised and given four litres of oxygen gas per minute. Lucas was exhausted. He could not talk any longer. The test result showed that he had purulent phlegm, a sustainable thick mucus with blood, in his airways. He was cyanotic[11] and was admitted to the Department for Infectious Diseases for parental antibiotic therapy and bilevel positive airway pressure as breathing support.

1 June 2011 – About ten months after his initial diagnosis, Lucas passed away in the hospital.

INTRODUCTION

Everybody born will die. "The same attention and care we give those that enter life, the newborn, we should also give those that are leaving life, the elderly and those with known incurable diseases" (Stjernswärd 2004, p. 40).

For many, the end of life is a time of agony due to a lack of either availability of or access to palliative care and pain relief.

Lucas's case provokes numerous questions regarding health systems. What obligations does the state have with regard to palliative care? What rights does the patient have? What ethical concerns are at play? What choices regarding therapy and care should the patient be offered? Should the patient play a role in deciding his treatment? If so, how does this affect the overall health system? Before analysing Lucas's case, the chapter will provide a brief introduction to palliative care. It will then explore the issue of pain relief, highlight the barriers to accessing palliative care, and discuss two practical examples from Spain and India that demonstrate the successful implementation of palliative care programmes. The chapter will conclude by analysing Lucas's case and highlighting future challenges regarding palliative care.

DEFINITION OF PALLIATIVE CARE

Palliative care has its origins in hospice care and has long been associated with terminal cancer. Today, palliative care should be offered to all patients in need, irrespective of diagnosis or age.

According to the World Health Organization (WHO), palliative care "relieves suffering and improves quality of life for both patients and for their families throughout an illness experience, not just at the end-of-life," and "palliative care and pain treatment are an essential—not optional—component of care" (1990, p. 11). WHO specifies that palliative care does the following:

- provides relief from pain and other distressing symptoms
- affirms life and regards dying as a normal process
- intends neither to hasten nor postpone death
- integrates the psychological and spiritual aspects of patient care
- offers a support system to help patients live as actively as possible until death
- offers a support system to help family members cope during the patient's illness and in their own bereavement

- uses a team approach to address the needs of patients and their families, including bereavement counselling, if indicated
- will enhance quality of life and may also positively influence the course of illness
- is applicable early in the course of illness, in conjunction with other therapies that are intended to prolong life (1990, figure 2; 2002, p. 84)

WHO's definition of palliative care for children is closely related to that of adult palliative care (see box 11.1).

BOX 11.1

PALLIATIVE CARE FOR CHILDREN

Palliative care begins when illness is diagnosed and continues regardless of whether or not a child receives treatment directed at the disease; it is a care in which health providers must evaluate and alleviate a child's physical, psychological, and social distress; and it is an active total care of a child's body, mind, and spirit that also involves supporting the child's family.

Source: WHO (2002, p. 85)

Palliative care requires a multidisciplinary approach that takes the patient's family into account and makes use of available community resources. It can be delivered in different settings, including hospitals, tertiary care facilities, outpatient clinics, residential hospices, nursing homes, community health centres, and the patient's home. Palliative care can be successfully implemented in resource-poor settings (WHO 2002).

THE SIZE OF THE PROBLEM

Of the fifty-eight million people who presently die worldwide each year, thirty-three million require palliative care (Stjernswärd 2008, p. 2). In the 1980s, WHO's cancer chief declared pain relief and care for the incurable a public health problem, especially in developing countries, where 80% of cancer patients were incurable and without such services (Stjernswärd 1985,

p. 555; 1993, p. 809; 2007; Stjernswärd and Gómez-Batiste 2008; Stjernswärd, Stanley, and Tschekovski 1986; Stjernswärd et al. 1996, p. 66; Swerdlow and Stjernswärd 1982, p. 327; WHO 1984).

Recently, WHO reiterated that 50% of cancer patients in developed countries and at least 80% of cancer patients in developing countries need palliative care (2002, p. 86). Of the twelve million new cancer cases each year, seven million will die of their disease. In 2007, three million people died from AIDS-related deaths; if preventative measures do not work, it is estimated that annual deaths from AIDS-related causes will grow to four million by 2015 and six million by 2030 (Stjernswärd and Gómez-Batiste 2008, table 1.1). Data indicate that up to 80% of patients in the final stage of the illness experience significant pain (Open Society Foundations 2010, p. 11).

Given the shifting distribution of death and disease from younger to older generations, an increasing and ageing world population, and a change in disease patterns from infectious, perinatal, and maternal causes to non-communicable diseases (Stjernswärd 1993, p. 807; WHO 2008), an increasing number of people will need palliative care in the coming years. For example, it is estimated that by 2025 there will be 1.2 billion people aged sixty and older, doubling from today's 600 million, and that the incidence of new cancer cases will more than double before 2050, from an annual ten million today to twenty-four million (Stjernswärd 2007, p. 44). By 2050, it is estimated that the world will have about two billion people over the age of sixty, 85% of whom will be living in urban areas of what are today's developing countries (WHO 2008, p. 8). As a result of the demographic shift, UN Special Rapporteur on the Right to Health, Anand Grover, urges states to re-evaluate and act on these changes.[12]

With these developments, people in need of palliative care will have a wide range of chronic and potentially fatal disorders, underlining the importance of cooperation between cancer, HIV, and non-communicable diseases programmes in the development and support of palliative care initiatives (Gómez-Batiste et al. 1996; WHO 2002).[13]

The remainder of this section will explore the concept of pain (one of the most common symptoms that palliative care must address); barriers to accessing palliative care and the related consequences; and two successful palliative care initiatives in Spain and India.

PALLIATIVE CARE AND TOTAL PAIN

Total Pain: Palliative Care and Pain Relief

<u>Brief history.</u> Pain is one of the most prevalent symptoms addressed by palliative care and can be used as an indicator for monitoring the effective implementation of palliative care. In the 1950s and 1960s, Cicely Saunders—founder of the modern hospice movement and professionally trained in nursing, medicine, and social work—emphasised the need to understand pain as the key that "unlocks other problems" (Clark 1999, p. 727). Saunders coined the term "total pain" to capture the multiple dimensions of pain. Around the same time, Elisabeth Kubler-Ross, a Swiss-born doctor with experience working with concentration camp survivors, stressed the need for an integrated approach in order to be able to cover the combination of physical symptoms, mental distress, and emotional and social problems (Kubler-Ross 1970). This later came to be referred to as a "holistic" approach.

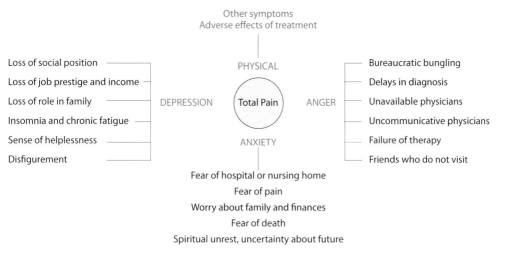

FIGURE 11.1 Total pain: Factors influencing a patient's perception of pain.

Reproduced by permission from WHO (1990).

Total pain became a central element of WHO's definition of palliative care (WHO 1990, p. 21; see figure 11.1). WHO member states were encouraged to recognise the singular importance of home care for patients with advanced cancer and to ensure that hospitals could offer appropriate backup and support for home care (WHO 1990, p. 65).

The impact of pain and chronic pain. Chronic pain, according to WHO, is one of the most underestimated health-care problems in the world today. Although the final stage of life is unique for each person, it is common to first experience physical pain and then psychosocial pain; the latter includes stages such as denial, anger, and depression (Kubler-Ross 1970). When those stages have passed, the "good death" emerges—a person experiences existential anxiety and pain in which a number of questions come to mind: What is the reason for this illness? What is the meaning of life? How long do I have to live? What happens when I die? Feelings of guilt and loneliness often emerge when death becomes a reality. In the case of HIV, many also fear revealing their HIV status, due to the associated stigma and discrimination (UNAIDS 2000). Even if one is surrounded by friends and family, a person is alone in facing his or her own death. This existential and emotional pain can be just as real and hurt just as much as physiological pain.

Diagnosis of a terminal illness and suffering from pain can also lead to questions of euthanasia. While euthanasia is beyond the scope of this chapter, it is worth mentioning briefly. In parts of Europe, such as Belgium and the Netherlands, active euthanasia is legally permitted for people who are terminally ill. Sweden is also presently debating whether to follow suit. This debate is emerging partly as a result of advocacy around people's right to self-determination and their right to participate in determining their treatment and care. Many people do not want to experience total pain and be kept alive only through the assistance of machines—they wish to be able to determine their life outcome themselves. With increasing patient participation and decision making in treatment and care, as well as today's demographic and disease changes, this discussion will likely become significant in the coming years.

Impact on the family and society. Total pain not only affects the person who is ill but also places a major burden on caregivers—who may experience difficulties in pursuing their normal work, participating in social activities, and caring for their children or other family members—and on the entire health system (WHO 1990, 2002). The questions raised by a terminally ill person also affect that person's caregivers, as many may not have experienced death before, at least not in their own homes.

What to do. Saunders stressed that health professionals need particular clinical skills in order for "listening … to develop into real hearing" and highlighted that "pain demands the same analysis and consideration as an illness itself" (Clark 1999, pp. 732–733). Further, multidisciplinary palliative care teams are critical, given the complexity, range of associated emotions, and different stages of an illness (Gómez-Batiste et al. 2008, 2011).

It is important not to forget that those close to the patient are the ones who often inform him or her of developments—for example, regarding how much time the patient has left to live, what he or she can expect to happen, what support is available, and what the patient's options are. They are also there to listen to how the patient wants to use his or her remaining time.

Total pain thus moves away from a purely medical approach, making the health professional look at the patient holistically and not only as a medical case. However, many people who are in need and might wish for palliative care and are hindered by numerous barriers, including a lack of palliative care experts and services. Some of these obstacles are highlighted below.

Barriers to Accessing Palliative Care and the Related Consequences

Numerous barriers prevent people in need from accessing palliative care, including a lack of recognition, knowledge, and availability of palliative care services. To come to terms with such barriers, WHO recommends addressing three areas in particular: (1) governmental policy, (2) education, and (3) the accessibility and availability of essential drugs, such as pain relief (1990, pp. 65–66).

Governmental policy: International law and national practice. Throughout the world, governments, medical and nursing societies, and non-governmental organisations have expressed strong support for WHO's definition of palliative care and have endorsed the integration of these principles into public health and disease control programmes. A country cannot claim to have comprehensive national disease control plans for the elderly, for patients with cancer and non-communicable diseases, or for people living with HIV unless these programmes have an identifiable palliative care component (WHO 2002).

Additionally, a majority of the world's countries have ratified the International Covenant on Economic, Social and Cultural Rights (ICESCR) and have consequently committed themselves to realising the right to health, which encompasses the right to palliative care.[14] Despite these ratifications, there is a palpable gap between rhetoric and reality—or, more specifically, between international law and national practice. Governmental policies on palliative care, with a few exceptions, are usually absent.

A lack of governmental policy leads to palliative care not being recognised as part of the overall health system by planners, donors, and citizens, and thus it is often not included in countries' national health plans. As a result, countries often experience shortages of palliative care resources (Stjernswärd and Clark 2004; WHO 2002).

An additional problem is that people are not always aware of their right to health or of the fact that it encompasses palliative care, and consequently do not demand it.

The last decade has witnessed some changes related to human rights and palliative care. The international health-care community has begun to recognise the dying as a "vulnerable population" and palliative care as one of this population's basic needs, therefore calling for a decent death and freedom from suffering as a human right (Stjernswärd and Backman 2009). Nevertheless, palliative care as a human right is less established than other rights, even if there has been positive progress in recent years. For example, the Korean Declaration on Hospice and Palliative Care[15] highlights that governments should ensure access to hospice and palliative care a human right; the International Guidelines on HIV/AIDS and Human Rights note that "States should also take measures necessary to ensure for all persons, on a sustained and equal basis, the availability and accessibility of ... preventive, curative and palliative care of HIV and related opportunistic infections and conditions" (OHCHR and UNAIDS 2006, guideline 6); and the 2008 Joint Declaration and Statement of Commitment on Palliative Care and Pain Treatment as Human Rights calls on governments to recognise their human rights commitments to ensure that palliative care and pain treatment are available and accessible to everyone.[16]

The former Special Rapporteur on the Right to Health urged states to pay more attention to palliative care, and the present Special Rapporteur has reinforced his predecessor's recommendations in a recent report on the elderly, submitted to the Human Rights Council, which contains a section devoted to palliative care as part of the right to health and encourages increased attention to the issue.[17] Moreover, in 2011, the UNAIDS Reference Group on HIV and Human Rights issued a statement encouraging UN member states to reaffirm their focus on human rights and their commitment to treatment, prevention, and palliative care for people living with HIV (UNAIDS 2011a). Other organisations, such as Human Rights Watch (2009a) and the Open Society Foundations (2011), also call for the recognition of palliative care as a human right. However, palliative care has not created the same sense of ownership among the cancer population or any other group in need of palliative care; thus, these groups have not used human rights as a tool to demand access to palliative care and pain relief. This stands in stark contrast to HIV, where people living with and affected by HIV use human rights as a vehicle to realise their demands (see, for example, discussion of the *Treatment Action Campaign* case in chapter 9).

Education. Palliative care is not seen as a specialty within medicine, and positions are not available allowing a career in palliative care. This has led to shortages of human resources for delivering palliative care. Furthermore, palliative care and pain relief are often not included in the training curricula for health workers, resulting in poor quality of service (Human Rights Watch 2010; Stjernswärd and Pampallona 1998; WHO 2002). To remedy this, palliative care should be included in the curricula for all future health and social workers; the training should be a combination of theoretical and practical work and should be eligible for exam. Such a curriculum change is essential, considering that thirty-three million of the fifty-eight million people who die each year would experience an improved quality of life and death through access to palliative care (Stjernswärd 2007, p. 44).

If palliative care comes to rely on volunteers and is created as a structure parallel to the health system, there is a danger of governments and the medical profession not taking it seriously.

Pain relief: Essential medicine. In palliative care, pain relief must be available and accessible. Pain relief is included in WHO's essential medicines list[18] and includes strong painkillers, such as morphine—the gold standard of severe pain that is vital to the function of palliative care (WHO 1986, 1990, 2002).

Essential medicines are defined as those that "satisfy the health-care needs of the majority of the population" and should therefore "be available at all times in adequate amounts" (WHO 2011, p. 2). Millennium Development Goal 8 stipulates that all countries should work to ensure access to essential medicines for everyone. The provision of essential drugs as defined under the WHO Action Programme on Essential Drugs is also a core obligation of the right to health.[19] Morphine, although classified as an essential medicine, is also classified as an opioid analgesic (narcotic) by the International Narcotics Control Board and is therefore subject to international control. This is one of the reasons why morphine is not available in many countries. Importantly, however, the Board stipulates that "the medical use of narcotics continues to be indispensable for the relief of pain and suffering and adequate provision must be made to ensure the availability of narcotic drugs for such purposes."[20] Despite this, access to and use of morphine is still severely restricted in many parts of the world. The reasons, which are complex and numerous, include a lack of information and understanding, inadequate training of health workers, bureaucratic obstacles (e.g., stringent national drug regulations), cost, industrial greed by not making generic affordable morphine tablets easily available, poor health systems structures, lack of appropriate health policies and strategies, and plain human ignorance (Angell 2005; Stjernswärd 1993, 2004, 2010; WHO 1990, 2002). Nevertheless, for a national palliative care programme to fulfil the requirement of drug availability, a country must both have and effectively implement a national drug policy and an essential medicines list (WHO 2002, p. 87).

Barriers to palliative care and pain relief lead to unnecessary drug-related morbidity at a high cost, as well as increased costs for the overall health system. Limited access to pain relief disproportionally affects developing countries. Globally, over the past two decades, morphine consumption (an indicator of access to pain treatment) has increased, but mainly in a small number of developed countries. In 2007, six developed countries accounted for 79% of global morphine consumption (Austria, the United States, Canada, Denmark,

Portugal, and Australia) (WHO 2011, pp. 1, 5). Developing countries, which make up approximately 80% of the world's population, accounted for just 6% of global morphine consumption (WHO 2011, p. 1). In 2007, the discrepancy persisted, with 132 of 160 countries reporting consumption below the global mean (WHO 2011, pp. 1, 4).

Furthermore, barriers to palliative care can lead to violations of people's human rights, including the right to health and the right to be free from torture, inhuman, and degrading treatment. The former UN Special Rapporteur on Torture[21] has stated that "the denial of access to pain relief raises questions as to whether [states] have adequately discharged this obligation [to protect people under their jurisdiction from inhuman and degrading treatment]."[22]

The WHO measures need to be grounded in human rights law, which in turn should be incorporated into a country's constitution so that the measures are not merely optional.[23] It is also important that every country's policy formation and service delivery be based on the local context and include public participation (see figure 11.2).

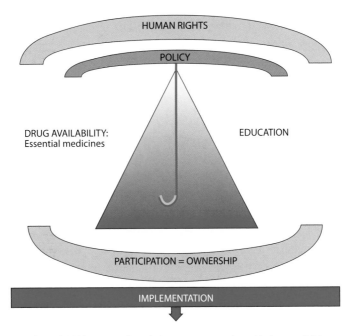

FIGURE 11.2 Adjusted WHO strategy foundation measures anchored in human rights.
Adapted from WHO (1990).

In the 1980s, WHO pointed out that the lack of pain management is a solvable public health problem and produced guidelines for simple, effective, and scientifically valid methods for pain control that are applicable, affordable, and maintainable at the community level (WHO 1986; Stjernswärd 2004). These guidelines were accompanied by recommendations to governments on strategies and priorities for implementation (WHO 1990, 1995, 2002), as well as the development of WHO demonstration projects that comprehensively addressed the barriers to palliative care (Stjernswärd, Colleau, and Ventafridda 1996).

Catalonia, Spain, and Kerala, India, are two of these demonstration projects.[24] While numerous other projects have been important, WHO's demonstration projects are particularly worth noting because they have been monitored and evaluated for over two decades. They have demonstrated the instrumental and practical application of human rights, even if the use of human rights language has not always been explicit. As these projects show, ensuring collaboration between civil society and the health sector can be a successful tool for addressing obstacles to palliative care and questions of sustainability. Ultimately, all terminally ill patients could benefit from this public health approach, using the same methods, principles, and policies (Stjernswärd, Colleau, and Ventafridda 1996).

From Rhetoric to Practice: Catalonia and Kerala

The Catalonia WHO demonstration project. In 1989, Catalonia, a Spanish province of seven million people, was the site of the first WHO demonstration project designed to achieve long-term palliative care outcomes. This is the first case documented to show that it is possible to reach the majority of those in need of pain relief and palliative care, independent of disease. From its outset, the project adopted high ethical standards and aimed to reach all people without discrimination—elderly patients, cancer patients, people living with HIV, and others in need of palliative care. The project started by making palliative care a people's movement, and thereafter both the people and the government took ownership of it. It successfully incorporated palliative care into the province's health plan, established a Catalonian palliative care policy, and mobilised resources for the policy's successful implementation. Evidence showed that palliative care was successfully integrated into all levels of the Catalonian health-care system; opioid consumption rose to acceptable levels

(21 kg per million inhabitants per year), 75% of which was morphine (compared with opioid consumption of 3.5 kg per million inhabitants per year at the start of the project). The results also showed considerable cost savings when palliative care was introduced into the health-care system, mainly by patients not requiring expensive accident and emergency department services and beds. Additionally, increased patient and family satisfaction were documented (Gómez-Batiste et al. 1996, 2007, 2008, 2011). Catalonia is estimated to have saved about 48 million euros in 2005 as a result of the programme (Gómez-Batiste et al. 2007). Furthermore, studies in Spain generally and Catalonia specifically indicate that the average savings per cancer patient admitted to a specialised palliative care unit was 2,250 euros (Gómez-Batiste et al. 2007).

The Kerala WHO demonstration project. This project in India developed a community-based approach to ensuring acceptable coverage. It has the promise of becoming one of the most realistic and relevant models for two-thirds of the world's population—namely, those residing in low- and middle-income countries (for more on community approaches, see chapters 1, 3, and 4). As a result of the project, Kerala successfully integrated palliative care into existing health-care services (Ajithakumari, Sureshkumar, and Rajagopal 1997; Kumar 2004, 2006; Neighborhood Network in Palliative Care 2004; Paleri 2008; Stjernswärd 2005). Figure 11.3 illustrates the structure of palliative care in Kerala.

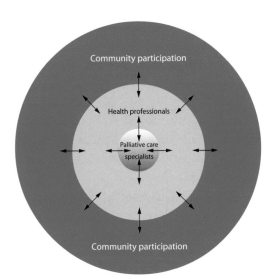

FIGURE 11.3 Palliative care for all: A community-based approach.

Adapted from Stjernswärd (2005).

This community approach is also in line with the 1978 Alma-Ata Declaration,[25] which underlines the importance of community participation and ownership; WHO's recommendations for public health and primary health care, as outlined in its *World Health Report 2008*; and the right to health, for which the UN Committee on Economic, Social and Cultural Rights (ESCR Committee) has highlighted the importance of participation in all health-related decision making at the community, national, and international levels (see chapters 3 and 4).[26] The Kerala community approach is important for a number of reasons (Stjernswärd 2005, 2009):

- It succeeded in encouraging people to assume responsibility for and ownership of the care of the terminally ill.
- It established high ethical standards aiming to extend palliative care coverage to all people in need of palliative care, independent of disease.
- It demonstrated an alternative to the existing over-medicalised, over-specialised, institutionalised, and ultimately unaffordable care of the dying.
- It demonstrated the practical application of human rights and its success.
- It showed financial self-sustainability.
- It demonstrated that social and psychological support, nursing care, and partial medical management can be performed by the community.

Kerala is also interesting from the perspective of accountability, which is a critical component of all human rights that has, in recent years, been highlighted as important for the health sector as well (see chapter 3). The people petitioned the Kerala State Human Rights Commission for access to palliative care in public hospitals, and in turn the Commission directed the government to take steps to include palliative medicine in the curricula for nursing and undergraduate medicine, as well as in public and private hospitals. Since then, palliative care services have been established in every district (Paleri 2008).

India, home to one-sixth of the world's population, still has fewer than one hundred palliative care specialists. The majority of India's terminally ill patients reside administratively in districts, with populations of two to five million people each. It is in these home districts that patients should receive palliative care, as opposed to large specialised centres located in urban areas

(Stjernswärd 2005, p. 111). Kerala has shown that regardless of diagnosis or disease, the majority of those in need of palliative care can be reached and that specialised hospitals are not the only solution. The project showed that four principles were critical for delivering good palliative care through a community-based approach, including home care: (1) social support, (2) psychosocial and spiritual support, (3) nursing care and medical clinical management, and (4) application of human rights.

The following section will analyse Lucas's case from medical/public health, ethical and legal, and right-to-health perspectives.

MEDICAL/PUBLIC HEALTH ASPECTS

Medicine has always emphasised early recognition of a problem in order to alleviate or prevent its full development. Lucas utilised state-of-the-art diagnostic tools and therapies, resulting in a reduction of his symptoms. He was administered chemotherapy, shrinking but not eliminating the primary tumour. Despite the merits of these interventions, they did not cure him. Approximately ten months following his initial diagnosis, Lucas died.

Just like medicine, palliative care should be recognised as an exercise in prevention, as it prevents suffering through the prioritisation of diagnosis and management of sources of distress at the earliest possible moment. This, however, cannot be fulfilled unless palliative care has priority status within public health and disease control programmes (WHO 2002). In 1990, WHO made inclusion of palliative care one of the four pillars of national cancer control programmes and a condition for cancer centres to be recognised as comprehensive (WHO 1990, 1995). It has been established based on WHO principles in several countries, including Georgia, India, Jordan, Mongolia, Spain, and Uganda, among others (Gómez-Batiste et al. 1996; Mongolian Ministry of Health, National Cancer Center, and WHO 2007; Odontuya et al. 2007; Stjernswärd 2002, 2006; Stjernswärd, Foley, and Ferris 2007; Stjernswärd et al. 2007). As part of a "common sense strategy," WHO also recommended introducing palliative care at the time of diagnosis of an incurable cancer and not just when a patient is diagnosed as terminally ill (Stjernswärd 1993, 2010; WHO 1990). This strategy has recently been confirmed to improve patients' quality of life and even prolong life, as discussed below.

PEOPLE-CENTRED APPROACH

Lucas's treatment and care plan should have been developed with the involvement of Lucas and his family. Doctors should have paid specific attention to assessing Lucas's physical and psychosocial symptoms; establishing goals of care; assisting in decision making regarding different treatment options, including palliative care; ensuring that Lucas was aware that chemotherapy would not cure his cancer but would only reduce the tumour size; and coordinating care on the basis of Lucas's needs (National Consensus Project for Quality Palliative Care 2009; WHO 1990, figure 2). Training for palliative care specialists should encompass tools on how to inform patients of their situation. While most in the older generation of medical professionals have not been trained in palliative care, including how to break bad news, it is gradually becoming part of the education for today's generation of physicians and nurses (Buckman 1992).

Once a patient's prognosis is revealed, the patient has the rights to be informed about his or her situation in an individually adjusted way and to be offered palliative care (if incurable) or proven curative therapy (if curable).

Lucas should have been told that while the prescribed drugs in his case would shrink the tumour, they would also have side effects and would not be curative. He should have also been offered palliative care up front as an alternative or in conjunction with proposed therapies. Yet, studies have shown that communications between doctors and patients are often fraught. Many doctors focus only on tests and therapy, and often use ambiguous words; for example, Dr. Johansson told Lucas that there was a "treatment" available. Treatment often has a more positive meaning for patients than for doctors: "treatment for the doctors means that there is a treatment that can prolong life, while for a patient it is often interpreted as 'Something can be done about it'" (The et al. 2000, p. 1379). In addition, it has been documented that uncertainty based on false hopes—for example, repeated information about surrogate endpoints, such as tumour shrinkage—can be stressful for patients and can contribute to depression. On the other hand, telling a patient exactly what the prognosis is has been shown to be reassuring to the patient and to lead to better outcomes, including an improved quality of life, a more positive attitude, and a longer life (Temel et al. 2010).

Although it can be distressing for health workers, carers, and patients alike to discuss emotional and practical issues regarding a person's death, making plans can reduce anxiety and be beneficial for all. Practical issues that may need to be discussed before death include child custody, family support, making a will, funeral arrangements, and costs such as children's education. A will can prevent family conflict and ensure that partners and children are not left destitute.

Emotional issues to be discussed before death might involve resolving old quarrels, telling family members or friends that they are loved, sharing hopes for the future (especially for children who will be left behind), and saying goodbye to family and friends.

Had Lucas been fully informed, told the truth, and offered various alternatives, he might have opted for a longer vacation with his wife. Knowing his prognosis would have given him more time to close the chapters with loved ones and to prepare for his death, which came only seven months after he initiated his first chemotherapy cycle. He died in an expensive, highly specialised hospital bed the day after he was admitted; whether he was prepared for his death, whether dying at home was his wish, and whether he died alone or surrounded by his family, the story does not tell. In many cultures, Lucas's death would not be considered a good death—and in others, it would even be considered a shameful one. In terms of cost-effectiveness, it was expensive. It is documented that patients often experience a greater sense of community, solidarity, and meaningfulness when dying in the home where one is a family member. In an institution, the person is a patient, and thus partly excluded from family life.

HEALTH SYSTEMS: HUMAN RESOURCES AND FINANCES

For any cancer centre or cancer control programme to be labelled "comprehensive," a palliative care team must be available (WHO 1996, 2002). Despite being a patient at a specialised university centre, Lucas was not offered palliative care. Furthermore, there does not appear to have been any continuity of care between the hospital, community, and home settings.

New drugs are often very expensive and difficult to afford, even in wealthy countries; a nine months' supply of chemotherapy drugs can cost up to 100,000 euros. The cost of health care is a topic of frequent discussion, and many studies have documented end-of-life health care to be extremely costly. To take an extreme example, in the United States, most of the money spent on caring for a cancer patient is paid during the patient's last year, mainly on therapy but also on the resuscitation of terminally ill patients with incurable tumours (Stjernsward 1993, p. 810); it is estimated that 12% of Medicare money is spent on end-of-life health-care treatment (Open Society Foundations 2010, pp. 33–34).

Besides chemotherapy, Lucas underwent numerous expensive, highly specialised diagnostic tests that were necessary for proving the ultimately unsuccessful effect of his chemotherapy. This use of (over)diagnostics can eat up a country's often limited resources for, to take an example, the early diagnosis of other patients who may be curable if diagnosed at an early stage of disease.

Using taxpayer or out-of-pocket money for routine chemotherapy for terminal patients detracts from the development of other initiatives, such as the establishment of nationwide palliative care programmes, routine care for the elderly, smoking prevention programmes, or advocacy for healthy lifestyles.

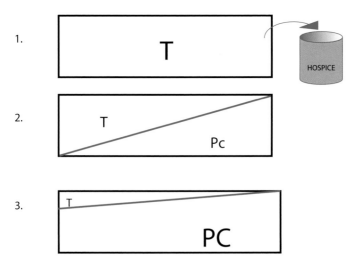

FIGURE 11.4 Integrating palliative care.
Note: T = therapies; PC = palliative care

Adapted from WHO (1990); Stjernsward (1993).

WHO's longtime common-sense strategy of offering palliative care up front at the time of diagnosis of an incurable cancer and not only in the terminal phase was recently confirmed in a randomised study in which 151 patients with metastatic non-small-cell lung cancer received either early palliative care and chemotherapy or chemotherapy alone. The results showed that the patients receiving palliative care had a better quality of life, were less depressed, and lived longer. The median survival was even longer among patients receiving palliative care: 11.6 months versus 8.9 months (Temel et al. 2010, p. 733). Further, palliative care resources achieve optimal cost-effectiveness when introduced up front as opposed to only in the terminal stage, as is often practised today.

WHO's common-sense strategy would help to solve the dilemma of over-promising, over-diagnosing, and over-treating cancer patients with often unaffordable new cancer drugs. The present use of new cancer drugs as drugs of "false hope"—in place of palliative care—(Lancet Oncology Commission 2011; Stjernswärd 2010) is both an economic and an ethical

Description to figure 11.4.

Box 1 shows how palliative care often is practised: palliative care is offered only in the terminal stage when the patient clearly is dying, and usually by a separate unit (a hospice). However, palliative care would achieve a bigger effect and be more cost-effective if introduced at time of diagnosis of incurable patients, as shown in box 2, in high-income countries. In this scenario, the patient's quality of life and quality of death are improved significantly, as health-care professionals pay specific attention to assessing the patient's physical and psychosocial symptoms, establishing goals of care, assisting with decision making regarding treatments, and coordinating care that respects the individual needs of the patient and his autonomy to choose how best to live his now-known limited lifespan. Box 3 shows the same the strategy for low- and middle-income countries, where most patients are already in a late stage of disease when diagnosed, and their countries' very limited resources are often wasted on treatments with no life-prolonging effect for clearly incurable patients and often with severe physical and economic side effects for the patient and the family. Instead, therapy resources should be focused on the curable early-stage patients, and palliative care should be a therapy alternative for the numerous incurable patients.

In the PC boxes, palliative care is incorporated at all levels in a country's health-care system—central hospitals, district hospitals, community health centres, home care, and, when available, hospices.

WHO discourages countries from practising palliative as shown in box 1, which, lamentably, is still the approach used in most countries. Instead, WHO recommends that high-income countries follow box 2 and that low- and middle-income countries follow box 3.

problem. WHO has tried to address this problem by establishing essential drug policies for cancer drugs (Sikora et al. 1999; WHO 1985, 1994), but these policies have had few takers. Resources are not unlimited, and the escalating amounts spent on new cancer drugs with marginal effects could have a much greater effect if spent on integrating palliative care as therapy at the time of diagnosis (see figure 11.5). This would offer a solution for high-income countries and especially for low- and middle-income countries, which are home to the majority of the world's incurable patients and where palliative care would be the most human, ethical, and realistic course of action.

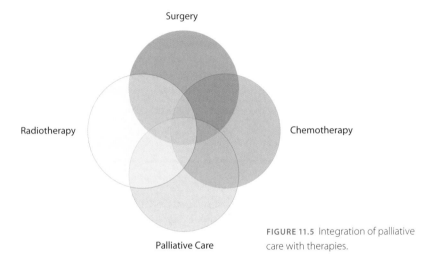

Surgery

Radiotherapy

Chemotherapy

Palliative Care

FIGURE 11.5 Integration of palliative care with therapies.

Thus, offering palliative care up front improves the quality of a patient's remaining life time, and it is more cost-effective and has a greater impact than when given only when clearly terminally ill—or not at all, as in the case of Lucas.

ETHICAL AND LEGAL PERSPECTVES

ETHICAL DILEMMAS AND CONCERNS

The old saying "To sometimes cure, often relieve, and always comfort" is still valid today.

The Swedish government has formulated three principles to form the basis for prioritising between cases: human dignity, solidarity, and cost-effectiveness.[27] Lucas was not offered comprehensive palliative care, despite the fact that, as highlighted above, it has been documented to be more cost-effective, improve quality of care, and even prolong life; instead, his doctor offered him chemotherapy, which did not provide any curative outcome for Lucas. By giving Lucas false hope and not telling the truth, his doctor also violated key ethical principles of respecting patients' autonomy and doing no harm.

According to the World Medical Association's Declaration of Lisbon on the Rights of the Patient, "the patient shall always be treated in accordance with his/her best interests."[28] This does not imply that Lucas should not be offered therapy—rather, it suggests that he should also be offered palliative care up front.

LEGAL CONTEXT

Chapter II of the Instrument of Government (*Regeringsformen*) is part of Sweden's Constitution. Despite being entitled "Fundamental Rights and Freedoms," this chapter does not enshrine the right to health. However, chapter I, "Principles for Public Life," stipulates that "the personal, economic and cultural welfare of the private person shall be fundamental aims of public activity. In particular, it shall be incumbent upon the public institutions to secure the right to health, employment, housing and education, and to promote social care and social security."[29]

The Health and Medical Services Act (*Hälso- och Sjukvårdslagen*)30 establishes that the goals of health and medical services are to ensure that Sweden's population is provided with good health care on equal terms.[31] Health care shall be based on respect for patients' decisions and integrity.[32] The law also applies to care provided to patients at the end of life, including palliative care (Kallenberg 2011). However, Lucas did not participate in developing his health care, and no attempts were made to include him.

It is important to note, however, that Sweden is decentralised in such a manner that county councils (*landstingen*) and municipalities are responsible for implementing the law. Consequently, the quality of palliative care varies widely across the country; for example, it can vary between county councils, between municipalities, and even between different parts of a city (Kallenberg 2011). Sweden's National Guidelines for Lung Cancer Care and Treatment illuminate those areas where the need for direction and guidance are greatest, owing to differences in practice, unequal levels of care across the country, or the existence of controversial issues (Socialstyrelsen 2011).

In 2003, the Council of Europe adopted recommendations provided by its Committee of Ministers, which encouraged governments to adopt laws and policies that ensure a coherent and comprehensive national framework for palliative care.[33] To improve the services offered, the hospital in which Lucas was treated should offer palliative care services at the point when diagnosed with an incurable disease and should ensure patients' involvement in developing these services. Sweden needs to have a palliative care strategy or policy in place, which will then be implemented at the central, county, and municipal levels.

The state provided Emilia with compensation (in the form of compassionate leave) for taking care of Lucas at home and in the hospital, but only after she broke down and took sick leave. She should have been informed of these allowances from the outset. This might have prevented her from falling ill or permitted her to share the Lucas's care more equitably with her sons, who were also eligible for compassionate leave. Compassionate leave is available in Sweden to individuals who are willing and able to care for terminally ill or hospitalised family members (Försäkringskassan 2010).

APPLICATION OF THE RIGHT TO HEALTH IN PRACTICE

Sweden has ratified numerous international human rights treaties, such as the ICESCR; the International Covenant on Civil and Political Rights; the Convention of the Right of the Child; the Convention on the Elimination of All Forms of Discrimination against Women; and the International Convention on the Elimination of All Forms of Racial Discrimination.[34] It has also ratified regional instruments, such as the European Convention on Human Rights, the revised European Social Charter, and the European Convention on Social and Medical Assistance.[35] The ratifications of international and regional human rights treaties give rise to obligations that are binding under international law. However, international obligations will have legal force in Sweden only if incorporated into national law, and Sweden has not incorporated any international human rights treaties into the Swedish Constitution. Importantly, though, Sweden has incorporated one of the regional instruments—the European Convention on Human Rights—into Swedish law, and regulations issued by European Union institutions have immediate application in Sweden.[36] However, the European Convention on Human Rights does not include the right to health, and regulations issued by the European Union to date have not addressed the right to health. At a first glance, this might not seem to imply much, but it gives less protection under the right to health at the domestic level and consequently it is harder to hold the Swedish state accountable for its provision (or lack thereof). The former Special Rapporteur on the Right to Health, during his visit to Sweden in 2006, encouraged Sweden "to incorporate international and regional treaties protecting the right to health into domestic law."[37]

DETAILED HEALTH PLAN/POLICY: A CORE OBLIGATION

Although the right to health is a progressive right, some components of this right—such as adopting and implementing a national public health plan; ensuring access to health facilities, goods, and services on a non-discriminatory basis; and providing essential drugs as defined by WHO—are core obligations that require immediate implementation by all states that are signatories to the ICESCR, irrespective of resources (see chapters 1 and 9).[38]

The ESCR Committee also underlines that formerly unknown diseases (such as HIV) and others that have become more widespread (such as cancer), as well as the rapid growth of the world population, have created new obstacles for the realisation of the right to health and need to be taken into account when interpreting article 12.[39] Interpreting the ICESCR and General Comment 14 in the context of palliative care would oblige governments to adopt and implement national health plans encompassing palliative care (for details of what a national health plan should encompass, see chapter 4).

A country's health plan needs to be costed, and both the plan and budget should be transparent and accessible to everyone, so that the public can see and monitor what the state has promised and hold it to account if necessary. The ESCR Committee has highlighted that investments should not disproportionately favour expensive curative health services, as "inappropriate health resource allocation ... can lead to discrimination that may not be overt" (see chapter 4).[40] In Lucas's case, the focus was on curative health services (i.e., expensive treatments).

Sweden does not have a comprehensive national health plan, policy, or strategy. As the ESCR Committee has noted, a health plan is a core obligation of the right to health: "it should be stressed ... that a State party cannot, under any circumstances whatsoever, justify its non-compliance with the core obligations set out in paragraph 43 above, which are non-derogable."[41]

MONITORING, ACCOUNTABILITY, AND REDRESS

Monitoring of palliative care requires effective and accessible accountability mechanisms. Accountability is especially important with regard to health systems. It should be stressed, however, that accountability is more than "naming and shaming" and litigation—there are different types of accountability, including administrative, quasi-judicial, social, political, and legal accountability (Potts 2008; see chapter 1). Sweden has numerous accountability mechanisms, such as patients' rights charters and ombudspersons. However, the right to health is not fully encompassed within the different mandates of the ombudspersons, and Sweden does not have a national human rights institution, which is important for protecting the entire spectrum of civil, political, economic, social, and cultural rights.[42] In addition, in order for people to be able to monitor, seek accountability, and request redress, they need to be aware of their human rights, including the right to health. In Sweden, there is generally a weak understanding of the right to health and its practical meaning, reflected in the absence of the right to health in domestic law. Yet, there has been recent progress; in April 2011, an evaluation of the Swedish government's action plan on human rights was presented by the Department of Labour. Further, as of July 2011, Sweden's educational system will encompass human rights.[43]

AVAILABLE, ACCESSIBLE, ACCEPTABLE, AND OF GOOD QUALITY

Improving the accessibility of palliative care in Sweden, or in any other country for that matter, is not only about holding relevant actors to account and demanding a scaling up of palliative care services. Rather, it is critical also to look at the overall functioning and planning of the health system and to review both national laws and overall economic, social, and cultural aspects in order to ensure that health services are available, accessible, acceptable, and of good quality (AAAQ). In relation to Lucas's case, this section will briefly look at availability, one aspect of accessibility (information accessibility), and quality.

Lucas was not offered palliative care. From a human rights perspective, the state needs to firstly explain, if asked, the reasons for that Lucas was not offered palliative care; secondly, if palliative care is available in the country, the state needs to explain why it was not accessible to Lucas. In Sweden, the availability, accessibility, acceptability, and quality of services vary, as there are no clear directives explaining how county councils and municipalities should implement the domestic laws.

The former Special Rapporteur on the Right to Health confirmed this in his 2007 report to Sweden:

> The Special Rapporteur was concerned about reports of unsatisfactory coordination between the counties and municipalities with respect to health care and related support services. He urges central, county and municipal authorities to take steps to improve coordination, with a view to the better protection of the right to health and implementation of the goals of the Health and Medical Services Act.[44]

With regard to information accessibility, the state is obligated to ensure that patients are informed of the availability and accessibility of services and that they can make educated decisions about their treatment and care.[45] This was not done for Lucas. The reasons for this are not clear from the case. It could be that palliative care was not available in his municipality or country council, or that there were poor referrals between different departments.

To be able to request or demand information and specific care, Lucas needed to know that he had a right to demand such information. However, with the terminally ill, as discussed earlier, some patients do not want to know their status or health outcome and thus do not ask. If they do not know their health outcome, they cannot ask what their treatment options are and consequently cannot demand them.

For health services to be of good quality, skilled personnel are required and services must be acceptable, among other things.[46] While Lucas was offered the best technologies and medical support, delivered by specialised staff, he as not offered palliative care. However, the provision of palliative care is required for comprehensive cancer treatment and for realisation of the right to health.

For Sweden to ensure that palliative care is made available, accessible, acceptable, and of good quality to everyone, without discrimination, the government needs to make some systemic changes. The National Board of Health and Welfare in Sweden has noted that changes in diagnostics, curative treatment, and palliative treatment have great consequences in economic and organisational terms, as they demand changes in health and medical services, and investment in human resources and competence (Socialstyrelsen 2011). The right to health understands this and does not demand that change take place overnight; it does, however, expect a health plan with time frames, indicators, and benchmarks to be in place outlining how Sweden will progressively ensure the realisation of AAAQ of palliative care throughout the whole country.

EQUALITY AND NON-DISCRIMINATION

Equality and non-discrimination is a core obligation of the right to health.[47] In order to be able to determine whether any group is being discriminated against, health information must therefore be disaggregated on grounds such as sex, age, rural/urban, income, and ethnicity. In Sweden, disaggregation on the grounds of race and ethnicity is a sensitive issue, as such data run the risk of being misused; however, it is also difficult to monitor realisation of the right to health if data are not disaggregated.[48] The ESCR Committee has noted that special attention should be paid to older persons and to chronically and terminally ill persons, sparing them avoidable pain and enabling them to die with dignity.[49] The current Special Rapporteur on the Right to Health has highlighted that there is not enough palliative care for the world's elderly, despite the fact that the right to health clearly proscribes discrimination on the basis of age, including within palliative care services.[50] The Committee has also stated that governments must ensure "the equitable distribution of all health facilities, goods and services."[51] In Lucas's case, this did not take place.

A health system lies at the core of the right to health. Palliative care should be part of the overall health system and not a parallel structure. This is obvious if looking at the required structure of the realisation of palliative care, which encompasses essential medicines, qualified health professionals of all cadres (e.g., palliative care specialists, physical and mental health workers, nutritionists, physiotherapists, managers, oncologists, and geriatric specialists), services, health information, referral systems, leadership, and finances. Palliative care services should also have a good working relationship with other sectors, such as patients' organisations and religious leaders. Yet for palliative care to be part of the overall health system structure and for services to be available, accessible, acceptable, and of good quality, the government must have a national health plan in place and ensure that its decisions reflect commitments made at the regional and international levels.

PARTICIPATION

The right to health is interested not just in outcomes but also in processes. Health outcomes can be improved only if there is participation of the affected groups and persons (WHO 2008),[52] including patients' groups. Such participation must be an integral component of any policy, programme, or strategy, as in the example of Kerala. The community should participate in setting priorities, making decisions, planning, implementing policies, and evaluating strategies to achieve better health.[53] Lucas should have participated in devising his health-care plan. In addition, if health professionals did not ensure his participation, he needed to know that he had a right to ask for it. By including patients' input, health services will also be culturally acceptable, thus improving access and quality, all of which are essential for realising the right to health.[54]

However, it is also important that health workers participate in developing a country's palliative care plan, which should be linked to the national health plan. If there is no national health plan, health workers should demand one—something that they can do if they are aware that it is a right-to-health obligation. In Sweden, it is also critical that district and regional managers participate, as they often have no influence in deciding budget allocations or health priorities related to the delivery of their health services.

CONCLUSION AND FUTURE CONSIDERATIONS

The same attention that is given to those who are entering life should be given to those who are leaving life: the elderly and the incurably ill. The tragedy of palliative care and pain relief is that it is often accessible only to a lucky few. This is despite the fact that palliative care is part of the right to health and that it has been documented to improve the quality of both life and death for patients and their families, while being cost-effective. Adequate pain relief is an essential medicine and a core obligation of the right to health, which implies that it is non-derogable. While WHO has provided guidance on how to make palliative care accessible and available, worldwide still too few can access it. To better reach those who need it, palliative care must be incorporated into national constitutions and into all levels of health-care services, including the home-care level. It must be "people centred"—that is, owned by the people. A rights-based health plan offers the best approach for translating knowledge and skills into evidence-based and cost-effective interventions that can reach everyone without discrimination. As a legal instrument, the right to health offers a crucial and constructive tool for the health sector to provide the best care for patients. It also provides support and guidance for health workers in their work and offers a tool for holding national governments and other stakeholders to account.

REFERENCES

Ajithakumari, K., K. Sureshkumar, and M. R. Rajagopal. 1997. "Palliative Home Care: The Calicut experience." *Palliative Medicine* 11:451–454.

Angell, M. 2005. *The Truth About Drug Companies: How They Deceive Us and What to Do about It.* 2nd ed. New York: Random House.

Backman, G., P. Hunt, R. Khosla, et al. 2008. "Health Systems and the Right to Health an Assessment of 194 Countries." *The Lancet* 372 (9655): 2047–2085.

Buckman, R. 1992. *How to Break Bad News: A Guide for Health-Care Professionals.* London: Pan Books.

Clark, D. 1999. "'Total Pain', Disciplinary Power and the Body in the Work of Cicely Saunders, 1958–1967." *Social Science and Medicine* 49:727–736.

Council of Europe. 2003. *Rekommendation Rec (2003) 24 av medlemsstaternas ministerkommitté till medlemsstaterna om organisation av palliativ vård. Antagen av Europarådets ministerkommitté den 12 november 2003 på*

ministrarnas 860:e fullmäktigemöte.
http://www.nationellaradetforpalliativvard.se/blanketter/publikationer/
Europarådets%20rekommendationer.pdf.

Försäkringskassan. 2010. "Om någon närstående blir svårt sjuk." Accessed 12
October 2011. http://www.forsakringskassan.se/privatpers/sjuk/om_nagon_
narstaende_blir_svart_sjuk.

Gómez-Batiste, X., J. M. Borrás, M. D. Fontanals, et al. 1996. "Palliative Care in
Catalonia 1990-95." *Palliative Medicine* 6:321–327.

Gómez-Batiste, X., C. Caja, J. Espinoze, et al. 2011. "The Catalonia WHO
Demonstration Project for Palliative Care Implementation: Quantitative and
Qualitative Results at 20 Years." *Journal of Pain and Symptom Management*
(in press).

Gómez-Batiste, X., J. Porta-Sales, A. Pascual, et al. 2007. "Catalonia WHO
Palliative Care Demonstration Project at 15 Years (2005)." *Journal of Pain and
Symptom Management* 33 (5): 584–590.

Gómez-Batiste, X., J. Porta-Sales, P. Paz, et al. 2008. "Models of Organization."
In *Palliative Medicine*, ed. D. Walsh, A. T. Caraceni, R. Fainsinger, et al.,
23–29. Philadelphia: Elsevier.

Human Rights Watch. 2009a. *Please do not make us suffer any more: Access to
Pain Treatment as a Human Right.* New York: Human Rights Watch.

—. 2009b. *Unbearable Pain: India's Obligation to Ensure Palliative Care.*
New York: Human Rights Watch.

—. 2010. *Needless Pain: Government Failure to Provide Palliative Care for
Children in Kenya.* New York: Human Rights Watch.

Hunt, P. 2008. Statement by Paul Hunt, the UN Special Rapporteur on the
Right to Health, to the UN Human Rights Council. 11 March. http://www.
essex.ac.uk/human_rights_centre/research/rth/docs/oralRemarks_to_hrc_
march_2008.doc.

Kallenberg, J. 2011. "Palliativ vård präglas av helhetssyn." Last modified 26 April.
http://www.1177.se/Vastra-Gotaland/Fakta-och-rad/Mer-om/Palliativ-vard-
praglas-av-helhetssyn.

Kubler-Ross, E. 1970. *On Death and Dying.* London: Tavistock Publications.

Kumar, S. 2004. "Palliative Care Can Be Delivered through Neighbourhood
Networks." *British Medical Journal* 329:1184.

—. 2006. "The Chronically and Incurable Ill: Barriers to Care."
In *The Commonwealth Health Ministers Reference*, 2–5. London:
The Commonwealth Secretariat.

Lancet Oncology Commission. 2011. "Delivering Affordable Cancer Care in
High-Income Countries." *The Lancet Oncology* 12 (10): 933–980.

Mongolian Ministry of Health, National Cancer Center, and WHO (World Health Organization). 2007. *National Cancer Control Program 2007–2017.* Ulaanbaatar, Mongolia: WHO.

National Consensus Project for Quality Palliative Care. 2009. *Clinical Practice Guidelines for Quality Palliative Care.* 2nd ed. Pittsburgh, PA: National Consensus Project. http://www.nationalconsensusproject.org/guideline.pdf.

Neighborhood Network in Palliative Care. 2004. *Work Book: International Workshop on Community Participation in Palliative Care.* Kerala, 26–28 November.

Odontuya, D., J. Stjernswärd, M. Callaway, et al. 2007. "Mongolia: Establishing a National Palliative Care Program." *Journal of Pain and Symptom Management* 33 (5): 568–572.

OHCHR (Office of the UN High Commissioner for Human Rights) and UNAIDS (Joint UN Programme on HIV/AIDS). 2006. *International Guidelines on HIV/AIDS and Human Rights.* Geneva: UNAIDS.

Open Society Foundations. 2010. *Easing the Pain: Success and Challenges in International Palliative Care.* New York: Open Society Foundations.

—. 2011. "Palliative Care as a Human Right: Public Health Fact Sheet." Accessed 12 October 2011. http://www.soros.org/initiatives/health/focus/ipci/articles_ publications/publications/palliative-care-human-right-20110524/palliative-care-human-right-20110524.pdf.

Paleri, A. K. 2008. "Showing the Way Forward: Pain and Palliative Care Policy of the Government of Kerala." *Indian Journal of Palliative Care* 14 (1): 51–54.

Potts, H. 2008. *Accountability and the Right to the Highest Attainable Standard of Health.* Essex: Univ. of Essex. http://www.essex.ac.uk/human_rights_centre/ research/rth/docs/HRC_Accountability_Mar08.pdf.

Sikora, K., S. Advani, V. Koroltchouk, et al. 1999. "Essential Drugs for Cancer Chemotherapy: A World Health Organization Consultation." *Annals of Oncology* 10 (4): 385–390.

Socialstyrelsen. 2011. "National Guidelines for Lung Cancer Care and Treatment: Summary." Accessed 12 October 2011. http://www.socialstyrelsen.se/ nationalguidelines/nationalguidelinesforlungcancercareandtreatment.

Stjernswärd, J. 1985. "Cancer Pain Relief: An Important Global Public Health Problem." In *Advances in Pain Research and Therapy* (vol. 9), ed. H. L. Fields et al., 555–558. New York: Raven Press.

—. 1993. "Palliative Medicine: The Global Perspective." In *Oxford Text Book of Palliative Medicine,* ed. D. Doyle, G. Hanks, and N. Macdonald, 805–816. New York: Oxford Univ. Press.

—. 2002. "Uganda: Initiating a Government Public Health Approach to Pain Relief and Palliative Care." *Journal of Pain and Symptom Management* 24 (2): 257–264.

—. 2004. "Innovation in Pain Management." In *Wellcome Witnesses to Twentieth Century Medicine*, ed. L. A. Reynolds and E. M. Tansey, 83–84. London: Wellcome Trust Centre for the History of Medicine at University College.

—. 2005. "Community Participation in Palliative Care." *Indian Journal of Palliative Care* 11 (2): 111–117.

—. 2006. *Georgia: National Palliative Care Program.* Tbilisi: Parliament. http://www.parliament.ge/files/619_8111_336972_Paliativi-Eng.pdf.

—. 2007. "Palliative Care: The Public Health Strategy." *The Journal of Public Health Policy* 28:42–55.

—. 2010. "The Importance of Proper Integration of Palliative Care in the Health Care System(s)." Presented at *Palliative Care: Facing the End with Dignity*, Forum Against Cancer Europe, Brussels, 16 November.

Stjernswärd, J., and G. Backman. 2009. "Total Pain: Our Might of the Patient Right." In *Freedom from Pain*, ed. S. Bahtnagar, 47–54. New Delhi: International Publishing House Pvt Ltd.

Stjernswärd, J., and D. Clark. 2004. "Palliative Medicine: A Global Perspective." In *Oxford Textbook of Palliative Medicine* (3rd ed.), ed. D. Doyle, G. Hanks, and N. Macdonald, 1197–1224 New York: Oxford Univ. Press.

Stjernswärd, J., S. Colleau, and V. Ventafridda. 1996. "The World Health Organization Cancer Pain and Palliative Care Program: Past, Present and Future." *Journal of Pain and Symptom Management* 12 (2): 65–72.

Stjernswärd, J., F. Ferris, N. Khleif, et al. 2007. "Jordan Palliative Care Initiative" *Journal of Pain and Symptom Management* 33 (5): 628–633.

Stjernswärd J., K. Foley, and F. Ferris. 2007. "Integrating Palliative Care into National Policies." *Journal of Pain and Symptom Management* 33 (5): 514–518.

Stjernswärd, J., and X. Gómez- Batiste. 2008. "Palliative Medicine: The Global Perspective; Closing the Know-Do Gap." In *Palliative Medicine*, ed. E Walsh, 2–8. Philadelphia: Elsevier.

Stjernswärd, J., and S. Pampallona. 1998. "Palliative Medicine: The Global Perspective." In *Oxford Textbook of Palliative Medicine* (2nd ed.), ed. D. Doyle, G. Hanks, and N. Macdonald, 1025–1244. New York: Oxford Univ. Press.

Stjernswärd, J., K. Stanley, and M. Tsechkovski. 1986. "Cancer Pain Relief: An Urgent Public Health Problem in India." *Indian Journal of Pain* 1 (1): 8–17.

Swerdlow, M., and J. Stjernswärd. 1982. "Cancer Pain Relief: An Urgent Problem." *World Health Forum* 3 (3): 325–330.

Temel, J. S., J. A. Greer, A. Muzikansky, et al. 2010. "Early Palliative Care for Patients with Metastatic Non-Small-Cell Lung Cancer." *The New England Journal of Medicine* 363 (8): 733–742.

The, A-M., T. Hak, G. Koeter, et al. 2000. "Collusion in Doctor-Patient Communication about Imminent Death: An Ethnographic Study." *British Medical Journal* 321:1376–1381.

UNAIDS (Joint UN Programme on HIV/AIDS). 2000. *AIDS: Palliative Care; UNAIDS Technical Update*. Geneva: UNAIDS.

—. 2011a. "UNAIDS Reference Group on HIV and Human Rights Encourages UN Member States to Focus on Human Rights Ahead of High Level Meeting on AIDS." 12 April. http://www.unaids.org/en/resources/presscentre/featurestories/2011/april/20110412refgrouphr/.

—. 2011b. "UNAIDS Strategy Goals 2015: Women and Girls." Accessed 12 October 2011. http://www.unaids.org/en/strategygoalsby2015/womenandgirls/.

UNICEF (UN Children's Fund). 2009. *Taking Evidence to Impact: Making a Difference for Vulnerable Children Living with a World with HIV and AIDS*. New York: UNICEF.

WHO (World Health Organization). 1984. *Global Medium Term Program 1984–1989*. Geneva: WHO.

—. 1985. "Essential Drugs for Cancer Chemotherapy: Memorandum from a WHO Meeting." *Bulletin of the World Health Organization* 63 (6): 999–1002.

—. 1986. *Cancer Pain Relief*. Geneva: WHO.

—. 1990. *Cancer Pain Relief and Palliative Care*. Technical Report Series No. 804. Geneva: WHO.

—. 1994. "Essential Drugs for Cancer Chemotherapy: A WHO Consultation." *Bulletin of the World Health Organization* 72 (5): 693–698.

—. 1995. *National Cancer Control Programs: Policies and Managerial Guidelines*. 1st ed. Geneva: WHO.

—. 2002. *National Cancer Control Programmes: Policies and Managerial Guidelines*. 2nd ed. Geneva: WHO.

—. 2008. *The World Health Report: Primary Health Care; Now More Than Ever*. Geneva: WHO.

—. 2011. *The World Medicine Situation 2011: Access to Controlled Medicines*. Geneva: WHO.

NOTES

1 Computer tomography is an imaging method that uses x-rays to create cross-sectional pictures of the chest and upper abdomen.

2 The cerebellum (Latin for "little brain") is a region of the brain that plays an important role in motor control. It is also involved in some cognitive functions, such as attention and language, and probably some emotional functions, such as regulating fear and pleasure responses.

3 Magnetic resonance imaging is a non-invasive medical test that produces detailed pictures of organs, soft tissues, bone, and virtually all other internal body structures—and, as a result, helps physicians diagnose medical conditions.

4 Commonly associated with lung cancer, adenocarcinoma is a type of cancer that develops in the cells lining glandular organs, such as the lungs, breasts, colon, prostate, stomach, pancreas, and cervix.

5 Lymph nodes are oval-shaped organs of the immune system, distributed widely throughout the body, which act as filters or traps for foreign particles. They are important for proper functioning of the immune system. Lymph nodes also have clinical significance, as they become inflamed or enlarged with an infection. In the case of cancer, lymph nodes are significant and used for cancer staging, which decides the treatment to be employed, and for determining the prognosis.

6 Metastases are tumours that have spread from somewhere else in the body. For example, colon cancer sometimes spreads to the liver. When this happens, instead of calling it "liver cancer resulting from colon cancer," doctors refer to it as "liver metastasis."

7 EGFR is found at abnormally high levels on the surface of many types of cancer cells. The EGFR mutation test allows the physician to prescribe the most suitable therapy for patients with locally advanced or metastatic non-small-cell lung cancer.

8 Thrombocytes are essential for haemostasis. Haemostasis is a process that causes bleeding to stop, meant to keep blood within a damaged blood vessel; the opposite of haemostasis is haemorrhage.

9 Varicella zoster vesicles are small blisters associated with varicella zoster virus, one of eight herpes viruses known to infect humans and other vertebrates. The virus commonly causes chickenpox in children and both shingles and postherpetic neuralgia in adults.

10 Known as *närståendepenning* in Swedish.

11 Cyanotic refers to the skin having a bluish colour due to insufficient oxygen in the blood. It is frequently observed on lips and skin, as well as underneath the fingernails.

12 Anand Grover, Thematic study on the realization of the right to health of older persons by the Special Rapporteur on the right of everyone to the enjoyment of the highest attainable standard of physical and mental health, Human Rights Council, U.N. Doc. A/HRC/18/37 (2011) [hereinafter Grover Report].

13 Ibid.

14 Committee on Economic, Social and Cultural Rights, General Comment 14, U.N. Doc. E/C.12/2000/4 (2000), para. 34.

15 Korea Declaration on Hospice and Palliative Care, 2nd Global Summit of National Hospice and Palliative Care Associations, March 2005.

16 Joint Declaration and Statement on Palliative Care and Pain Treatment as Human Rights, 2008, http://www.hospicecare.com/resources/pain_pallcare_hr/docs/jdsc.pdf.

17 Grover Report, *supra* note 12.

18 According to WHO, examples of essential medicines listed under the international drug conventions include codeine, morphine, methadone, and buprenorphine. For further details, see WHO (2011, table 1.1).

19 General Comment 14, *supra* note 14, para. 43(d).

20 Single Convention on Narcotic Drugs, adopted 30 March 1961, preamble.

21 The full title is the UN Special Rapporteur on Torture and other cruel, inhumane or degrading treatment or punishment.

22 Manfred Nowak, Report of the Special Rapporteur on torture and other cruel, inhuman or degrading treatment or punishment, Human Rights Council, U.N. Doc. A/HRC/10/44 (2009).

23 International Covenant on Economic, Social and Cultural Rights, G.A. Res. 2200A (XXI), 21 U.N. GAOR Supp. (No. 16) at 49, U.N. Doc. A/6316 (1966), 993 U.N.T.S. 3, entered into force 3 January 1976, art. 12(2)(d) ("The creation of conditions which would assure to all medical service and medical attention in the event of sickness"). In addition, General Comment 14 (*supra* note 14, para. 17) states, "The creation of conditions which would assure to all medical service and medical attention in the event of sickness" (art. 12.2(d)), both physical and mental, includes the provision of equal and timely access to basic preventive, curative, rehabilitative health services and health education; regular screening programmes; appropriate treatment of prevalent diseases, illnesses, injuries and disabilities, preferably at community level; the provision of essential drugs … A further important aspect is the improvement and furtherance of participation of the population in the provision of preventive and curative health services.

24 Other WHO demonstration projects include Jordan, Mongolia, and Uganda.

25 Declaration of Alma-Ata, International Conference on Primary Health Care, Alma-Ata, USSR, 6–12 September 1978.

26 General Comment 14, *supra* note 14, para. 11.

27 Proposition 1996/97:60. In Swedish: "propositionen, Prioriteringar inom hälso- och sjukvården formulerade regeringen tre etiska principer som borde ligga till grund för prioriteringar inom vården: människovärdesprincipen, behovs- och solidaritetsprincipen samt kostnadseffektivitetsprincipen" (Sveriges Riksdag, 1996/97:60, Prioriteringar inom hälso och sjukvård, http://www.riksdagen.se/webbnav/?nid=37&dokid=GK0360).

28 World Medical Association Declaration of Lisbon on the Rights of the Patient, adopted by the 34th World Medical Assembly, Lisbon, Portugal, September/October 1981, principle 1(c).

29 SFS 1974:152, ch. I, art. 2.

30 Hälso- och sjukvårdslagen, SFS 1982:763, art. 2.

31 SFS 1982:763, sec. 2.

32 SFS 1982:763; SOSFS 2011:7, ch. 2, paras. 6, 7. In Swedish: Den som tillhör hälso- och sjukvårdspersonalen skall utföra sitt arbete i överensstämmelse med vetenskap och beprövad erfarenhet. En patient skall ges sakkunnig inom omsorgsfull hälso- och sjukvård som uppfyller dessa krav. Vården skall så långt som möjligt utformas och genomföras i samråd med patienten. Patienten skall visas omtanke och respekt. (SFS 1998:531, ch. 2(1))

33 In Swedish: "antar policies, lagstiftning och andra nödvändiga åtgärder för ett sammanhängande och omfattande nationellt ramverk för palliativ vård" (Council of Europe 2003).

34 International Covenant on Economic, Social and Cultural Rights, *supra* note 23; International Covenant on Civil and Political Rights, G.A. Res. 2200A (XXI), 21 U.N. GAOR Supp. (No. 16) at 52, U.N. Doc. A/6316 (1966), 999 U.N.T.S. 171, entered into force 23 March 1976; Convention on the Rights of the Child, G.A. Res. 44/25, Annex, 44 U.N. GAOR Supp. (No. 49) at 167, U.N. Doc. A/44/49 (1989), entered into force 2 September 1990; Convention on the Elimination of All Forms of Discrimination against Women, G.A. Res. 34/180, 34 U.N. GAOR Supp. (No. 46) at 193, U.N. Doc. A/34/46 (1979), entered into force 3 September 1981; International Convention on the Elimination of All Forms of Racial Discrimination, G.A. Res. 2106 (XX), Annex, 20 U.N. GAOR Supp. (No. 14) at 47, U.N. Doc. A/6014 (1966), 660 U.N.T.S. 195, entered into force 4 January 1969.

35 Convention for the Protection of Human Rights and Fundamental Freedoms, 213 U.N.T.S. 222, entered into force 3 September 1953; European Social Charter (revised), ETS No. 163, entered into force 7 January 1999; European Convention on Social and Medical Assistance, ETS No. 014, entered into force 1 July 1954.

36 Convention for the Protection of Human Rights and Fundamental Freedoms, 213 U.N.T.S. 222, entered into force 3 September 1953; Paul Hunt, Report of the UN Special Rapporteur on the right of everyone to the enjoyment of the highest attainable standard of physical and mental health, General Assembly, U.N. Doc. A/HRC/4/28/ Add.2 (2007), para. 18 [hereinafter Hunt Report].

37 Ibid., para. 18.

38 General Comment 14, *supra* note 14, para. 43(f).

39 Ibid., para. 8.

40 Ibid., para. 19.

41 Ibid., para. 47.

42 Hunt Report, *supra* note 36, para. 31.

43 Arbetsmarknadsdepartementet 2011, SOU 2011:29, *Samlat, genomtänkt och uthålligt? En utvärdering av regeringens nationella handlingsplan för mänskliga rättigheter 2006–2009*, 11 April.

44 Hunt Report, *supra* note 36, para. 20.

45 General Comment 14, *supra* note 14, paras. 12(b), 37.

46 Ibid., para. 12(d).

47 Ibid., paras. 18, 43(a).

48 Hunt Report, *supra* note 36, para. 120.

49 General Comment 14, *supra* note 14, para. 25.

50 Grover Report, *supra* note 12.

51 Ibid., para. 43(e).

52 Ibid., para. 54.

53 Grover Report, *supra* note 12, para. 59; General Comment 14, *supra* note 14, para. 25.

54 General Comment 14, *supra* note 14, para. 54.

CONCLUSION

CHAPTER 12

Human Rights, Health, and Development, or What the Future Holds

DANIEL TARANTOLA

This volume is rich in information spanning across a broad spectrum of topics—from the philosophical and historical roots, interpretations, and evolution of the "right to health" to its practical applications to public health policy and practice. Debates about the value of this human right from the perspectives of its contents, universality, and enforceability continue to be fuelled by the emergence of new issues on the global and national public health agenda, and by the multiplicity and diversity of actors—states, international institutions, foundations, civil society organisations, academia, and the commercial health industry—whose definitions of rights, entitlements, obligations, and duties vary widely. The debate will not and should not end with a consensus based on a least common denominator; rather, it should continue and be enriched by evidence supporting or challenging the view that human rights are greater drivers of public health than are market forces or self-interest.

Chapters in this volume have sought, quite successfully, to explore the relevance of the right to health to the revitalisation (if not the re-creation) of health systems that are effective, responsive, fair, and sustainable. This focus of attention is highly appropriate, given the widening health and economic disparities both within and across countries. High-income countries are questioning the capacity of their health systems to respond to an ever-expanding demand at a cost seen as no longer affordable. Uncertain, profit-making, private health-care enterprises, along with out-of-pocket expenditures on health, are expected to make up for the deepening public funding deficit while safety nets for the most vulnerable populations are loosely meshed, if available at all. In many low- and middle-income countries, unprecedented national and international investments in health have reached the limits of effectiveness as health systems can no longer bear the expanding burden of multiple, narrowly focused, poorly coordinated, and restrictively funded initiatives. The renewed worldwide interest in reforming or revitalising health systems stems from the recognition that while more money may be necessary, money alone will not be sufficient to produce better health; structural and systemic changes are urgently needed as well. These changes not only are called for in the health sector but should concern the broader spectrum of human development—that is, the transformation of the social, economic, and political conditions that determine people's living standards, life opportunities, and quality of life. Development is not necessarily "more" (growth) or "bigger" (larger scale). It is a change to "better," defined as an improvement in individual and social living standards and security (welfare and services) in general and improved access to resources (incomes and employment), life claims, and opportunities in particular. Realisation of the right to health is moving incessantly towards goalposts that are constantly becoming more distant as new health issues are recognised, new technologies are developed, and new demands have to be met. The fulfilment of this right implies a comprehensive understanding of how better health can be induced by health systems that are in greater harmony with human development aspirations and capacity.

This chapter aims to suggest areas where the practice and testing of health and human rights principles, norms, and standards can contribute to progress in both of these fields—and beyond, to human development—as well as ways in which the next generation of scholars and students can make a difference. This chapter considers the implications of the right to health and related rights governing the determinants and production of health, some of which are specifically referred to in General Comment 14[1]—but the chapter also invokes the reverse contribution of the fulfilment of this right to human development, on which General Comment 14 does not elaborate. For this and other reasons, this chapter uses the term "health and human rights" instead of "right to health." By necessity, the suggested directions for the future are selective and incomplete; but, as underscored in the third section of this chapter, increasing attention ought to be brought to the reciprocal relationships between health, human rights, and development. This new perspective has given rise to a growing body of literature to which the reader's contribution is warmly encouraged.

Every chapter of this volume contains abundant indications of how the connections between public health and human rights have been exposed, as well as how they are defined by and affect human development goals. Several chapters underscore the critical role played in this regard by more effective acquisition and dissemination of evidence informing public policy and generated through practice and research.

In hindsight, there has been no quiet time between the promulgation of the Universal Declaration of Human Rights; the entry into force of its two covenants three decades later; the recognition of the reciprocal interaction between health and human rights during these and the following decades; the expanding response to the global HIV epidemic in the past thirty years; and, more recently, the application of human rights principles, norms, and standards to an ever-growing array of public health issues. This evolution has not happened by chance or simply goodwill. It has resulted from the juxtaposition and occasional convergence of several movements: a human rights-focused advocacy that initially centred on civil and political rights but became more encompassing after the emergence of HIV, as the epidemic showed the critical importance of social and economic drivers of HIV transmission and denial of care; a public health approach that evolved from an international to a global[2] perspective better suited to bring out the evidence of worldwide disparities in the enjoyment of health and rights; and the growth of civil society organisations as increasingly valued interlocutors and actors on the local, national, international, and global scenes.

In the twenty-first century, the gains achieved through dialogue between the public health and human rights disciplines have reached a point where the question of *why* should attention be paid to the interface between these two disciplines has revealed the other critical question of *how* such an interface could be efficiently and universally achieved. Yet, both questions remain valid, as gains in human rights and public health are never permanent, given the constraints imposed on health systems and their users in response to the current global economic crisis. To protect the accumulated gains and move the health and human rights agendas forward, health and rights actors—that is, civil society organisations and state actors substantially engaged in interpreting, monitoring, raising awareness around, and providing rights-based health services—may take advantage of three opportunities for change. In an attempt to offer a perspective for the future, this chapter will touch on three sets of opportunities and challenges: (1) generating and managing knowledge; (2) moving from concept to practice; and (3) seeking new synergies. The chapter also includes a suggestion to readers as to how to completely engage in this work.

GENERATING AND MANAGING KNOWLEDGE[3]

Contemporary public health upholds the value of scientifically demonstrated "evidence" that commonly attaches greater significance to biomedical and epidemiological quantitative data than to principles and standards that should guide their collection, interpretation, and application. In recent years, demands for evidence to support claims that human rights and rights-based approaches to health add power to public health have been growing. Such demands have been prompted by some public health practitioners on the premises that human rights may create obstacles to public health.[4] The human rights framework's seemingly individual focus is alleged to hamper the realisation of a public good. Tension prevails, for example, between the widespread practice of mandatory HIV testing of individuals at greater risk of infection (typically, sex workers, injecting drug users, men who have sex with men, and prison populations) and the view that such mandatory testing is a poorly effective public health approach that violates the autonomy and the dignity of the person, while voluntariness of testing is inherent to the respect of the human rights of the individuals concerned and a precondition for their effective participation in prevention, care, and support. To resolve this tension, those who argue in favour of mandatory HIV testing challenge their opponents to produce evidence showing that, from a population perspective, testing is more effective when voluntary than when mandated. Drawing over-extended analogies between HIV and other sexually-transmitted infections for which tests are routinely performed—disregarding the fact that these other infections are curable and less associated with exclusion, discrimination, and violence—the same proponents devolve the burden of proof onto those who voice human rights concerns. Responding to demands for evidence can be helpful to the advancement of health and human rights in at least one way and problematic in two others.

Positively, monitoring and evaluating health and human rights policies and practice can generate useful knowledge about "how best" the convergence between health and rights can work in specific settings. In fact, much of the evidence supporting and explicating the reciprocal impacts of health and human rights does not have to be generated anew and can be drawn from existing databases. For example, evidence has already been accumulated linking access to health services and outcomes to structural, economic, and social determinants. However, linkages between these determinants and human rights have not been systematically made explicit. The added value of extending such analyses would be to establish the degree to which public health policies comply with human rights norms and standards, thereby documenting progress made—or lack thereof—by states and non-state actors towards fulfilling their respective obligations and duties. Rearranging and restructuring the available evidence through the application of human rights norms and standards would help formulate national and international policies and programmes seeking to advance health and human rights simultaneously.

Evidence building, however, can be problematic when it does not address the right question. Critically, new knowledge does not have to justify "why" rights-based approaches should be preferred to others labelled inappropriately as "public health approaches" by some authors. This question was answered even before human rights principles were enunciated and international treaties ratified in response to massive abuses perpetrated during World War II, and no reasonable individual will challenge the evidence that human rights violations were hugely detrimental to human dignity and the attainment of justice, peace, security, and health. The tragically abundant *a contrario* evidence should suffice to convince detractors that policies and practices promoting and protecting public health and human rights are the default value. As human rights constitute a set of internationally recognised norms and standards that most states have committed themselves to abide by, the burden of proof falls on those who wish to restrict rights and not on those who are trying to promote and protect human rights in health policy and practice. Detractors should therefore bear the burden of proof that deviating from these principles is humanely acceptable and sound from a dual public health and human rights perspective. For example, withholding the enjoyment of a human right in order to gauge the effects of such a measure on health or development, or observing prospectively these effects in a community whose human rights are being violated, would fail to comply with ethical requirements. Study designs could, however, consider retrospectively comparing the adequacy and outcome of an intervention or a programme where human rights have been violated. For example, behavioural patterns in young people may be affected when information relevant to a desired behaviour change has been denied, as would be the case where the right to information on sexuality and sexual and reproductive health is withheld from young people. As another example, ensuring compliance of health systems with the right to health could build on the pragmatic and largely documented recognition that discrimination, non-participation, denial of services, and socially and culturally inappropriate services are not sound premises for the production of health. Taking stock of insufficiencies in existing systems and probing best practices and their impacts prospectively on health-seeking behaviours may add further evidence that can inform policies and programmes.

Public health and human rights are the concerns of a wide variety of disciplines and actors. Yet, this great opportunity to broaden the scope of action and enrol new energies towards knowledge generation is not without problems. Indeed, all of the different disciplines engaged in health and human rights work have their own perception of and requirements for evidence. Some expect that evidence consists in a relationship between cause (such as a violation of a particular human right) and effect (for example, on a particular health issue), concluding to a statistically valid probability of causation. Others defend the view that the plausibility of such a relationship (i.e., whereby evidence converges towards a plausible conclusion without inferring causation) would be the mainstay of evidence building. Research design in this field is contingent on compliance with ethical and technical imperatives precluding experimental (i.e., with randomisation of comparison groups) and quasi-experimental (i.e., without randomisation of comparison groups) designs. The differences in perception of which evidence would be "good enough" from different disciplinary vantage points stems less from disagreement on methodology than disputes over semantic issues. To illustrate this point, clinicians may consider randomised clinical trials as the gold standard in evidence production; epidemiologists recognise the value of evidence arising from pre- and post-research and the evaluation of public health interventions; while human rights practitioners may consider individual satisfaction that needs are now being met as plausible evidence of the fulfilment of one or more human rights.

In all, evidence building and dissemination are important drivers of progress in health, human rights, and development terms. This process calls for greater understanding, methodological work, empathy, and mutual support across disciplinary boundaries.[5]

MOVING FROM CONCEPT TO PRACTICE

The chapters in this volume illustrate the need to accelerate the translation of health and human rights concepts and principles into practice. Rights-based approaches (RBAs) have been heralded as logical pathways in this direction, and examples are now forthcoming about their practicality and value, as well as the barriers (structural, political, social, economic, and cultural) that they have to surmount. Yet there are different interpretations of RBAs, as they constitute an evolving and dynamic field.

The UN's definition of RBAs through its Common Understanding on Human Rights-Based Approaches to Development Cooperation, was adopted by the UN Development Group in 2003 in the context of UN reform.[6] Since then, many other interpretations have been put forward by different actors (governments, international official development assistance agencies, research institutions, non-governmental organisations, and academic groups), in different disciplines (health, education, justice, fisheries, and agriculture, among others), and with a focus on different populations (e.g., women, children, the elderly, migrants, people with disabilities, and refugees). In the absence of a universally agreed-upon definition of RBAs— which may be premature, as ongoing experiences have yet to inform such an agreement—an essential requirement for all interpretations of RBAs is to be very clear about what and whose specific human rights are being considered and what specific health and/or development approach, output, outcome, or impact is being studied in relation to these rights. For example, the principle of "participation" and the need for community involvement in every stage of research and programme design and implementation are commonly seen as pivotal components of RBAs. How to achieve a deeper understanding of power relations in participatory processes in RBAs remains an essential research question, one that can be best answered through a combination of multidisciplinary research, tight monitoring, and systematic evaluation of policies and programmes. RBA monitoring calls for proven methods and tools, some of which have been produced by scholars and international organisations but require more field testing, and all of which suffer from insufficient use. Evaluation, for which methods and tools continue to be lacking, should be systematically applied to ongoing policies and programmes. It should also be used prospectively to project the likely impact of such policies and programmes through "health and human rights impact assessments," often promoted but seldom carried out and practically absent in the literature.

In moving from concept to practice in an actively debated field, health and human rights practitioners run the risk of focusing their attention excessively on differences between various concepts and methods rather than on their commonalities. Practitioners need a simple framework to introduce shared concepts to policy makers and other decision makers. The simplest graphic representation of what constitutes a common goal, regardless of differences in opinions about methodologies, was offered by Mann and collaborators in the 1990s (see figure 12.1). It may be useful to reintroduce the "two-by-two table"—which could be more appropriately credited to its lead author as the "Jonathan Mann Quadrant." Most practitioners who have been introduced to this framework have kept a vivid memory of this simple diagram. Even though it does not pretend to reflect the complexity of ways and means to achieve the highest possible impacts of policies and programmes in health and human rights terms, this quadrant has the great merit of illustrating the reciprocal relationship between health and rights and demonstrating a pathway for all practitioners to engage in these fields collaboratively towards a common goal. Readers contemplating policy options relevant to health systems, for example, may wish to examine how this simple diagram can help shape choices. In this quadrant, where would a gender-insensitive policy on access to services be situated? Where would an isolated scheme of mandatory HIV testing of at-risk communities be located? Where would voluntary, confidential, provider-initiated HIV testing with guaranteed access to counselling, care, and support be positioned?

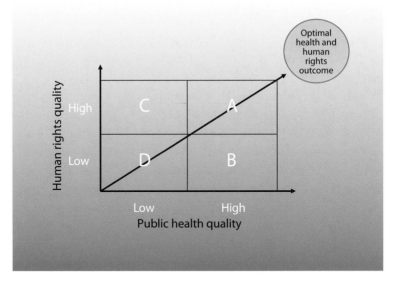

FIGURE 12.1 Optimising health and human rights: The "Jonathan Mann Quadrant".

Adapted from FXB Center for Health and Human Rights and IFRC (1995, pp. 42–43).

Description to figure 12.1.

As a way to visualise the intersection of health and human rights, this diagram places **human rights quality** on the y-axis and **public health quality** on the x-axis. The levels or rank of both measures are graphically displayed at some point in the Cartesian plane. The goal is to optimise policies and practices that may belong to area D of the quadrant (i.e., those with zero or low potential for improving the realisation of public health and human rights) to area A by acting on both their public health and human right qualities, thereby achieving the highest possible outcome.

In summary, translating concepts into practice requires simplicity and clarity in laying out the rationale for transformation and ways in which it can and should be effected. In all likelihood, RBAs will contribute greatly to this transformation. The success of these approaches will be contingent on our collective ability to present them simply and to increase literacy amongst policy makers, deciders, and other actors. This volume is a valuable step in this direction.

CREATING SYNERGIES: HEALTH, DEVELOPMENT, AND HUMAN RIGHTS

The interactions between human rights and health include the realisation of the "right to health," which is necessary but not sufficient for human development.

If both the 1993 Vienna Declaration[7] and General Comment 14 brought some clarity to the interdependence of human rights, the Millennium Development Goals (MDGs) have been criticised for seemingly setting a reductionist vision of the relationship between health, development, and human rights.[8] Typically, MDGs 4, 5, and 6 are seen as being "health focused" while others are deferred to other sectors of the development agenda. All MDGs are in fact dependent on progress in health while, in turn, their attainment will affect health. The MDGs on poverty alleviation, education, gender equality, environmental sustainability, and global partnerships are closely connected to health and, as an earlier chapter argues, to human rights. Thus, there is a bidirectional inference of the right to health on all other human rights governing human development. To decipher and take advantage of these complex relationships implies concerted actions across sectors of development—whether under the purview of government, civil society, or the private sector—whereby health agendas should not be merely imposed on those whose primary concerns lie outside the field of health but whose sectoral goals, concerns, responsibilities, and accountability should be supported by a human rights agenda inclusive of health. Health then provides an indication of where development efforts need to focus primarily; it is seen as a critical requisite for and contributor to effective development in other sectors; and it is used to monitor their progress and possible shortcomings.

Human development can be measured individually and collectively in various, and potentially problematic, ways: as status (e.g., measured as income or health status), capacity (e.g., as human capital in the form of knowledge and skills), participation (e.g., as individuals' access to employment and capacity to engage with institutions), and possibilities (e.g., as the presence of pathways to future development). There may be a risk of dilution of efforts and accountability involved in the broadening of the interface between health and rights to encompass other dimensions of human development. Yet, such a perspective expands opportunities for partnerships with the aim of not only achieving the highest possible realisation of rights, health, or development but of amplifying the synergies between them, resulting in overall benefits substantially greater than the sum of the parts. Recognising these reciprocal relationships and synergies does not imply that *any* policy or action in *any* of the three domains will positively affect the others. For example, an untested development programme may have negative effects on health systems or outcomes, or on the environment; the protection of the right to health without attention to other human rights may be harmful to some individuals or communities; and disproportionate investments in a narrowly targeted health intervention may temporarily constrain progress in other health and social areas.

The basic premise underlying a combined health, development, and human rights approach is that optimal policies and programmes must simultaneously consider the implications—both positive and negative— for health, development, and human rights opportunities and outcomes, maximising overall benefit and minimising pitfalls and potential harms. This adds a third dimension to Mann's quadrant, as illustrated in figure 12.2. Bringing together health, development, and human rights means examining the context in which they function, seeking to identify opportunities for the elaboration of sound policy and programmes, and recognising and addressing the tensions and pitfalls in their interactions. It requires ensuring that the processes of policy and programme development, implementation, and monitoring are informed by best knowledge and practice relevant to the three domains. Ideally, this provides a vision of human development where policies and programmes achieve the highest possible outcome and where impact is measured and accounted for in health, development, and human rights terms. To this end, the challenge is to determine not only how all sectors of development can contribute to health but also how health can be defended as a prerequisite of human development and the enjoyment of all human rights. Synergies across state and non-state actors committed to building a better future cannot be exclusively guided by health imperatives— they must also be guided by mutual gains, including those enlisted in each sector of development against its own goal, whereby health becomes a means to achieving this end.

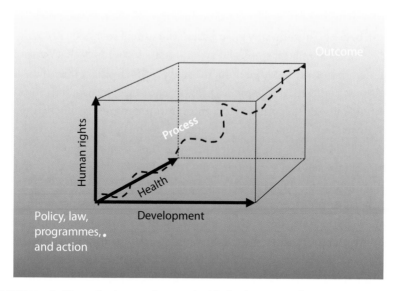

FIGURE 12.2 Seeking optimal synergy between health, development, and human rights: Context, process, and outcome.

Adapted from Tarantola et al. (2008).

Description to figure 12.2.

Bringing human rights, health, and development together means examining the **context** in which they function, seeking to identify opportunities for the elaboration of sound policies and programmes, and recognising and addressing the tensions and pitfalls in their interactions. It requires ensuring that the **processes** of policy and programme development, implementation, and monitoring are informed by best knowledge and practice relevant to the three domains. This analysis can provide a vision of human development whereby policies and programmes achieve the highest possible **outcome**, measured and accounted for in health, development, and human rights terms.

A PERSONAL MESSAGE TO READERS: WHAT THE FUTURE HOLDS IS WHAT YOU MAKE OF IT

Equipped with new knowledge, you, readers of this volume, are about to engage in or pursue a career in health and human rights. As you close this book (to reopen it often, it is hoped), your life is going to be not only very exciting but also fairly busy going forward! Please consider the following modest agenda as you plan your career in this area:

- ➢ On Mondays, you will create new concepts and approaches for bridging the growing economic and social gaps between the "haves" and the "have-nots" of this world and for combating inequality, injustice, and discrimination.
- ➢ On Tuesdays, you will discover new pathways for our society to better foresee and mitigate the societal impact of climate changes that have resulted from our adverse individual and collective behaviours.
- ➢ On Wednesdays, you will develop innovative approaches to respond to both old and new demands for improving health and rights, such as those imposed by HIV, influenza, diabetes, maternal mortality, and Alzheimer's disease. In determining how to prevent and control them more effectively, you will ensure that vulnerable communities are not merely passive objects but active subjects of preparedness and responses.
- ➢ On Thursdays, you will undertake to decipher the patterns of human mobility and their social, economic, and cultural roots and impacts. You will search for ways to alleviate the trauma that migrants, displaced persons, asylum seekers, and refugees often have to experience.
- ➢ On Fridays, you will explore facets of the burgeoning economic globalisation in an attempt to magnify its positive impacts while suppressing its deleterious effects on individuals, communities, and nations.
- ➢ On Saturdays, wondering how on earth the above can be achieved, you will find that international human rights declarations, treaties, and machinery—in spite of their imperfections and limitations—can help you frame these issues towards a greater balance of power, more effective and transparent governance, and respect for the rights and dignity of your fellow human beings.

➢ On Sundays, a day of rest for many, you will be grateful for being able to spend time with your loved ones, satisfied that you have discovered and nurtured the relevance and value of human rights, and not just because they give you the right to rest and leisure.

On the eve of choosing the path of your own future as a privileged and educated human being, a member of your community, a citizen of your nation, and a passenger on this planet, you have an enormous opportunity to bring a human face to the panoply of ideological and technological forces that are now reshaping our world. Do not miss this opportunity. If you run out of inspiration or energy, read again the Universal Declaration of Human Rights and remind yourself that the enjoyment of human rights matters even more to those who do not have them than to those who do.

REFERENCES

Alston P. 2005. "Ships Passing in the Night: The Current State of the Human Rights and Development Debate seen through the Lens of the Millennium Development Goals." *Human Rights Quarterly* 27 (3): 755–829.

FXB (François-Xavier Bagnoud) Center for Health and Human Rights and IFRC (International Federation of the Red Cross). 1995. *AIDS, Health, and Human Rights.* Cambridge, MA: Harvard School of Public Health.

Gruskin, S., and D. Tarantola. 2001. "Health and Human Rights." In *Oxford Textbook on Public Health*, ed. R. Detels and R. Beaglehole, 311–335. New York: Oxford Univ. Press.

Mann, J. M. 2002. "Medicine and Public Health, Ethics, and Human Rights." In *Public Health Law and Ethics: A Reader*, ed. L. Gostin, 113–115. New York: Milbank Memorial Fund.

Mann, J. M., L. Gostin, S. Gruskin, et al. 1994. "Health and Human Rights." *Health and Human Rights* 1 (1): 6–23.

Tarantola, D. 2005. "Global Health and National Governance." *American Journal of Public Health* 95 (1): 8.

Tarantola, D., A. Byrnes, M. Johnson, et al. 2008. "Human Rights, Health and Development." *Australian Journal of Human Rights* 13 (2): 1–32.

UN Development Group. 2003. "The Human Rights Based Approach to Development Cooperation Towards a Common Understanding Among UN Agencies." Accessed 24 October 2011. http://www.undg.org/archive_docs/6959-The_Human_Rights_Based_Approach_to_Development_Cooperation_Towards_a_Common_Understanding_among_UN.pdf.

NOTES

1 General Comment 14 maps out some of the drivers of health from a dual public health and human rights perspective (U.N. Doc. E/C.12/2000/4 (2000), Committee on Economic, Social and Cultural Rights). The study of the social determinants of health, which was given prominence in the literature during the following decade, did not explore the interdependence between social and economic factors affecting health and the realisation of related human rights. This remains a rich area of research and policy development.

2 While the term "international" has framed much of the work in health across countries over the past decades, the term "global" has become more politically viable in that it elevates the vision of health to the whole planet, moving beyond geopolitical boundaries and including not only governments but nongovernmental stakeholders and actors. See, for example, Tarantola (2005).

3 This section draws partly from the outcome of the Research Symposium on Realising the Rights to Health and Development for All, Hanoi, Vietnam, 30 October 2009, Daniel Tarantola, Dao Duy Quat, and Cao Duc Thai, co-chairs (unpublished report available at http://globalhealth.usc.edu/en/Resources/Pages/GHHR%20Resources%20and%20Databases.aspx).

4 For a discussion of the definitions of public health and medicine and the relationships between these two disciplines and human rights, see, for example, Gruskin and Tarantola (2001).

5 In 1995, a student in Jonathan Mann's class at the Harvard School of Public Health humorously noted, "Public health spends too much time on 'p' values of biostatistics and not enough time on values" (Mann 2002, p. 114). Subsequently to the 1994 seminal article by Mann et al., many authors and actors have argued that the upholding of these other values—human rights in particular—is at the core of the new public health of the twenty-first century. A similar argument is defended with specific reference to health systems in chapter 4 of this volume.

6 The Statement of Common Understanding specifically refers to a rights-based approach to development cooperation by UN agencies (UN Development Group 2003). The statement laid out key principles for development programming later interpreted diversely by UN entities, official development assistance agencies, and

non-governmental organisations to suit their respective constituencies, missions, and mandates.

7   The 1993 Vienna Declaration and Programme of Action states that "all human rights are universal, indivisible and interdependent and interrelated" and "reaffirms that the universal and inalienable right to development, as established in the Declaration on the Right to Development, must be implemented and realized" (World Conference on Human Rights, 25 June 1993, U.N. Doc A/Conf.157/23 (1993), pt. 1, paras. 5, 72).

8   A provocative perspective on the interface between the MDGs and human rights is proposed by Alston (2005).